Clinical Research
for the Doctor *of*
Nursing Practice

SECOND EDITION

ALLISON J. TERRY, PhD, MSN, RN

Assistant Dean of Clinical Practice
Associate Professor of Nursing
Auburn University at Montgomery
Montgomery, Alabama

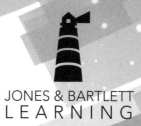

JONES & BARTLETT
LEARNING

World Headquarters
Jones & Bartlett Learning
5 Wall Street
Burlington, MA 01803
978-443-5000
info@jblearning.com
www.jblearning.com

Jones & Bartlett Learning books and products are available through most bookstores and online booksellers. To contact Jones & Bartlett Learning directly, call 800-832-0034, fax 978-443-8000, or visit our website, www.jblearning.com.

Substantial discounts on bulk quantities of Jones & Bartlett Learning publications are available to corporations, professional associations, and other qualified organizations. For details and specific discount information, contact the special sales department at Jones & Bartlett Learning via the above contact information or send an email to specialsales@jblearning.com.

The content, statements, views, and opinions herein are the sole expression of the respective authors and not that of Jones & Bartlett Learning, LLC. Reference herein to any specific commercial product, process, or service by trade name, trademark, manufacturer, or otherwise does not constitute or imply its endorsement or recommendation by Jones & Bartlett Learning, LLC and such reference shall not be used for advertising or product endorsement purposes. All trademarks displayed are the trademarks of the parties noted herein. *Clinical Research for the Doctor of Nursing Practice, Second Edition* is an independent publication and has not been authorized, sponsored, or otherwise approved by the owners of the trademarks or service marks referenced in this product.

There may be images in this book that feature models; these models do not necessarily endorse, represent, or participate in the activities represented in the images. Any screenshots in this product are for educational and instructive purposes only. Any individuals and scenarios featured in the case studies throughout this product may be real or fictitious, but are used for instructional purposes only.

The authors, editor, and publisher have made every effort to provide accurate information. However, they are not responsible for errors, omissions, or for any outcomes related to the use of the contents of this book and take no responsibility for the use of the products and procedures described. Treatments and side effects described in this book may not be applicable to all people; likewise, some people may require a dose or experience a side effect that is not described herein. Drugs and medical devices are discussed that may have limited availability controlled by the Food and Drug Administration (FDA) for use only in a research study or clinical trial. Research, clinical practice, and government regulations often change the accepted standard in this field. When consideration is being given to use of any drug in the clinical setting, the healthcare provider or reader is responsible for determining FDA status of the drug, reading the package insert, and reviewing prescribing information for the most up-to-date recommendations on dose, precautions, and contraindications, and determining the appropriate usage for the product. This is especially important in the case of drugs that are new or seldom used.

Production Credits
Executive Publisher: William Brottmiller
Executive Editor: Amanda Martin
Associate Acquisitions Editor: Rebecca Myrick
Production Editor: Keith Henry
Senior Marketing Manager: Jennifer Stiles
VP, Manufacturing and Inventory
    Control: Therese Connell
Manager of Photo Research, Rights &
    Permissions: Lauren Miller
Composition: Cenveo Publisher Services
Cover Design: Kristin E. Parker
Cover Image: © echo3005/ShutterStock, Inc.
Printing and Binding: Edwards Brothers Malloy
Cover Printing: Edwards Brothers Malloy

Library of Congress Cataloging-in-Publication Data
Terry, Allison J., author.
  Clinical research for the doctor of nursing practice / Allison J. Terry.—Second edition.
    p. ; cm.
  Includes bibliographical references and index.
  ISBN 978-1-284-04593-2
  I. Title.
  [DNLM: 1. Education, Nursing, Graduate—methods. 2. Nurse Clinicians—education. 3. Nursing Research—methods.
4. Research Design. WY 18.5]
  RT75
  610.73071'1—dc23
                        2014022038
6048

Printed in the United States of America
18 17 16 15 14   10 9 8 7 6 5 4 3 2

Contents

Preface   *xi*

UNIT I   **Preparing for Your Capstone Project**   **1**

Chapter 1   **The Importance of Research in the Doctor
of Nursing Practice Degree**   **3**

Introduction to the Doctor of Nursing Practice Degree   4

The DNP Graduate as an Agent for
Quality Improvement   10

The DNP Graduate as an Advocate for Health Care
Through Use of Healthcare Policy   12

The DNP Graduate as an Advanced Practice Nurse   14

The DNP Graduate as a User of Information
Systems and Technology   15

The DNP Graduate With an Aggregate Focus   16

The DNP Graduate's Clinical Scholarship and
Evidence-Based Practice   16

The DNP Graduate's Participation in Evidence-Based
Decision Making   20
The Process of Translating Evidence Into
Clinical Practice   21
Learning Enhancement Tools   23

Chapter 2   Developing the Researchable Problem   27

Selection of the Research Problem and
Development of the Research Question   28
Appropriate Use of a Research Question   31
Appropriate Use of a Hypothesis   32
Developing a Testable Hypothesis   32
Use of a Theoretical or Conceptual Framework   36
Learning Enhancement Tools   38

Chapter 3   Conducting a Literature Review   47

Purpose of the Literature Review   48
Structuring the Literature Review   49
Critical Appraisal of the Literature   50
Collecting Data Sources   52
Learning Enhancement Tools   60

Chapter 4   Ethics in Clinical Research   61

Ethical Principles   62
Informed Consent   63
Rights of Participants in a Research Study   64
Confidentiality   65
Health Insurance Portability and Accountability
Act Compliance   66
Institutional Review Boards   68
Learning Enhancement Tools   75

UNIT II Choosing a Design for Your Capstone Project   79

Chapter 5 Designing a Clinically Based Quantitative Capstone Research Project   81

Basic Types of Quantitative Research   82
Advantages and Limitations of Quantitative Research   83
Experimental Research Designs   83
Nonexperimental Research Designs   87
Quasi-Experimental Research Designs   90
Learning Enhancement Tools   95

Chapter 6 Designing a Clinically Based Qualitative Capstone Research Project   99

Basic Types of Qualitative Research   100
Advantages and Limitations of Qualitative Research   103
Qualitative Research Designs   105
Selecting a Qualitative Research Design   113
Learning Enhancement Tools   114

Chapter 7 Designing a Clinically Based Mixed Method Capstone Research Project   119

Introduction to Mixed Method Research   120
Advantages and Limitations of Mixed Method Research   120
Deciding to Utilize a Mixed Method Approach   122
Mixed Research Approaches   122
Specific Mixed Research Designs   124
Selecting a Type of Mixed Research Design   129
Stages of the Mixed Research Process   130
Learning Enhancement Tools   132

UNIT III Implementing Your Capstone Project   137

Chapter 8   Sampling   139

Introduction to the Process of Sampling   140
Quantitative Sampling Designs   140
Random Selection and Random Assignment   146
Determining Sample Size   146
Qualitative Sampling Designs   148
Qualitative Sampling Strategy   149
Learning Enhancement Tools   152

Chapter 9   Data Collection   157

Introduction to the Process of Data Collection   158
Types of Data Collection Methods   159
Data Collection in Mixed Method Research   172
Learning Enhancement Tools   172

Chapter 10 Issues Related to Survey Data Collection   177

Introduction to Survey Data Collection   178
Recruiting the Sample for Survey Research   181
Planning the Content of a Survey Instrument   182
Sampling During Survey Research   188
Designs in Survey Research   190
Learning Enhancement Tools   191

Chapter 11 Data Analysis   197

Introduction to the Process of Data Analysis   198
Quantitative Research   198
Qualitative Research   202
Learning Enhancement Tools   206

Chapter 12 Writing the Research Report for Potential Publication   **211**

     Initiating the Writing Process   211

     Choosing a Journal for Manuscript Submission   215

     Formatting the Manuscript   218

Appendix 12A Critique of Clinically Based Research   **221**

     Abstract   221

     Introduction   221

     Conceptual Framework   222

     Literature Review   223

     Methodology   224

     Limitations   225

     Implications   225

     Conclusion   227

     Model for the Enhancement of Job Satisfaction of LPNs in Rural Alabama Counties   228

UNIT IV   Examples of Studies/Projects   **231**

Chapter 13 Reducing 30-Day Hospital Readmission of the Heart Failure Patient   **233**

     Institute of Medicine Six Aims   236

     Needs Assessment   236

     Quality Improvement   238

     Evidence-Based Model   240

     Review of the Evidence   240

     Phases of the Project   242

     Plan for Evaluation   244

     Identification of Performance Measures   245

     Retrieval of Data   245

     Data Analysis   246

Appendix 13A SWOT Analysis   **251**

Appendix 13B Gap Analysis   **252**

Appendix 13C Protocol for Quality Improvement Project   **253**

Appendix 13D Plan, Do, Study, Act Model   **254**

   Plan   254

   Do   255

   Study   255

   Act   255

Appendix 13E Project Planning Model   **256**

Appendix 13F Review of the Literature   **257**

Appendix 13G Grading System Used by New Zealand Guideline Group in Cardiac Rehabilitation Guideline   **266**

Appendix 13H Heart Failure Education Packet   **268**

   Table of Contents   268

   Section One: What Is Heart Failure?   268

   Section Two: Warning Signs and Symptoms and Whom to Contact   270

   Section Three: Weighing Every Day   270

   Section Four: Your Medication   271

   Section Five: Diet   272

   Section Six: Activity   273

   Section Seven: Questions for My Healthcare Provider   274

Appendix 13I Telephone Survey   **276**

Appendix 13J Balance Scorecard   **278**

Appendix 13K Evaluation Grid   **279**

Chapter 14 A Community–Academic Collaboration to Impact Childhood Obesity   **283**

   Abstract   283

   Background   285

   Project Overview   289

Method 290

Data Collection 291

Data Analysis 293

Results 293

Value Propositions 295

Limitations 296

Conclusion and Implications 297

Appendix 14A Pretest/Posttest **304**

Appendix 14B Collaboration Survey **307**

Chapter 15 The Impact of Evidence-Based Design **311**

Abstract 311

The Impact of Evidence-Based Design 312

Background and Significance 313

A Proposed Project 314

Theoretical Framework 315

Catalyst 315

Assessing 316

Asking 317

Acquiring 317

Appraising 318

Applying 324

Needs Assessment 324

Implementation 326

Analyzing 332

Adopting and Advancing 338

Discussion 339

Findings 340

Conclusion 342

Appendix 15A Evidence Analysis Grid **346**

Appendix 15B Small Test of Change Timeline **354**

**Appendix 15C Assessment for Quality Improvement
Project** **356**

Appendix 15D Evidence-Based Design Project Budget   357

Appendix 15E The Timeline for the Red Zone Project   358

Appendix 15F Outline of Needs Assessment, Implementation, and Process Outcomes   360

Chapter 16 The Lived Experience of Chronic Pain in Nurse Educators   **363**

Abstract   363

Introduction   364

Review of the Literature   380

Research Design and Methodology   397

Research Findings   409

Discussion, Limitations, and Recommendations   437

Glossary   *471*

Index   *487*

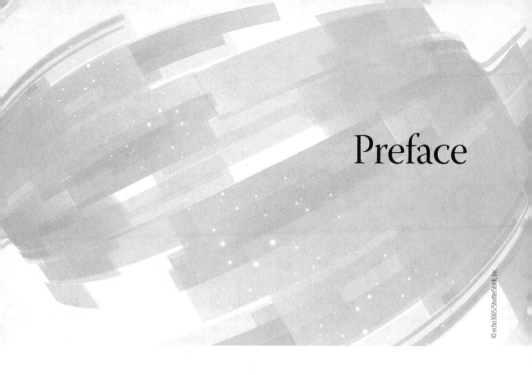

Preface

Today's modern society is changing so rapidly that in many ways it seems to be more virtual than reality, thanks in part to ever-expanding technology that allows us to make the community grow from our backyard into the neighboring country. When these aspects are combined with a patient's ever-changing healthcare need, the result can be bewildering for nurses trying to prepare themselves as leaders in the healthcare arena. That preparation can come from a combination of evidence-based practice and the education preparation that is found in the doctor of nursing practice (DNP) degree.

For the nurse who has been dedicated to a bedside practice and now is conscientious enough to seek the additional validation derived from the DNP degree, the capstone project can be a source of anxiety. It is the hope that this text will serve as a guidebook for the nurse who is navigating through that process, a compass that will assist in avoiding obstacles, developing realistic timelines, and setting achievable goals.

The second edition of the book has the capstone project as its central focus, with the text being divided into four units. Unit

I centers on the preparation required for the project, while Unit II reviews the various designs that are possible for the project and how to select the one that will best achieve the objectives of the DNP student. Unit III discusses the nuts-and-bolts issues involved in implementation of the project, and Unit IV contains actual examples of both studies and capstone projects that have been completed to allow the DNP student to see examples of what could be accomplished.

It is the hope of the author that this text will assist the DNP student who is intending to serve as a catalyst for change in the healthcare community. May it serve as a compass for the nurse who is uncertain as to which fork in the road to the capstone project will be most helpful.

UNIT I

Preparing for Your Capstone Project

Chapter 1: *The Importance of Research in the Doctor of Nursing Practice Degree*

Chapter 2: *Developing the Researchable Problem*

Chapter 3: *Conducting a Literature Review*

Chapter 4: *Ethics in Clinical Research*

The Importance of Research in the Doctor of Nursing Practice Degree

Objectives

Upon completion of this chapter, the reader should be prepared to:

1. Describe the fundamental differences between a practice-oriented doctorate and the traditional research-focused doctorate.
2. Discuss the seven primary areas of content that the American Association of Colleges of Nursing (AACN) has recommended be included in all doctor of nursing practice (DNP) programs.
3. Review the time line that led to the development of the DNP degree.
4. Discuss the concerns that have arisen regarding implementation of the DNP degree.
5. Review the primary areas of content of any DNP program.
6. Describe how the DNP graduate should be prepared to function as an agent for quality improvement.
7. Describe how the DNP graduate should be prepared to act as an advocate for health care through use of healthcare policy.
8. Describe how the DNP graduate should be prepared to function as an advanced practice nurse in a specialty.

9. Describe how the DNP graduate should be prepared to utilize information systems and technology.
10. Describe how the DNP graduate functions while assuming an aggregate focus.
11. Discuss the relationship of the DNP graduate's clinical scholarship to evidence-based practice.
12. Differentiate between a systematic review and the development of clinical practice guidelines.
13. Describe the process of evidence-based decision making.
14. Be familiar with websites that can provide additional information related to evidence-based practice.

Introduction to the Doctor of Nursing Practice Degree

The doctor of nursing practice (DNP) degree is a terminal practice degree that has the goal of preparing nurses to assume leadership roles in clinical practice, clinical teaching environments, and action research arenas. It is a graduate degree that builds on the generalist foundation produced through the acquisition of a baccalaureate and master's degree in nursing (National Association of Neonatal Nurses, n.d.). The degree provides less emphasis on theoretical underpinnings and research initiation and greater emphasis on advanced clinical practice, utilization of research, and accurate evaluation of both practice and care delivery models (Association of Operating Room Nurses, 2011). According to the American Association of Colleges of Nursing (AACN), the DNP degree has tremendous momentum—whereas in 2005, eight programs were admitting DNP students and 80 institutions were considering the development of such programs, by 2013, 222 colleges had developed DNP programs and were accepting students (AACN, 2013).

TIME LINE FOR THE DEVELOPMENT OF THE DNP DEGREE

Although the concept of a practice doctorate in nursing is not a new one, the time line for the creation of the doctor of nursing practice degree extends more than 20 years. In fact, the first practice-focused nursing doctorate was offered in 1979 at Case Western Reserve University. The origins of the DNP degree can be traced back as far as the early 1900s, however, when nurses were first awarded a doctoral degree in education. Doctor of nursing science degree programs began to emerge by 1970. These programs required clinical competence and proficiency as well as scholarly research. Progress toward the ultimate development of the DNP degree continued as the doctor of nursing degree emerged in 1979 to prepare nurses who were assuming the role of the clinical leader.

The next step was the development of the doctorate of nursing practice degree, which was initially focused on nurse practitioners. This degree was first developed to prepare nurse practitioners for independent primary care roles in multiple settings but is proving to be valuable for all types of nurses in advanced practice settings. It focuses on direct care, with a concentration in research utilization to improve delivery of care, patient outcomes, and clinical systems management. The AACN has recommended that the DNP degree be the standard for entry into advanced practice for nurse practitioners, nurse–midwives, nurse anesthetists, and clinical nurse specialists by 2015. An anticipated benefit of the DNP degree is a higher rate of reimbursement for the services for advanced practice nurses in the previously mentioned specialties (National Association of Neonatal Nurses, n.d.).

As DNP programs have developed and continue to evolve, certain characteristics have begun to distinguish these practice-oriented programs. Such characteristics include:

- Less content focused on research methodology, focusing instead on the evaluation and usage of research rather than the implementation of the research process.
- Use of a capstone project in most DNP programs that is grounded in clinical practice and designed to solve problems in practice or to add new information to practice.
- Emphasis on clinical practice improvement, innovation and testing of interventions, testing of care delivery models, evaluation of healthcare outcomes, and the expertise to provide leadership in establishing clinical excellence (AACN, 2006).

These differences make the doctor of nursing practice degree the unique educational credential that it is, and they equip the graduate with the knowledge and skills needed to be an active participant in the research process.

THE CAPSTONE PROJECT

The previously mentioned capstone project that is used in the majority of practice-oriented doctorates is an integrative practice experience that results in a practice-focused, written document that will be subjected to peer and/or professional scrutiny. It is the DNP degree's alternative to the research-focused doctorate degree's dissertation. The capstone project is the culmination of the student's academic experience (Rutgers College of Nursing, 2007), and it should make a significant contribution to evidence-based nursing practice or indicate the solution to an existing problem in the healthcare delivery system. The capstone project is integral to the DNP degree because the hallmark of all doctoral education is the completion of a project that both illustrates the synthesis of the student's work and provides the foundation for future scholarship.

Some DNP programs prefer the capstone project to be a practice portfolio that documents the impact of practice initiatives or outcomes resulting from practice. Another frequently used format is that of a practice change initiative. This can consist of a pilot study, a program evaluation, a quality improvement project, an evaluation of a new practice model, or a consultation-type project. Although quantitative research is certainly possible for the DNP graduate and will be discussed in this text, many graduates gravitate toward qualitative research and thus qualify for the expedited category if using human subjects and approaching an institutional review board. An institutional review board will usually consider a research project to qualify for the expedited category if it poses little risk to the human subjects involved (Auburn University at Montgomery, 2009).

A qualitative research project focused on quality improvement can frequently be an excellent choice for a DNP student's capstone project, regardless of the practice setting. This text will focus on the planning, organizing, implementing, and evaluating of the capstone project, including the intricacies of navigating through the institutional review board (American Association of Colleges of Nursing, 2006).

Other examples of DNP capstone projects that have been utilized in these programs include the submission of manuscripts for publication, involvement in a large institution-wide research project, completion of systematic reviews, and the development of evidence-based clinical practice guidelines. Systematic reviews and clinical practice guidelines will be addressed in more detail later in this chapter.

Regardless of the form it assumes, the final DNP project will be derived from the practice experience of the student and reviewed and evaluated by an academic committee, much in the way that a research-focused doctoral candidate undergoes the defense of a dissertation. The underlying theme in any project should be the use of evidence to improve practice through either healthcare delivery or patient outcomes (AACN, 2006). Thus, it becomes clear that the DNP program cannot be separated from the concept of evidence-based practice and its foundation in research.

BENEFITS OF IMPLEMENTING THE DNP DEGREE

Implementing the DNP credential for advanced practice nurses may allow these nurses to become even more competent in the multiple roles of practice, faculty, and leadership. As these nurses enhance their knowledge

---

 TOOLBOX

Begin considering various topics that would be of interest to you as a focus for your capstone project. You'll want to begin this process by initially addressing some basic questions:

- Is there a clear need for an area to be changed or improved in your current work environment?
- Are there individuals in your current facility who would be supportive of a project in this area?
- Are there resources that could be made available to assist you, such as personnel or funding?
- Is this idea manageable and realistic? (Determine this by mapping a timeline.)
- Can you verbalize what you would be attempting to achieve by implementing the project?

If you can answer these questions, then you are well on the way to developing your topic for your project. If you cannot answer the questions, don't be concerned; you have initiated the important process of determining your project focus. The development of the capstone project will be addressed in further detail later in the text.

base, they will have the ability to improve their nursing practice as well as their patient outcomes through improved healthcare delivery. Their nursing practice will also be strengthened by their enhanced leadership skills. Nurse educators have identified that the current educational curriculum is inadequate for preparation of advanced practice nurses in light of health care's increasingly complex skill set, which incorporates new knowledge in the areas of information systems, technology, healthcare policy development, and epidemiology. At least six areas of practice have been identified as being inadequately addressed in current nursing curricula for advanced practice nurses:

1. Practice management
2. Health policy
3. Use of information technology
4. Risk management
5. Evaluation of evidence
6. Advanced diagnosis and management of the disease process (Apold, 2008)

These can be incorporated into DNP programs to prepare the new generation of clinicians.

CONCERNS REGARDING IMPLEMENTATION OF THE DNP DEGREE

As would be expected, concerns arose regarding the implementation of this new degree. A primary source of anxiety for clinicians was that of the title for the graduate of a DNP program. The DNP degree is intended to be a practice doctorate, so discussion has arisen over the use of the title of "doctor." In reality, if credentials are clearly displayed by the graduate, there should be no confusion on the part of patients, the public, or practitioners. Advanced practice nurses who complete such a program will retain their specialized credentials but will simply have the enhanced knowledge and leadership skills unique to the DNP program (National Association of Neonatal Nurses, n.d.).

A second concern that has been raised, particularly by practicing nurse practitioners, is the reaction of state boards of nursing if the DNP degree becomes the entry-level degree for nurse practitioner education. This should not be a source of anxiety for any candidate for a DNP program, because no certification agency currently requires the practice-oriented doctorate as an eligibility requirement, and regulatory bodies have not drafted a plan to require all nurse practitioners in current practice to obtain the DNP degree (National Association of Neonatal Nurses, n.d.).

A third concern with very practical overtones is that of the job market for the DNP graduate. What will be the demand for DNP-prepared advanced practice nurses, and would their pay be adequate to justify the expense of the additional education? Research has shown a link between higher levels of nursing education and more positive patient outcomes, so it is believed that DNP-prepared clinicians will prove their worth through their leadership skills, honed critical thinking ability, and heightened economic and public policy knowledge, in addition to their superior clinical skills (National Association of Neonatal Nurses, n.d.).

In addition, there is a concern that nurses who have acquired the DNP credential may have difficulty finding tenure-track faculty positions, because the PhD has traditionally been considered the entry-level degree for an assistant professor in academia. Because tenure provides professors with unique rights, status, and privileges in addition to implied longevity in the current position, it will be the responsibility of nursing leaders in academia to ensure that DNP-prepared faculty are not only prepared to apply for tenure but also are thoroughly incorporated into the overall university environment, including committee participation. The DNP graduate who opts to move into a career in academia must select his or her academic appointment carefully to ensure that the position assumed is one that enhances the recently acquired degree rather than diminishes it (Apold, 2008). Many DNP-prepared nurses are already being utilized in academia with great success.

RECOMMENDED CONTENT FOR DNP PROGRAMS

Because of the explosive growth in practice-oriented nursing doctoral programs, the AACN developed a task force that was charged with the examination of the current status of such programs. The task force recommended that practice-focused doctoral nursing programs include seven primary areas of content:

1. The scientific basis for practice
2. Advanced nursing practice
3. Organization and system leadership/management and quality improvement

4. Analytic methodologies related to practice evaluation and the application of evidence for nursing practice
5. Utilization of both technology and information for the improvement and transformation of health care
6. The development, implementation, and evaluation of health policy
7. Interdisciplinary collaboration for improving patient healthcare outcomes as well as healthcare outcomes for the greater population (AACN, 2006)

Review of these areas of content will reveal the importance of the research process to the doctor of nursing practice student. It is the intent of the DNP curriculum that graduates will have a broad scientific base that can be translated efficiently to influence healthcare delivery and patient outcomes. These outcomes encompass not only direct patient care, but also the needs of the family unit, the community, and ultimately, the global patient perspective. In order to be able to conceptualize new healthcare delivery models, graduates must be adept at working in both organizational and public policy arenas. The DNP graduate must be particularly proficient in quality management strategies and at functioning as a change agent at both the local organizational level and the greater policy level. He or she must be able to evaluate the cost-effectiveness of a particular aspect of care delivery and to have enough knowledge of finance and economics to design realistic, fiscally sound patient care delivery strategies. However, none of these strategies can be accomplished without the presence of a sound scientific base that can translate both effectively and efficiently into patient care delivery (AACN, 2006).

The DNP Graduate as an Agent for Quality Improvement

The concept of the DNP graduate being an agent for quality improvement in a facility through an emphasis on systems thinking is so important that the AACN considers it one of the essential hallmarks of a DNP curriculum. In fact, the AACN states that the DNP program should prepare a graduate to:

- Develop and evaluate patient care delivery approaches to meet both the current and anticipated need of patient populations; this development and evaluation process should be based on scientific findings in nursing as well as economic theory, political science, and organizational research.

- Ensure accountability for the quality of the health care delivered and the degree of safety of the patient populations with whom the graduate works.
- Use advanced communication skills and processes to lead quality improvement and patient safety initiative in a healthcare system; these advanced communication processes should include technological skills that would require the graduate to be adept with various forms of computerized communication.
- Use principles of business, finance, economics, and health policy to develop and implement plans to improve the quality of healthcare delivery; these plans may be at the practice level or the system level.
- Develop a budget for practice initiatives for improved delivery of patient care; this includes the ability to monitor the budget for efficient use of the funds.
- Analyze the cost-effectiveness of practice initiatives to improve healthcare outcomes, taking into account the risk involved to both the overall system and the patient population.
- Demonstrate sensitivity to diversity in both patients and providers, both at the cultural level and at the overall patient population level.
- Develop and/or evaluate effective strategies for management of ethical dilemmas that can occur in the course of healthcare delivery, whether in the healthcare organization itself or within the research process. Modified from American Association of Colleges of Nursing (2006). The essentials of doctoral education for advanced nursing practice. Retrieved September 26, 2009, from www.aacn.nche.edu/DNP/pdf/Essentials.pdf

An offshoot of the incorporation of quality improvement initiatives for the DNP student is clinical prevention and population health. The AACN defines clinical prevention as health promotion and risk reduction, as well as illness prevention for both individuals and families. Population health is considered to include aggregate, community, environmental, occupational, cultural, and socioeconomic dimensions of health, with aggregates being groups of individuals who can be defined by a shared characteristic such as gender (AACN, 2006). The DNP graduate is focused in the areas of clinical prevention and population health in an effort to improve the overall health status of the population of the United States while continuing to integrate nursing's long-standing emphasis on health promotion and disease prevention. These foci are also consistent with the

TOOLBOX

A quality improvement project is a great way to implement your capstone project. Because it frequently is something that a facility such as a hospital would be implementing as part of its overall quality initiative, it may be easy to obtain institutional support for the project. Typically, the more that a project is institutionally driven, the easier it is to move smoothly through the institutional review board (IRB) process. Can you think of a quality improvement initiative that would benefit your facility and also form a basis for a capstone project?

DNP graduate's focus on evidence-based practice and research because the student should be prepared to analyze epidemiological, biostatistical, occupational, and environmental data. Groundbreaking knowledge of infectious disease processes as well as disaster preparedness and triage also will be integrated into clinical prevention (AACN, 2006).

The DNP Graduate as an Advocate for Health Care Through Use of Healthcare Policy

The framework for delivery of healthcare services is provided by healthcare policy—whether through governmental regulations, institutional procedures, or the standards of a healthcare organization—and that framework can either enhance or impede healthcare delivery to patients. Although political activism and a commitment to policy development that will lead to delivery of the highest possible quality of health care for patients are integral to the role of the professional nurse, the DNP graduate will be uniquely qualified to assume a leadership role as advocate for both the public and the nursing profession. The DNP graduate will be prepared not only to design and implement new healthcare policies, but also to influence existing policies that will significantly affect the financing of health care, practice regulation, access to health care, safety in patient care, quality of care delivered, and efficacy in patient care outcomes. The DNP curriculum should prepare the graduate to analyze the policy process and competently influence policy formation. The graduate's analysis should occur from the perspectives of consumers, nursing, allied and ancillary healthcare professions, and the public, all of whom will be stakeholders in the policy development process. The graduate should be prepared to attempt to influence policy makers through participation on committees at every level, whether institutional or international, so that patients will receive improved delivery of health care and higher level outcomes. Finally, the DNP graduate will educate all stakeholders in conjunction with serving as an advocate for both the nursing profession and patients so the public is informed regarding the need for improved patient care outcomes (AACN, 2006).

Accurate evaluation of healthcare policy frequently occurs most effectively through interprofessional collaboration. The modern healthcare environment is dependent on the skills of individuals from multiple professions. This means that DNP graduates must have preparation in leadership of teams as well as the establishment of interprofessional teams. Regarding interprofessional collaboration, the DNP program should prepare the graduate to:

- Use effective communication and collaborative skills in both the development and implementation of practice models; these skills should also be utilized in peer review, practice guidelines, health policy, standards of care, and production of other scholarly works.
- Lead interprofessional teams to analyze complex practice and organizational issues.
- Use both consultative and leadership skills with intraprofessional and interprofessional teams to serve as change agents in healthcare delivery systems (AACN, 2006).

 TOOLBOX

Do you serve on any interprofessional committees in your facility or in your local healthcare community? If not, check on the availability of areas where you can serve in the role of advocate. Interprofessional collaboration will result and may also provide you with access to individuals who are ready to assist you as you implement the capstone project. Is the level of interprofessional collaboration in your own facility strong? If not, what could you do in your new role of DNP to strengthen this collaboration?

The DNP Graduate as an Advanced Practice Nurse

A hallmark of the DNP degree is preparation to practice in a specialized area within the larger, overriding umbrella of the nursing profession. Although in reality no nurse can demonstrate mastery of all advanced roles with a grasp of the knowledge required to function in each of them, DNP programs should prepare the nurse to practice within a distinct specialty that requires both expertise and an advanced knowledge base that includes legal and regulatory issues. In preparation for functioning in a specialty practice role, the DNP program will provide foundational practice competencies such as honed assessment skills and the application of biophysical, psychosocial, behavioral, sociopolitical, cultural, and economic knowledge in practice settings. The DNP graduate functioning as an advanced practice nurse utilizes a holistic perspective to assist patients, families, and communities in decision making, making positive lifestyle changes, and self-care. Because the advanced practice nurse assesses, manages, and evaluates patients at the most independent level of clinical nursing practice, the DNP student is required to take courses in advanced health, physical assessment, advanced physiology and pathophysiology, and advanced pharmacology. These courses will assist the DNP graduate who is practicing as an advanced practice nurse to identify developing practice trends, identify changes occurring at the systemic level, and make improvements in the care of patient populations within their practice systems. In their function as advanced practice nurses, DNP graduates should be adequately prepared to:

- Conduct a comprehensive, systematic assessment of health and illness parameters in complex situations; because these situations may involve individual patient populations, families, communities,

 TOOLBOX

What practice trends can you identify in your local, state, and regional healthcare communities? Do you view these trends as being beneficial and generating positive patient care outcomes, and do you see them as potentially harmful to consumers? Give the rationale for your answer.

nations, or even global populations, the graduate must be able to incorporate cultural sensitivity in diverse scenarios.
■ Use nursing science as well as other sciences to design, implement, and evaluate therapeutic interventions and the patient care outcomes that result from them (AACN, 2006).

The DNP Graduate as a User of Information Systems and Technology

The DNP graduate is distinguished by the ability to use information systems and technology to provide leadership within a healthcare system or an academic setting. The degree equips the graduate to design, select, and utilize information systems and technology to evaluate programs of healthcare delivery, outcomes of patient care, and systems of care. Incorporation of information systems and technology enables the graduate to use tools regarding budget and productivity as well as Internet-based tools to enhance patient care. The DNP graduate should be prepared to demonstrate both the conceptual ability and technical skills needed to develop and implement a plan for data extraction from databases containing practice information. Once such a plan is implemented, the graduate should be capable of categorizing the data extracted from such databases, using the appropriate computer program to generate statistics and then accurately interpreting those statistical results. In addition, the graduate should be proficient in using information systems and technological

 TOOLBOX

The public is more technologically adept today than ever before. Does the area where you practice maintain a list of websites that will provide patients with accurate information that they can access once they are discharged? If not, develop this and provide this to patients upon discharge. This will ensure that they absorb more accurate information during discharge teaching and also act as follow-up to answer questions that may arise. Are you familiar with the process that is typically used in your area of practice for discharge teaching? Would you change it if you could, and if so how?

resources as quality improvement initiatives are incorporated into the healthcare delivery system. Finally, the graduate should have knowledge of the standards and principles involved in the evaluation of patient care technology and the ethical, regulatory, and legal issues that surround such an evaluation (AACN, 2006).

The DNP Graduate With an Aggregate Focus

The DNP graduate who functions in an administrative, healthcare policy, informatics, or population-based specialty has an aggregate focus, which means the graduate directs his or her attention toward populations, systems, organizations, and state or national policies. Although these specialties may not have direct patient care responsibilities, there will still be the need for problem definition and the design of health interventions at the aggregate level. The DNP graduate who opts to have an aggregate focus will, out of necessity, be required to be competent in community assessment techniques so that aggregate health or system needs can be identified (AACN, 2006).

 TOOLBOX

Envision yourself functioning at the aggregate level and addressing public policy. Are there healthcare policies in your state or at the national level that you would like to address? If so, what are they, and how would you like to change them? How would these changes affect consumers of health care within the next 5 years?

The DNP Graduate's Clinical Scholarship and Evidence-Based Practice

It has been established that scholarly research is a hallmark of doctoral education. In the case of the DNP graduate, the nurse applies knowledge in the solution of a problem. This is known as the scholarship of practice in nursing. This form of scholarship highlights key activities of DNP graduates—namely, the translation of research into practice, as well as the dissemination and integration of new knowledge. Whereas research-focused nursing doctoral programs provide the research skills needed for discovery of new knowledge in the discipline, DNP programs provide the leadership skills needed for the graduate to engage in evidence-based practice. According to Pipe, Wellik, Buchda, Hansen, and Martyn (2005), evidence-based practice focuses on methods of critically appraising and applying available data and research to achieve a better understanding of clinical decision making. The method integrates research evidence with clinical expertise and patient values, which means that the best available evidence will be combined with clinical judgment. This necessitates competence in knowledge application, which consists of:

- Translating research into practice.
- Evaluating practice.
- Improving the reliability of healthcare practice and outcomes.
- Participating in collaborative research.

This means DNP programs focus on applying new science and evaluating new knowledge. In addition, DNP graduates use their practice to generate evidence that will serve as parameters in guiding improvements in practice and patient care outcomes (AACN, 2006). Evidence in health care most frequently consists of:

- *Quasi-experimental studies*—Often used because they do not require randomization or control of all variables.
- *Descriptive research*—Considered to be a systematic analysis of an area of interest to the researcher; often uses survey instruments and does not necessarily examine causation.
- *Ex post facto studies*—These can be used very effectively by the DNP graduate once a healthcare trend has been identified; they involve retrospective research that allows the cause-and-effect relationship to be discovered as variables are analyzed. Once the cause-and-effect relationship can be identified, a preventive strategy can be developed (Hanchett, 2005).

Regarding evidence-based practice, the DNP graduate will be prepared to perform a critical appraisal of existing literature, apply relevant findings in the development of practice guidelines, design and implement processes to evaluate practice outcomes, and design, implement, and evaluate quality improvement methodologies. Ultimately, the graduate should be able to:

- Collect appropriate data to generate evidence for nursing practice.
- Direct the design of databases to generate evidence for practice.
- Analyze data derived from practice.
- Design evidence-based nursing interventions.
- Predict and analyze patient care outcomes.
- Examine patterns of behavior and outcomes.
- Identify gaps in the evidence for practice (AACN, 2006).

The relationship of the DNP graduate to evidence-based practice is illustrated by the definition of this type of practice. The American Association of Neuroscience Nurses defines evidence-based practice as the integration of the best, most accurate evidence available; nursing expertise in the field; and the values as well as preference of the individuals who are served, or the families or even communities if they assume the client role. The idea of best practices means that care concepts, interventions, and techniques are grounded in research, and therefore will promote a higher quality of client care (Mcilvoy & Hinkle, 2008). The DNP graduate addresses this concept by performing systematic reviews. This means that the findings of all methodologically sound studies that address the same research question are summarized. The systematic review treats eligible research studies as a population to be sampled and surveyed. The individual study characteristics and results will then have an abstract developed, and results will be quantified, coded, and developed into a database that can be statistically analyzed (DiCenso et al., 2000).

The systematic review can be an outstanding research tool for the DNP clinician. As a graduate of a practice-focused doctoral program, the practitioner who conducts such a review is able to make an objective assessment of the available evidence, specifically of the outcomes of particular interventions that could be implemented. The evidence will be located, evaluated, and then consolidated into a comprehensive and unbiased summary. The comprehensive nature of the review allows literature to be sorted into low and high quality. If the sheer volume of available resources is overwhelming, the quantity of literature can be reduced by:

- Reducing the time frame of the search to within the past 5 years.
- Restricting the number of databases investigated.
- Narrowing the focus of the study by selecting specific research methods.
- Reducing the search to certain journals, although the DNP clinician should recognize that this may skew results.
- Limiting searches to studies published in certain nations.
- Excluding unpublished literature (also known as gray literature) (Forward, 2002).

The integration of the process of translating evidence into practice for the DNP clinician can best be illustrated by Carper's work, which identified four essential patterns of knowing in nursing: empirical, ethical, personal, and aesthetic patterns (Pipe et al., 2005). Empirical knowing was defined as relating to factual descriptions, explanations, and predictions; ethical knowing was thought to pertain to moral obligations, values, and desired results; personal knowing was defined as the genuine relationship that develops between each nurse and patient; and aesthetic knowing referred to the nurse's perception of the significant areas in the patient's behavior as well as the art involved in performing nursing skills. Evidence-based practice is believed to pertain most closely to empirical knowing, focusing on critical appraisal and application of available data and research in order to understand the process of clinical decision making more fully.

Evidence-based clinical practice guidelines developed as a means of influencing patient outcomes while bringing evidence-based practice into bedside nursing practice. Clinical practice guidelines are practice recommendations based on the analysis of the evidence available on a specific topic and a specific patient population (Mcilvoy & Hinkle, 2008). The guidelines are developed with representation from as many stakeholders as are interested in contributing, should be tested by healthcare professionals who were not involved in their development, and should be reviewed regularly and then modified as needed in order to incorporate new knowledge that is emerging in the field (DiCenso et al., 2000).

The concept of evidence-based nursing was consolidated by Flemming (1998) into five distinct stages:

1. Information needs are identified in current practice and are then translated into focused questions; the questions should be

searchable while still reflecting the focus on a specific patient, clinical situation, or managerial scenario.

2. Once a focused question has been identified, it is used as a basis for a literature search so that the relevant evidence from current research can be identified.

3. The relevant evidence that has been gathered undergoes critical appraisal to determine if validity is present; the extent of the generalizability of the research will also be appraised.

4. A plan of care is developed using the best available evidence and clinical expertise, as well as the patient's perspective.

5. A process of self-reflection, audit, and peer assessment is used to evaluate implementation of the designed plan of care.

Unless the focused question is framed correctly, the DNP graduate will have difficulty implementing evidence-based practice through the translation of evidence. An accurately framed question should consist of the clinical situation being addressed, the selected intervention, and the patient care outcome (Flemming, 1998).

 TOOLBOX

Think about your current area of practice in your facility. Are there areas that you know are being implemented daily but are not grounded in evidence-based practice? If so, why do you think that these areas have continued to be utilized? What could you do as a DNP to change them? How would you initiate the change process?

The DNP Graduate's Participation in Evidence-Based Decision Making

An integral part of evidence-based practice is evidence-based decision making, and the DNP graduate is uniquely qualified to fully participate in this process. Evidence-based decision making involves combining the knowledge the DNP graduate derives from clinical practice with patient preferences and research evidence that is weighted based on its internal and external validity. It is evidence-based decision making that will allow nurses who hold a practice doctorate to actively engage with research evidence as it is accessed, appraised, and incorporated into these clinicians' professional judgment and clinical decision making. There are several components of the process of evidence-based decision making:

- Formulate a focused clinical question once there is a recognized need for additional information; the DNP clinician's capacity to fulfill a variety of roles in a facility will allow this to occur easily.
- Search for the most appropriate evidence to meet the need that has been previously identified.
- Critically appraise the evidence that has been retrieved to meet the identified need.
- Incorporate the evidence that has been critically appraised into a strategy for action.
- Evaluate the effects of decisions that are made and actions that are taken; the DNP clinician's close ties to the clinical setting will allow such evaluation to occur easily (Thompson, Cullum, McCaughan, Sheldon, & Raynor, 2004).

Each component must be fully implemented to ensure the process that is occurring is one of evidence-based decision making.

 TOOLBOX

The previous toolbox asked you to identify areas in your practice area that you know are not based on evidence-based practice but have continued to be implemented. Once the change process has been initiated to ground these practices in current evidence, how do think that the overall change process would be implemented?

The Process of Translating Evidence Into Clinical Practice

As graduates of practice-focused doctoral programs, DNP students will be uniquely qualified to frequently progress through the process of reformulating evidence into clinical practice. As graduates of a practice-oriented doctoral program, these clinicians should be continually involved in the systematic review of research in preparation for designing a change in practice based on the validated evidence. Rosswurm and Larrabee's model proposed that six phases are involved in this process (1999):

1. *Assessing the need for a change in practice*—Determine whether there is sufficient evidence to warrant initiating the process of changing nursing practice; this is accomplished by collecting internal data about the current practice and then comparing it to the external data (Duffy, 2004).

2. *Linking the problem with nursing interventions and patient care outcomes*—Once the clinician has determined that evidence indicates a need for a change in nursing practice, he or she must identify the nursing interventions that could potentially create the change and the outcomes that would ideally result from that change.

3. *Synthesizing the best evidence*—Conduct an exhaustive literature search so the literature can be weighed and examined with a critical eye; although a large body of literature may be identified, unless it is of the highest quality, there may not be sufficient need to progress through the process of translating that evidence into practice. The DNP graduate can carry out this step through a systematic review, because once the clinical problem has been identified, it must be stated as a focused clinical question that can be answered by searching the literature. It is the focused clinical questions that will be used to select keywords and limits for the search in order to make it more precise. Potential benefits and risks to the patient must be identified prior to implementing a change in nursing practice (Duffy, 2004).

4. *Designing the practice change*—Involve stakeholders to identify strategies that will explore the original issue as much as possible and then be used to implement it into practice; often referred to as a clinical protocol, this change should take into account the practice environment, available resources, and stakeholder feedback. The less complex the new protocol, the more likely it is to be accepted by stakeholders. Conducting a pilot test of the new protocol can make the change more acceptable because it will allow stakeholders who are practitioners to influence the formation of the change to suit their needs (Duffy, 2004).

5. *Implementing the practice change*—If the evidence supports changing nursing practice, begin implementation of the strategies that were identified in the previous step, evaluating each carefully to ensure they are indeed evidence based. During this process, follow-up reinforcement of learning should occur, as should data collection of outcomes from stakeholders, analysis of the data, and interpretation of the results to determine whether the protocol was implemented as was originally intended and the effect of the new protocol on patient care outcomes (Duffy, 2004).

6. *Integrating and maintaining the change in practice*—Once the change in nursing practice has been integrated, maintain the change through development of evaluation criteria that allow for frequent reassessment of the change and the interventions that were used to implement it. Planned change principles should be used at this point, with administration providing the infrastructure and resources needed to implement the change (Duffy, 2004).

This chapter has illustrated the ever-strengthening relationship of the DNP clinician to the research process and patient care outcomes. This practitioner's educational background and capacity for fulfilling multiple roles in the nursing community prepare the DNP graduate to provide unique contributions to nursing research in all areas of the healthcare community. Subsequent chapters will break down the specific areas of the research process into reality-focused, manageable sections that can be implemented in any practice setting that is the focus of the DNP clinician.

Learning Enhancement Tools

1. Suppose you are a DNP graduate who is employed in a large hospital in the area of quality improvement. You have found that a large number of medication errors typically occur on a particular surgical floor when the unit admits more than six postoperative patients per shift.
   a. You are interested in developing a protocol to decrease the number of medication errors. How can this be addressed through a systematic review?

    b. After performing the systematic review, you opt to develop clinical practice guidelines. How should this process most appropriately occur?

2. Imagine you are a DNP graduate who is working in the area of risk management in a large medical practice. You find that evidence seems to indicate a need to manage preoperative anxiety more effectively in the patient population in order to achieve better postoperative patient outcomes. Describe the process of translating this evidence into clinical practice.

3. Imagine you are a DNP graduate who is functioning as a clinical coordinator in a large psychiatric facility that treats primarily adolescents. You note that a few of your patients seem to achieve a more manageable level of anxiety when they practice the technique of journaling. You are interested in determining whether this would be an effective technique to use with all of the adolescent patients who are experiencing a high level of anxiety. How would you want to frame the focused question regarding this clinical situation to accurately implement evidence-based nursing?

    a. Imagine further that you have developed the focused question, implemented the literature search, and begun the critical appraisal of the research evidence. You determine that validity is present, but the degree of generalizability to other patient populations will be smaller than you had originally envisioned. What should you do?

    b. Suppose you develop a plan based on the individual patient's input, available evidence, and clinical expertise. The plan is implemented, and performance is evaluated using a combination of audits and peer assessment. The evaluation indicates that the plan was not as effective as you had hoped it would be. What should you do?

4. Assume you are a DNP graduate who is functioning in an education position in a large teaching medical center that is university affiliated. You are concerned that the IV catheter insertion technique that is currently being used with new registered nurses is not as effective as other methods.

    a. How would you perform a systematic review of the evidence on this subject?

    b. Once the systematic review of the evidence is completed, how would you design new clinical practice guidelines for the facility?

Resources

American Association of Colleges of Nursing. (2006). DNP roadmap task force report. Retrieved from www.aacn.nche.edu/DNP/pdf /Essentials.pdf

Bellini, S., & Cusson, R. (2012). The doctor of nursing practice for entry into advanced practice. *Newborn and Infant Nursing Reviews, 12*(1), 12–16.

Lenz, E. (2005). The practice doctorate in nursing: An idea whose time has come. *Online Journal of Issues in Nursing, 10*(3). Retrieved from www.medscape.com/viewarticle/514543

Marion, L., O'Sullivan, A., Crabtree, K., Price, M., & Fontana S. (2003). Curriculum models for the practice doctorate in nursing. *Topics in Advanced Practice Nursing eJournal.* Retrieved from www.medscape .com/viewarticle/500742

Mundinger, M. (2005). Who's who in nursing: Bringing clarity to the doctor of nursing practice. *Nursing Outlook, 53,* 173–176.

PEW Health Professions Commission. (1995). *Reforming health care workforce regulation: Policy considerations for the 21st century.* San Francisco, CA: Pew Health Professions.

Wall, B., Novak, J., & Wilkerson, S. (2005). Doctor of nursing practice program development: Reengineering health care. *Journal of Nursing Education, 44*(5), 396–403.

References

American Association of Colleges of Nursing. (2006). *The essentials of doctoral education for advanced nursing practice.* Retrieved from www.aacn.nche.edu/DNP/pdf/Essentials.pdf

American Association of Colleges of Nursing. (2013). *Leading initiatives.* Retrieved from www.aacn.nche.edu/dnp/program-schools

Apold, S. (2008). The doctor of nursing practice: Looking back, moving forward. *Journal for Nurse Practitioners, 4*(2), 101–107.

Association of Operating Room Nurses.(2011). Criteria for the Evaluation of Master's, Practice Doctorate, and Post-Graduate Certificate Educational Programs. Retrieved from http://www.aorn.org/Clinical_Practice /Position_Statements/Position_Statements.aspx

Auburn University at Montgomery. (2009). *Institutional review board.* Retrieved March 26, 2010, from http://www.aum.edu/indexm _ektid8178.aspx

DiCenso, A., Ciliska, D., Marks, S., McKibbon, A., Cullum, N., & Thompson, C. (2000). *Evidence-based nursing.* Retrieved from www.cebm .utoronto.ca/syllabi/nur/print/whole.htm

Duffy, M. (2004). Resources for building a research utilization program. Retrieved from www.medscape.com/viewarticle/495915_print

Flemming, K. (1998). Asking answerable questions. *Evidence Based Nursing, 1,* 36–37.

Forward, L. (2002). A practical guide to conducting a systematic review. *Nursing Times, 98*(2), 36.

Hanchett, M. (2005). Infusion nursing's greatest barrier: The lack of evidence to support evidence-based practice. *Topics in Advanced Practice Nursing.* Retrieved from www.medscape.com/viewarticle/507908_print

Mcilvoy, L., & Hinkle, J. (2008). What is evidence-based neuroscience nursing practice? *Journal of Neuroscience Nursing.* Retrieved from http://findarticles.com/p/articles/mi_hb6374/is_6_40/ai_n31179123

National Association of Neonatal Nurses. (n.d.). *Understanding the doctor of nursing practice (DNP): Evolution, perceived benefits and challenges.* Retrieved September 25, 2009, from www.nann.org/pdf/DNPEntry .pdf

Pipe, T., Wellik, K., Buchda, V., Hansen, C., & Martyn, D. (2005). Implementing evidence-based nursing practice. *MedSurg Nursing.* Retrieved from http://ajm.sagepub.com/cgi/reprint/22/3/148.pdf

Rosswurm, M., & Larrabee, J. (1999). A model for change to evidence-based practice image. *Journal of Nursing Scholarship, 31*(4), 317–322.

Rutgers College of Nursing. (2007). *DNP program in nursing handbook for students.* Retrieved September 25, 2009, from www.nursing.rutgers .edu/files/DNPHandbook07.pdf

Thompson, C., Cullum, N., McCaughan, D., Sheldon, T., & Raynor, P. (2004). Nurses, information use, and clinical decision making—the real world potential for evidence-based decisions in nursing. *Evidence Based Nursing, 7,* 68–72.

CHAPTER 2

Developing the Researchable Problem

© echo3005/ShutterStock, Inc.

Objectives

Upon completion of this chapter, the reader should be prepared to:

1. Discuss the elements needed to formulate a research question, specifically discussing the PICOT process of developing a research question.
2. Utilize sample scenarios to formulate suitable research questions.
3. Discuss the development of a testable hypothesis.
4. Describe the different categories of hypotheses: research vs. statistical, directional vs. nondirectional.
5. Determine when it would be most appropriate to utilize a research question and when it would be most appropriate to utilize a hypothesis.
6. Discuss the difference between a directional hypothesis and a nondirectional hypothesis.
7. Discuss the difference between a research hypothesis and a statistical hypothesis.
8. Discuss the relationship of a hypothesis to the theoretical framework.

9. Distinguish between the conceptual framework and the theoretical framework.
10. Describe the different categories of nursing theories: grand, midrange, and microrange.
11. Describe the difference between inductive reasoning and deductive reasoning.
12. Discuss the process of selecting an appropriate theoretical framework.

Selection of the Research Problem and Development of the Research Question

The selection of the **research problem** is arguably the most important step in the research process, for if the problem is not viable and therefore testable, the entire process may be implemented in vain, wasting valuable man-hours and financial resources while generating nothing more than frustration for the researcher. For the DNP clinician, the research problem must above all relate to some area of practice. The germ of the idea can come directly from patients or colleagues or more indirectly from the auditing process if the clinician functions in quality management or nursing administration (Fitzpatrick, 2007).

The DNP clinician must select a research problem that will contribute to evidence-based practice and to the development of either a **hypothesis** or a **research question**. The development of hypotheses and their proper usage will be discussed in the next sections. According to Stillwell, Fineout-Overhold, Melnyk, and Williamson (2010), five components will indicate that the researcher has developed a research question that is rooted in an evidence-based practice problem:

1. The patient group or patient condition is clearly identified.
2. There is an issue or intervention that is being investigated, such as a method of patient care or a specific diagnostic test.
3. There is a specified way for a baseline measurement to be made as well as a method for comparison.
4. An outcome or result is indicated.
5. There is a time frame required for the intervention to achieve the outcome.

In order for the researcher to keep these elements in mind while developing the research question, the acronym PICOT frequently is utilized:

- P = the specified patient or target population
- I = the issue or intervention being investigated
- C = the comparison being made
- O = the outcome that may be the result
- T = time frame required to achieve the outcome (Stillwell, Fineout-Overhold, Melnyk, and Williamson, 2010).

An example of an acceptable evidence-based practice question would be: Does use of a pain scale reduce the patient's experience of pain post-operatively? In this case:

- P = Patient is undergoing a surgical procedure.
- I = Patient is taught how to measure pain using a pain scale.
- C = The pain level without using a pain scale is compared to the pain level when using a pain scale.
- O = The patient has verbalized or indicated experience of postoperative pain.
- T = The time frame is the postoperative time period.

The impetus for a researchable problem frequently may arise from a clinical situation the researcher notes. In addition, the DNP clinician may make an observation in his or her daily practice and wonder whether the clinical issue is coincidental or fact based. A researchable problem may arise from reading journal articles in the DNP graduate's field of practice. Research articles typically state areas for further study that have arisen from that particular manuscript. Often an article will state that a recommendation is made for replication of the original study with a different population of patients or using a different type of methodology (Beyea, 2000). As potential researchable problems arise during the course of a typical practice-oriented day, the researcher should maintain a pocket-sized notebook specifically to jot down such thoughts. At the end of the day, additional details can be recorded, and then Internet search engines can be used to review the literature that is readily available on the topic. This will aid in the decision of whether the problem is manageable for the researcher, practical to implement in the form of research, and of sufficient interest to the researcher to be the focus of a lengthy project (Van Cott & Smith, 2009).

The researcher should also consider several practical concerns while formulating the research question:

- Is the research question one that could be easily understood by readers who are not nurses? This will help ensure the research report can be formulated into an article that could be published, because the broader the audience, the more likely that publication will occur. Furthermore, the nature of the practice-oriented doctorate incorporates elements of multiple fields of study, including management, economics, finance, and psychology, to name only a few. It is important to strive to appeal to the wide audience of professionals who practice in these areas.
- Is the answer to the research question not immediately obvious? If the answer is clearly obvious, the problem has no researchable basis.
- Can the research question be answered in the time available to the researcher? If the question requires an indeterminately long period of time to be answered, it will not be practical as a researchable problem.
- Can the research question be answered using the financial and personnel resources available to the researcher? If the question would require more money and personnel than the researcher has available, it is not practical as a researchable problem (Learning Domain, 2009). The researcher must be brutally honest regarding his or her own skills and resources—if the project would require hiring additional personnel to fill in knowledge gaps, and funds for such

 TOOLBOX

Think about the current practice situation in your own facility. Can you name three factors in your own work area that would form the basis of a research question? Now think beyond your own work area into other departments. Can you name three factors that would involve collaboration with other departments and would also generate research questions?

personnel are lacking, the researcher must strongly consider either phrasing the research question in a different manner or selecting a new topic.

Appropriate Use of a Research Question

A research question is most often used instead of a hypothesis when an **exploratory** or **descriptive study** is being undertaken. This type of qualitative research design is frequently used when there is a lack of literature in an area of interest to the researcher. The descriptive findings that are often generated in qualitative studies can provide the basis for further research that will utilize hypotheses. As previously mentioned, the sole intention of exploratory research designs is to make the researcher more familiar with the phenomena being investigated so that additional, more precise research questions as well as hypotheses can be generated. These studies can be utilized when the researcher is working with a new phenomenon that has never been thoroughly investigated. Compare this research design to descriptive studies, which are intended to more accurately represent a phenomenon that may have already undergone some previous investigation so that additional research questions and potentially even hypotheses can be generated (Manheim, Rich, & Willnat, 2002). Recognizing that a research question should be written for an exploratory research design when the phenomenon being studied is one that has never been thoroughly investigated before, an acceptable research question could be, "Is the incidence of substance abuse greater in hospice nurses who have experienced cancer in their own families than in hospice nurses who have no firsthand experience with the disease?" Note that

 TOOLBOX

Put yourself in the position of a researcher who is contemplating a descriptive study. Think about a phenomenon that is related to your current work situation and has been already investigated but could warrant additional investigation. How could a research question be generated from this phenomenon?

there is no attempt to predict any relationship that might exist, although the question is specific enough to provide direction for the study.

Appropriate Use of a Hypothesis

As previously mentioned, research questions are typically used when an exploratory or descriptive research design is being undertaken. For the most part, hypotheses should be developed for all other types of research projects. A hypothesis can be considered to be a prediction that will help the researcher seek a solution to the research problem. Specifically, a hypothesis is a statement about the relationship between two or more variables, with variables being the properties the researcher is study-ing. Variables are designated as either the **independent variable** or the **dependent variable**. The independent variable leads to the effect pro-duced in the dependent variable. For example, if the researcher is studying the effect of caffeine intake and test anxiety in students, caffeine intake would be the independent variable leading to the effect, which in this case would be test anxiety or the dependent variable. The dependent vari-able is actually the one the researcher is primarily concerned with under-standing more thoroughly. It is important to understand that although the researcher recognizes that variability in the dependent variable is assumed to depend on changes in the independent variable, there is no implication that a causal relationship is occurring (LoBiondo-Wood & Haber, 2002).

TOOLBOX

Suppose you are an investigator who is interested in studying the effect of consumption of a high-fiber diet on nursing students' performance in the clinical setting. What would you designate as the independent variable? What would be the dependent variable?

Developing a Testable Hypothesis

Once the researcher has formulated a researchable problem and has determined that a hypothesis is more appropriate for the research proj-ect than a research question, the next step in the research process for the

DNP clinician involves developing the testable hypothesis. According to LoBiondo-Wood and Haber (2002), hypotheses serve three purposes for the researcher:

1. To provide a connection between theory and the real world of the patient
2. To advance knowledge of the researcher through potential new discoveries
3. To provide direction for a research project by identifying a possible anticipated outcome of the research

Hypotheses are generated by either **dependent variable** or **deductive reasoning**. If trial and error is used to construct a theory, the hypotheses may be produced by inductive generalization. Hypotheses generated inductively can be prominent in exploratory research, which can be used to construct theories, but they do not help explain phenomena. Once a theory has been stated relating variables in a logical system, hypotheses can be derived from the theory by deductive reasoning (Manheim et al., 2002).

Several characteristics make an acceptable hypothesis, one of which is a relationship statement, which identifies the predicted relationship between the variables. For example, a possible hypothesis for a research project could be "High school students who do not drink caffeinated sodas have a lesser degree of test anxiety in comparison to high school students who drink at least two caffeinated sodas daily." This is an acceptable hypothesis because it makes a predictive statement about the variables, specifically, that caffeine use in high school students has an effect on their level of test anxiety. Note that the direction of the predicted relationship is also specified, in this case, using the phrase *lesser degree* (LoBiondo-Wood & Haber, 2002). Furthermore, an appropriate hypothesis should specify the variables being investigated, the population being studied, and the predicted outcome.

Perhaps the most important characteristic of an acceptable hypothesis is its testability by the researcher. This means that the variables of the hypothesis can be observed, measured, and analyzed. Specifically, this indicates that once the data are collected and analyzed accurately, the hypothesis will be either supported or not supported. Once the hypothesis is tested, the outcome proposed by the hypothesis either will be congruent with the actual outcome that occurs or will be different. A hypothesis can fail to achieve testability if the researcher has not predicted the anticipated outcome, has not utilized observable or measurable variables, or has failed to use objective phrases in wording the hypothesis (LoBiondo-Wood & Haber, 2002).

If a research problem was proposed at the beginning of the research report, the hypothesis should directly respond to that problem. The variables of the hypothesis should be understandable to the reader. A criterion that is related to testability is the idea of the hypothesis being stated in such a way as to be clearly supported or not supported. Although the more evidence that is provided, the more likely it is for a hypothesis to be accepted, but hypotheses are ultimately never proven (LoBiondo-Wood & Haber, 2002).

A hypothesis can be formulated in such a way as to be directional or nondirectional. A **directional hypothesis** specifies the predicted direction of the relationship between the independent and dependent variables. Some proponents of directional hypotheses argue that researchers naturally have expectations about the outcomes of their research, and thus may be potentially biased. An example of a directional hypothesis would be, "An oncology floor staffed with at least 75 percent registered nurses is positively related to patients verbalizing a decreased level of pain and nausea." A hypothesis that is deductive and is derived from a **theoretical framework** is usually directional. This means that the theory will provide the rationale for proposing that a relationship between variables will have a particular outcome. If there is no theoretical framework to provide rationale, a **nondirectional hypothesis** may be more appropriately utilized. Even if a theoretical framework is used as a base for a nondirectional hypothesis, it usually is not as fully developed as a directional hypothesis would be. A nondirectional hypothesis indicates the existence of a relationship between variables but does not specify the predicted direction. An example would be, "There will be a difference in the level of anxiety reported by nursing faculty who participate in a weekly focus group on current research." Researchers who favor the nondirectional hypothesis believe that this format is more objective and impartial than the directional hypothesis (LoBiondo-Wood & Haber, 2002).

Just as a hypothesis can be categorized as directional or nondirectional, it can also be categorized as a **statistical hypothesis** or a **research hypothesis**. A research hypothesis is also called a **scientific hypothesis**. The research hypothesis consists of a statement about the expected relationship among the variables and indicates what the outcome of the study is expected to be. If statistically significant findings are obtained for a research hypothesis, the hypothesis is supported. The statistical hypothesis is also called the **null hypothesis**, and it states that there is no relationship between the independent and dependent variables. If a statistically significant relationship emerges between the variables at a specific level of significance, the null hypothesis is rejected, and consequently the research hypothesis is accepted. An example of a null hypothesis would be, "There will be no difference in the level of anxiety reported by nursing faculty who participate in a weekly focus group on current research and those nursing faculty who do not participate in such a focus group" (LoBiondo-Wood & Haber, 2002).

LoBiondo-Wood and Haber (2002) have provided specific steps that would indicate whether a research question or a hypothesis should be developed, and if a hypothesis is most appropriate, the type of hypothesis to formulate:

1. The literature review and theoretical framework are examined to determine the concepts to be studied.
2. The primary purpose of the study and the research problem are determined.
3. If the primary purpose is exploratory, descriptive, or hypothesis generating, then research questions should be generated.
4. If the primary purpose is to test causal or associative relationships, then hypotheses should be generated.

An additional characteristic of a sound hypothesis is its consistency with an existing body of knowledge and its basis on sound scientific rationale. The reader of the research study should be able to trace the flow of an idea from the researchable problem to the research question or hypothesis, which also has a direct route to the literature review and the theoretical framework (LoBiondo-Wood & Haber, 2002). The **theoretical or conceptual framework** will be discussed in more detail later in this chapter, and the literature review that will generate the theoretical framework will be discussed elsewhere in this text. To reiterate, at this point in the research process, the DNP clinician should have:

- Selected a researchable problem that is realistic based on available resources, both financial and personnel, and on the accessible patient population.

- Sketched out a rough enough outline of what is being investigated so as to determine if an exploratory or descriptive research design is needed.
- Determined whether a research question or a hypothesis is more appropriate for the project.

The next step in the process will be to determine a theoretical framework for the project, and that will guide the wording of the hypothesis, assuming that a hypothesis is more appropriate for the project than a research question. The theoretical framework will assist the DNP clinician in determining whether the hypothesis should be directional or nondirectional, statistical, or research in nature.

 TOOLBOX

A significant part of having a realistic researchable problem is the determination of available resources and an accessible patient population. Think about a current situation existing in your work environment that would generate a potential research question. Are there resources that would help fuel an investigation of this question? If so, what type of resources exist? Financial? Personnel? Knowledge and expertise? Do you have access to a patient population to utilize in your investigation?

Use of a Theoretical or Conceptual Framework

It is important to recognize the link that exists among nursing theory, practice, and research. Just as nursing theory guides nursing practice, it is practice that tends to generate the questions that will ultimately form research questions or hypotheses, and it is research that will aid in the development of guidelines for practice. The terms *conceptual framework* and *theoretical framework* are frequently used interchangeably, although it is important to remember that whereas a concept is a mental image of an idea, theories are made up of interrelated concepts. For example, anxiety is a concept, and a theory could use the concepts of testing and anxiety to attempt to predict how test anxiety can fluctuate in junior year nursing students. The different categories of nursing theories will be discussed briefly in the following paragraphs prior to discussing the process of selecting a theoretical framework to guide the research project.

Nursing literature frequently uses the terms *grand theory, midrange theory*, and *microrange theory* to categorize nursing theories. A **grand theory** is the most abstract level of theory that establishes a knowledge base for nursing. Such a theory tends to include concepts such as *person, health*, and *environment*. Grand theories include those proposed by the great nursing theorists such as Dorothea Orem, Martha Rogers, and Imogene King, to name only a few (LoBiondo-Wood & Haber, 2002). In comparison, **midrange theories** incorporate nursing practice and research into ideas that are integral to the discipline. Finally, a low-level **microrange theory** could actually be synonymous with a hypothesis. It contains concrete concepts that are linked to form a statement that will be examined in practice and research. The beauty of the microrange theory is that DNP clinicians, because of their unique relationship to both practice and research due to the nature of the practice doctorate, are in a position every day to generate such low-level theories (LoBiondo-Wood & Haber, 2002).

Once the DNP clinician understands the types of nursing theories that make up theoretical frameworks, the next step in the research process involves selection of a framework that is appropriate for the research project and will provide direction and organization for the study. In order to select the appropriate framework, the researcher must determine whether inductive or deductive reasoning will be used throughout the process. It is the choice of inductive or deductive reasoning that will determine whether a conceptual framework or a more structured theoretical framework should be used to guide the project. If the DNP clinician chooses to use **inductive reasoning** when developing his or her research project, he or she will need to start with the details of experience with nursing practice and move toward a general picture. In comparison, deductive reasoning can also be used to develop the project. This involves starting with the general picture or theory and moving toward a direction for nursing practice (LoBiondo-Wood & Haber, 2002).

LoBiondo-Wood and Haber (2002) developed a decision tree that can be broken down to provide direction for the novice researcher on how to decide whether a conceptual or theoretical framework is more appropriate for the research project:

1. The researcher must initially decide whether deductive or inductive reasoning will be used to guide and organize the project:
   - Is the goal to create a structure that will guide the research? If so, deductive reasoning is being used, and a conceptual framework should be utilized.
   - Is the goal to identify a structure that will guide the research? If so, deductive reasoning is still being used, but a theoretical framework should be utilized instead.
   - Is the goal to begin to collect data to address a research question or hypothesis? If so, inductive reasoning is being used, and a framework does not have to be specified at this point because it will be based on the data collected and the literature review.
2. If a theoretical framework is judged to be most appropriate for this project, then the researcher must select the type of theory that will serve as the basis of the framework: grand, midrange, or microrange.

Once the type of reasoning that will guide the project has been determined, the researcher needs to specify a framework and determine whether a conceptual or theoretical framework will be used. If he or she decides that inductive reasoning will be used and there is not a need to specify the type of framework to be used at this point, then the researcher should proceed with the literature review, which will be the focus of another chapter.

Learning Enhancement Tools

1. Suppose you are a DNP graduate who is functioning in a management position. You want to find out if using 8-hour shifts rather than 12-hour shifts in an intensive care unit will lead to a decreased number of medication errors. Formulate a research question for this inquiry, specifying each element of the PICOT acronym.
2. Imagine you are a DNP graduate who is functioning in a nurse manager position. You want to find out if using a differently designed medication cart will lead to a decreased number of medication

errors on a medical-surgical floor. Formulate a research question for this inquiry, specifying each element of the PICOT acronym.

3. Assume you are a DNP student who is interested in performing a research project on nurses' perceptions of nurse coworkers who continue to function in their current job role while undergoing treatment for cancer.

    a. Do you think that a research question or a hypothesis would be more appropriate for this study? Give the rationale for your answer.

    b. Write either a research question or a hypothesis for this project based on your answer.

    c. As the researcher, suppose you opt to use a hypothesis for this research project. Write both a directional and a nondirectional hypothesis for the project.

    d. Write a statistical hypothesis for the research project.

4. Suppose you are a DNP student who is interested in performing a research project on whether cancer patients' level of pain is affected by being cared for by nurses who use prayer as their primary coping method.

    a. Do you think that a research question or a hypothesis would be more appropriate for this study? Give the rationale for your answer.

    b. Write either a research question or a hypothesis for this project based on your answer.

    c. As the researcher, suppose you opt to use a hypothesis for this research project. Write both a directional and a nondirectional hypothesis for the project.

    d. Write a statistical hypothesis for the research project.

5. Imagine you are a DNP student who is interested in performing a research project on whether the children of hospice nurses tend to engage in substance abuse to a greater extent than the children of nurses who work in other areas of patient care.

    a. Do you think that a research question or a hypothesis would be more appropriate for this study? Give the rationale for your answer.

    b. Write either a research question or a hypothesis for this project based on your answer.

    c. Write both a directional and a nondirectional hypothesis for the project in the event that as the researcher, you opt to use a hypothesis for this research project.

    d. Write a statistical hypothesis for the research project.

6. Read the passage in the box that follows and determine if research questions or hypotheses are embedded in the material.

    a. Do you think that they were appropriate for the selection?

    b. If not, explain your answer and write new ones for the material, writing both directional and nondirectional hypotheses, as well as research and statistical hypotheses.

    c. Can you determine if inductive or deductive reasoning was the basis for the study's organization? Examine your answer.

    d. Can you identify a conceptual or theoretical framework that was utilized?

    e. If you can identify a framework, do you think that the conceptual or theoretical framework that was used was appropriate for the type of study performed? Explain your answer.

 TOOLBOX

The recent paradigm shift in higher education has directly impacted nursing academia. The shift from teacher-centered teaching to learner-centered learning has resulted in a nursing educational environment that is student driven "where the faculty guides the individual development of students as needed" (Billings & Halstead, 2005, p. xiii). Nurse educators must consider the unique needs of the individual student and the theoretical constructs of self-directed learning, self-regulation, and learning motivation and the use of educational strategies and support methods to promote and enhance student integration of content value and progression toward intrinsic motivation. Academic learning activities focus on the development of critical thinking skills, autonomous decision making, clinical competence, case management skills, and teaching strategies focused on health promotion and disease management (Billings & Halstead, 2005; Ahern & Wink, 2010; Allen & Seaman, 2011; American Association of Colleges of Nursing, 2012; Jones & Wolf, 2010).

Multiple studies on academic self-regulation have been conducted in nursing education (Ali, Carlton, & Ryan, 2004; Ausburn, 2004; Beitz & Snarponis, 2006; Billings & Halstead, 2005; Fearing & Riley, 2005; Forrest, 2004; Knapp, 2004; Parker, Riza, Tierney, & Barrett, 2005; Peterson & Berns, 2005; Phillips, 2006; Ryan, Carlton, & Ali, 2005); however, a review of the literature revealed that no study has been conducted in nursing education to determine the presence or absence of academic motivation differences between groups of nursing students.

Resources

Alligood, M., & Marriner-Tomey, A. (2009). *Nursing theory: Utilization and application.* (7th ed.), St. Louis, MO: Mosby.

Barrett, E. (2002). The nurse theorists: 21st-century updates—Callista Roy. *Nursing Science Quarterly, 15,* 308–310.

Clarke, P., Killeen, M., Messmer, P., & Sieloff, C. (2008). Practitioner as theorist: A reprise. *Nursing Science Quarterly, 21,* 315–321.

Cody, W. (Ed.). (2006). *Philosophical and theoretical perspectives for advanced nursing.* Sudbury, MA: Jones and Bartlett.

Fawcett, J. (2002). The nurse theorists: 21st-century updates—Jean Watson. *Nursing Science Quarterly, 15,* 214–219.

Fawcett, J. (2003). The nurse theorists: 21st century updates—Martha E. Rogers. *Nursing Science Quarterly, 16,* 44–51.

Fawcett, J. (2005). *Analysis and evaluation of contemporary nursing knowledge: Nursing models and theories.* Philadelphia, PA: F.A. Davis Company.

Fawcett, J. (2007). Envisioning nursing in 2050 through the eyes of nurse theorists: King, Neuman, and Roy. *Nursing Science Quarterly, 20,* 108.

Fawcett, J. (2012). *Contemporary nursing knowledge: Analysis and evaluation of nursing models and theories* (3rd ed.), Philadelphia, PA: F.A. Davis Company.

Fitzpatrick, J., & Whall, A. (2005). *Conceptual models of nursing: Analysis and application.* Upper Saddle River, NJ: Pearson Prentice Hall.

Leininger, M., & McFarland, M. (Eds.). (2006). *Culture care diversity and universality: A worldwide nursing theory.* Sudbury, MA: Jones and Bartlett.

Madrid, M. (1997). *Patterns of Rogerian knowing.* New York, NY: NLN Press.

Neumann, B., & Fawcett, J. (2010). *The Neumann systems model* (5th ed.), Upper Saddle River, NJ: Prentice Hall.

Pilkington, F. (2003). Conceptual models of nursing: International in scope and substance? The case of the Roy adaptation model. *Nursing Science Quarterly, 16,* 315–318.

Pilkington, F. (2007). Envisioning nursing in 2050 through the eyes of nurse theorists: Katie Eriksson and Margaret Newman. *Nursing Science Quarterly, 20,* 200.

Pilkington, F. (2007). Envisioning nursing in 2050 through the eyes of nurse theorists: Leininger and Watson. *Nursing Science Quarterly, 20,* 8.

Pilkington, F. (2007). Envisioning nursing in 2050 through the eyes of nurse theorists: Rosemarie Rizzo Parse and Martha E. Rogers. *Nursing Science Quarterly, 20,* 307–308.

Polifroni, E., & Welch, M. (1999). *Perspectives on philosophy of science in nursing.* Philadelphia, PA: Lippincott.

Powers, B., & Knapp, T. (2010). *Dictionary of nursing theory and research* (4th ed.), Philadelphia, PA: Springer.

Reed, P. (2002). What is nursing science? *Nursing Science Quarterly, 15,* 51–60.

Reed, P. (2004). Conceptual models of nursing: International in scope and substance? The case of the Neumann systems model. *Nursing Science Quarterly, 17,* 50–54.

Renpenning, K., & Taylor, S. (2003). *Self care theory in nursing.* Philadelphia, PA: Springer.

Sitzman, K., & Eichelberger, L. (2010). *Understanding the work of nurse theorists: A creative beginning* (2nd ed.), Sudbury, MA: Jones and Bartlett.

TOOLBOX

A decision tree can be utilized when determining your researchable problem.

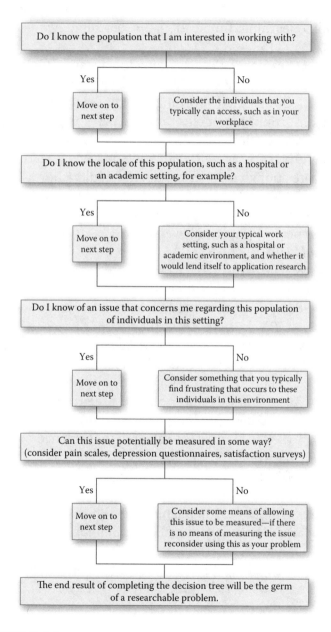

Do I know the population that I am interested in working with?

Yes — Move on to next step

No — Consider the individuals that you typically can access, such as in your workplace

Do I know the locale of this population, such as a hospital or an academic setting, for example?

Yes — Move on to next step

No — Consider your typical work setting, such as a hospital or academic environment, and whether it would lend itself to application research

Do I know of an issue that concerns me regarding this population of individuals in this setting?

Yes — Move on to next step

No — Consider something that you typically find frustrating that occurs to these individuals in this environment

Can this issue potentially be measured in some way? (consider pain scales, depression questionnaires, satisfaction surveys)

Yes — Move on to next step

No — Consider some means of allowing this issue to be measured—if there is no means of measuring the issue reconsider using this as your problem

The end result of completing the decision tree will be the germ of a researchable problem.

References

Ahern, N., & Wink, D. M. (2010). Virtual learning environments: Second life. *Nurse educator, 35*(6), 225–227. doi:10.1097/NNE.0b013e3181f7e943

Ali, N. S., Carlton, K. H., & Ryan, M. (2004). Students' perceptions of online learning: Implications for teaching. *Nurse Educator, 29*(3), 111–115.

Allen, I. E., & Seaman, J. (2011). Going the distance: Online education in the United States, 2011 (Sloan Consortium). Washington, DC: U.S. Government Printing Office. Retrieved from http://sloanconsortium.org/publications/survey/going_distance_2011

American Association of Colleges of Nursing. (2012). Nursing faculty shortage. Retrieved from www.aacn.nche.edu/media-relations/fact-sheets/nursing-faculty-shortage

Ausburn, L. J. (2004). Course design elements most valued by adult learners in blended online education environments: An American perspective [Electronic version]. *Educational Media International, 41*(4), 327–337.

Beitz, J. M., & Snarponis, J. A. (2006). Strategies for online teaching and learning. *Nurse Educator, 31*(1), 20–25.

Beyea, S. (2000). Getting started in nursing research and tips for success. *AORN Journal, 72*(6), 1061–1062.

Billings, D. M., & Halstead, J. A. (2005). *Teaching in nursing: A guide for faculty* (2nd ed.). St. Louis, MO: Elsevier Saunders.

Fearing, A., & Riley, M. (2005). Graduate students' perceptions of online teaching and relationships to preferred learning styles [Electronic version]. *Medsurg Nursing, 14*(6), 383–389.

Fitzpatrick, J. (2007). Finding the research for evidence-based practice. *Nursing Times, 103*(17), 32–33.

Forrest, S. (2004). Learning and teaching: The reciprocal link. *Journal of Continuing Education in Nursing, 35*(2), 74–79.

Jones, D., & Wolf, D. (2010). Shaping the future of nursing education today using distant education technology. *The ABNF Journal, 44*–47.

Knapp, B. (2004). Competency: An essential component of caring in nursing. *Nursing Administration Quarterly, 28*(4), 285–287.

Learning Domain. (2009). *Module 2: Stating the research problem.* Retrieved from http://www.learningdomain.com/module_2 .stating.problem.doc

LoBiondo-Wood, G., & Haber, J. (2002). *Nursing research: Methods, critical appraisal, and utilization.* St. Louis, MO: Elsevier.

Manheim, J., Rich, R., & Willnat, L. (2002). *Empirical political analysis: Research methods in political science.* New York, NY: Addison Wesley Longman.

Parker, E. B., Riza, L., Tierney, S., & Barrett, A. (2005). Interdisciplinary collaboration: An effective approach for developing Web-based courses [Electronic version]. *Computers, Informatics, Nursing, 23*(6), 308–313.

Peterson, R., & Berns, S. (2005). Establishing standards for intranet on-line education [Electronic version]. *Nursing Economics, 23*(5), 268–270.

Phillips, J. M. (2006). Preparing preceptors through online education. *Journal for Nurses in Staff Development, 22*(3), 150–156.

Ryan, M., Carlton, K. H., & Ali, N. S. (2005). A model for faculty teaching online: Confirmation of a dimensional matrix. *Journal of Nursing Education, 44*(8), 357–365.

Stillwell, S., Fineout-Overhold, E., Melnyk, B., and Williamson, K. (2010). Evidence-based practice, step by step: Asking the clinical question, *110*(3), 58-61.

Van Cott, A., & Smith, M. (2009). Nursing research: Tips and tools to simplify the process. *Dermatology Nursing, 21*(3), 138–140.

CHAPTER **3**

Conducting a Literature Review

Objectives

Upon completion of this chapter, the reader should be prepared to:

1. Discuss the process of critically analyzing data sources.
2. Identify databases that may be useful in locating data sources to include in a literature review.
3. Identify the purpose of the literature review.
4. Discuss important characteristics of a research article's Introduction section.
5. Discuss important characteristics of a research article's Methods section.
6. Discuss important characteristics of a research article's Discussion/Conclusion section.
7. Describe the importance of reliability to the research appraiser.
8. Describe the importance of statistical significance to the research appraiser.
9. Discuss the importance of external validity to the research appraiser.
10. Discuss the difference between a primary data source and a secondary data source.

Purpose of the Literature Review

As mentioned in the previous chapter, the reader of a research study should be able to trace the flow of an idea from the researchable problem to the research question or hypothesis, which also has a direct route to the **literature review** and the theoretical framework. This chapter will discuss the development of the literature review. A literature review is literally an account of what has been published on a topic by researchers, critically appraising each data source included for its relevance rather than simply summarizing what the author originally stated. The literature review is guided by the research question or the hypothesis. A literature review should discuss conceptual theories or models from nursing as well as other fields that will be used to examine the problem at hand. Because the review will reveal inconsistencies or unanswered questions about a subject, a correctly formulated literature review will allow for the research question or hypothesis to be further refined, if necessary (LoBiondo-Wood & Haber, 2009).

Apart from merely seeking out the literature that is available on a topic, the literature review must be formed using the researcher's critical appraisal skills. This means the researcher is able to apply principles of analysis to identify unbiased research studies, accurately assessing the data sources so that the strengths and weaknesses of each are discussed. If the literature review is developed appropriately, the reader should find it to be relevant, appropriate, and useful. The review should never deteriorate into simply a list summarizing one document after another (Taylor & Procter, 2009).

Ultimately, the purpose of the literature review is to establish the value of previous research on the study topic. The literature review should:

- Address a question not investigated in the literature previously and generate new research questions.
- Fill in a knowledge gap that has been found to exist in previously conducted research or reveal the existence of a knowledge gap in the field for the first time.
- Test an existing model under previously untested conditions or using a different patient population.
- Correct for errors in previously conducted research, or reveal existing errors for the first time.

- Resolve research findings that appear to be contradicting each other and determine the accuracy of reported findings (Taylor & Procter, 2009).

 TOOLBOX

Think about your own work environment. Can you think of a question related to that environment that has not been investigated and might generate new research questions?

Structuring the Literature Review

A literature review most commonly uses one of three formats. First is a discussion and evaluation of previous research beginning in chronological order. This would be used when the doctor of nursing practice (DNP) researcher is utilizing studies that are evaluated beginning with the earliest published report and moving chronologically until the most recently reported is discussed. Second is a literature review organized around a central concept. An example of this type of organization would be when the researcher is studying the patient's pain experience as the overall research concept. The literature review would then organize studies according to instruments used to operationalize or measure the degree of pain the patient experienced, treatments utilized for relief of pain, and the long-term effects of chronic pain. Finally, the literature review can be organized to first discuss an evaluation of studies that apply to the general research topic and then move toward the more narrowly defined research topic of the researcher (O'Sullivan, Rassel, & Berner, 2007). This could be used if a researcher first evaluated studies on the topic of the patient's pain experience and then moved to the more narrow focus of the experience of pain in cancer patients under the age of 21. In addition to these types of reviews, a derivation of a literature review that is frequently utilized is a meta-analysis. This consists of the use of quantitative procedures to statistically combine the results of studies. A small meta-analysis is considered to use no more than 50 articles (American Psychological Association, 2010).

As the author is developing the literature review, locating sources, and beginning the process of initial evaluation of data sources, he or she should consider the following:

- Are there gaps in the knowledge available on this subject? If so, identify the specific areas that are lacking. This will generate new research questions and potentially new research studies.
- Are there areas of further study that have been identified by other scholars that may serve as sources of additional research for a DNP researcher?
- How could these areas of further study impact the research project currently under way?
- Do potential relationships exist between concepts that would generate additional researchable hypotheses?
- How have other researchers defined and measured key concepts that will be used in the current research project? Do these definitions and measurements appear to be accurate and reliable?
- Have other researchers used data sources including topic-specific websites that the DNP researcher was not aware of?
- What keywords can be identified to help guide the researcher's search for information?
- How does the current research project relate to the work already generated by other researchers (F.D. Bluford Library, 2013)?

 TOOLBOX

Think about your own work environment. Based on your experience, are there gaps in the knowledge that is available on either the services provided to patients in your work area or on the patient population served?

Critical Appraisal of the Literature

Because of the nature of the DNP researcher's practice-oriented doctoral program, the DNP student must be particularly scrupulous in ensuring that each source included as part of the literature review contributes in some manner to evidence-based nursing practice. In order to ensure that the literature review is the result of a critical appraisal on the part of the researcher, Taylor and Procter (2009) have developed a series of questions the researcher should ask him- or herself regarding each data source undergoing critical evaluation:

- Has the author clearly formulated a problem statement? If not, is it at least clearly implied?
- Is the problem's significance established in terms of scope, severity, and relevance to the nursing profession?
- Could the defined problem have been approached more effectively from another perspective? If so, what perspective could have been selected?
- If the data source is a research study, what was the author's research design? Was the design appropriate for the type of research study implemented?
- What is the theoretical framework? Was it appropriate, or should a conceptual framework have been used instead?
- Is there a relationship between the theoretical or conceptual framework and research question or hypothesis, or is a disconnect evident?
- If a research study is being evaluated, can the study population, interventions, and outcomes be clearly identified?
- How accurate and valid are the measurements utilized—do they measure what they were intended to measure? Would the same results be obtained if the study was replicated?
- Is the analysis of the data that was performed in the study both accurate and relevant to the research question or hypothesis?
- Are the conclusions appropriately based on the analysis of the data?
- How does the data source contribute to the understanding of the problem under scrutiny, and how does it contribute to evidence-based practice?
- What are the strengths as well as the limitations of the research article? Do the limitations outweigh any benefits derived from the implementation of the research?
- How does the data source relate to the researcher's research question or hypothesis?

Collecting Data Sources

As the DNP researcher begins the process of searching out data sources that will be critically appraised for possible inclusion in the literature review, he or she should initially ensure that the topic that is the central focus of the research question or hypothesis is absolutely clear. The researcher should remain focused on the practice-related topic as well as the basic patient population being studied.

Next, the researcher should identify terms that are unique to the study. For example, if the study uses the research question, "Is the incidence of substance abuse greater in hospice nurses who have experienced cancer in their own families than in hospice nurses who have no firsthand experience with the disease?" then the unique terms that will be researched will be *substance abuse*, *hospice*, and *nurses*. As the researcher uses these terms to initiate a computerized search for data sources, broad-spectrum medical/nursing databases should initially be utilized, such as Cumulative Index to Nursing and Allied Health Literature (CINAHL), Index Medicus (MEDLINE), and Educational Resources Information Center (ERIC). This will provide the researcher with a large volume of articles that can then undergo critical appraisal. In addition, the use of multiple databases increases the researcher's access to multiple sources, allows for searching of the key terms selected, provides for ease of document retrieval, and increases the credibility of the search (LoBiondo-Wood & Haber, 2009).

Steps to Include in the Critique of a Research Article

1. Determine if the research is believable.
   ___ Is it well organized?
   ___ Is it grammatically correct?
   ___ Are terms that are used appropriate?
   ___ Do researchers have qualifications indicating they have sufficient knowledge of the topic?
   ___ Does the title indicate the topic?
   ___ Does the abstract provide a clear overview of the research problem, technique used to sample the population, methodology utilized, results achieved, and recommendations for further study?

2. Determine if the research problem is clearly identified.
3. Determine if the research question or the hypothesis is clearly stated and is appropriate.
4. Determine if the literature review is sufficiently extensive for the topic and includes primary sources no more than 5 years old.
5. Determine if the article identified a theoretical or conceptual framework that is appropriate for the research.
6. Determine if the research article described the method utilized to sample the population.
   ___ Is the sample size specified?
   ___ Was the sample utilized adequate for the research project?
7. Were research participants adequately informed about the research project?
   ___ Were research participants sufficiently protected from harm during the project?
   ___ What level of institutional review board permission was granted for the project (exempt, expedited, full)?
8. Are the terms and concepts used in the article clearly defined and understandable to the reader?
9. Is the research design clearly identified in the article?
   ___ Was the design appropriate for the research project?
   ___ Was an instrument used for data collection, and was it appropriate for the project?
   ___ Was reliability discussed in the article?
   ___ Was validity discussed in the article?
10. Does the article describe how the data were analyzed?
11. Does the article describe the statistical results of the analysis that was performed?
12. Does the article describe the strengths and limitations of the research project?
   ___ Did the article describe recommendations for further research?
   ___ Did the article generated either answer the research question or support the hypothesis?
13. Did the article discuss the implications of the research project?
14. Were the references included in the study appropriately cited (Ryan, Coughlin, & Cronin, 2007; Coughlin, 2007)?

INITIATING THE PROCESS OF CRITICAL APPRAISAL

A crucial skill that the DNP researcher must practice as part of the process of formulating a literature review that contains credible data sources is that of critical appraisal of the research. Wooten and Ross (2005) recommend breaking a journal article down into its component parts in order to appraise it efficiently. Initially, the DNP researcher should look for a journal article that is contained in a publication that is peer reviewed. This means the study underwent a prepublication review by experts in the specialty field to ensure the information it contained was both unbiased and accurate. The researcher must identify whether the source is primary or secondary. A **primary source** is one that was written by the person who either developed a theory or conducted the research being reported. A **secondary source** is written by someone other than the person who developed the theory or conducted the research (LoBiondo-Wood & Haber, 2009). A literature review should contain a majority of primary sources.

Next, the DNP researcher should look at the authors' qualifications. Are the authors' credentials appropriate for the topic being researched? Have they published other studies on similar subjects? For example, if the research is written using a population of intensive care patients, is the author a nurse with an intensive care practice background? If not, the author may lack credibility. Also, look at any funding sources the author used. Can it be determined if the research is biased in such a way as to reflect favorably on the funding organization?

 TOOLBOX

Initiate a search of the literature that is readily available on a topic related to your current work environment. Try to locate at least three primary sources and three secondary sources. Are the authors' credentials appropriate for the topic being researched? Why or why not?

CRITICAL APPRAISAL OF THE ABSTRACT

Once the DNP researcher has determined that the article in question is included in a peer-reviewed journal and that the author has sufficient qualifications to generate the research, he or she should take a cursory look at the study's **secondary source**, bearing in mind that the study cannot be accurately evaluated based on its **abstract** alone. The researcher should read the abstract to find a summary of the purpose; problem under investigation; participants; procedures utilized including a brief mention of the sample size, outcome measures, data gathering procedures, and research design; as well as results and the author's conclusions (American Psychological Association, 2010). This abstract appraisal may indicate the need to pursue a more detailed review of the article or may show that the article is not needed for inclusion in the literature review (Wooten & Ross, 2005).

CRITICAL APPRAISAL OF THE INTRODUCTION

The next step in the critical appraisal of the literature involves breaking down the article into its individual parts that form the "skeleton" of the research report: the introduction, methods, results, and discussion and/or conclusions. The **introduction** section should include the author's research question or hypothesis that clearly states the population being studied, the intervention being proposed, the comparison that will occur, and the expected outcome. The study should be based on research that has previously been conducted on the same topic or one very similar, so there should also be a discussion of previously conducted studies and a review of their findings. A well-crafted introduction should tell the reader:

- *Why the problem is important*—The reader should be able to understand the importance of the topic both to the individual nurse and to the nursing profession.
- *How the study relates to previous work in the area*—This will show a clear connection with the theoretical or conceptual framework.
- *If other aspects of the study have been reported prior to this study, how this report differs from the previous reports*—The study should be able to indicate what it will provide to the reader that other studies have not.
- *How the study relates to previous work in the area.*
- *The relationship of the hypotheses and research design to each other.*
- *The theoretical and practical implications of the study that have been identified* (American Psychological Association, 2010).

If the introduction section doesn't include a clearly stated research question or hypothesis, the novice researcher should consider it a poor addition to his or her own literature review for the project (Wooten & Ross, 2005).

CRITICAL APPRAISAL OF THE METHODS SECTION

When the DNP student begins appraisal of the **methods** section of an article, he or she will find that this is arguably the most important section in a research report, because it should contain the author's description of exactly what was done in the research as well as how it was implemented. It is the methods section that tells the DNP student about the reliability of the research being scrutinized—if this study were replicated, would the same results be achieved? If not, then the research has a very low degree of reliability and should not be included in the literature review.

The methods section should include a concise description of the procedure for data collection. If the author designed an instrument for data collection, such as a questionnaire or other tool that participants used during the research, then a copy should be included in this section. If statistical calculations are needed to make this section's description of the author's procedures more clear, were they included? This section should also include a detailed description of the population of research subjects, including how they were selected. Major demographic characteristics, level of education, socioeconomic status, and topic-specific characteristics should be included, such as number of years actively licensed as a registered nurse. Participant characteristics may help the researcher determine the extent to which findings can be generalized, or applied, to other populations (American Psychological Association, 2010).

The methods section should include a discussion of the technique used to determine sample size and randomization of subjects, if probability sampling was utilized. If nonprobability sampling was utilized and this randomization of subjects did not occur, the author should clearly state this and the reasoning for opting not to randomize. The methods section should also contain criteria for including subjects in the study population. Was the population studied large enough to validate the research on the problem being studied? If the author presented findings on a population of randomized subjects that yielded a group of five participants, the results of the research, and possibly the credibility of the researcher, will very likely be called into question. The methods section should include information on any agreements that were made with participants as well as any incentives they received for participating. This can include a tangible incentive such as receiving a payment as well as a more esoteric incentive such as awarding continuing education units.

The procedures used for data collection, such as administration of questionnaires, online surveys, or interviews, or conducting of focus groups, as well as any training that was provided to researchers implementing the study, should be described. If data are missing, such as would occur if participants failed to complete every question in a questionnaire, procedures designed to deal with the missing information should be discussed (American Psychological Association, 2010). The author should include information on the procedure used to approach an institutional review board (IRB) if there was manipulation of human subjects, the agreement made with the IRB, the procedures used to meet ethical standards, and safety monitoring methods instituted (American Psychological Association). In addition, the author should be able to describe the design of the study. Polit and Beck (2006) describe several characteristics of an acceptable design for a research project:

- The research design should suit the research question or the hypothesis; for example, if the researcher is interested in investigating four variables or areas being studied, then four groups of participants should be used.
- The design should not be biased; if groups of study participants are formed in a nonrandom manner, the threat of bias is always present. Therefore, the article's authors should state how the threat of bias was handled.
- The statistical procedures for analysis of the findings should be appropriate for the research design. If a quantitative research design was selected, were statistics used for analysis appropriate for such a design, or were the statistics primarily descriptive, such as might be used for a qualitative design?

The study should state if subjects were manipulated or randomly selected to specific groups. If control groups were used, they should be described, as well as any interventions that were applied (American Psychological Association, 2010). If the DNP student feels that the methods section presents nebulous details that don't describe how the research was implemented, the article should not be utilized as a reputable source in the literature review (Wooten & Ross, 2005).

CRITICAL APPRAISAL OF THE RESULTS SECTION

After a detailed appraisal of the methods section, the DNP student should move to a review of the research article's **results** section. This is a presentation of the author's findings. If the author used a hypothesis as part of the research study, he or she should be able to state that the hypothesis was accepted or rejected on the basis of statistically significant findings. This means it can be shown that the findings the author obtained are not likely to have resulted from chance at a specific degree of probability. If the hypothesis was rejected, it should be due to a nonsignificant outcome, meaning the findings were shown to possibly result from chance. The study should include all results obtained, even if they do not support the author's original hypothesis or are contrary to the research question. If findings are presented in the form of charts or tables, they should be scrutinized to determine if they are congruent with the rest of the research report. All participants should be accounted for at the conclusion of the study, including those who chose to opt out of the study before its conclusion. When participants choose not to complete a research project, it is known as attrition. The author should present findings that have statistical significance, but they should also have clinical significance in some way. This will be particularly important to the DNP student who is preparing a research project that relates to evidence-based practice. The results section should include some measure of the effect size generated in order for the reader to grasp the importance of the study's findings. If serious consequences occurred after interventions were applied, these should be detailed in this section (American Psychological Association, 2010). If the author appears to contradict his or her own findings, the DNP researcher should not include this source in the literature review (Wooten & Ross, 2005).

CRITICAL APPRAISAL OF THE DISCUSSION/CONCLUSIONS SECTION

The DNP student should analyze the **discussion** and **conclusions** section of the article. Findings should be traced back in a logical manner to the research question or hypothesis that was investigated. The researcher should evaluate the author's interpretation of findings carefully, looking for feasibility and clinical significance. The discussion and conclusions section should allow the researcher to evaluate and interpret the implications of the results presented in the previous section. If hypotheses were not supported, explanations should be offered. Are the findings meaningful to the audience originally targeted? Were unexpected findings revealed during the course of the study? Were the findings that were uncovered of insufficient magnitude as to be meaningful to readers? The author should include any potential limitations of the research project as well as the generalizability or external validity of the findings. These would include any problems with bias, sample size or inability to random sample, or the type of study design utilized. The author should be able to discuss how the research could be improved upon were it to be replicated (American Psychological Association, 2010).

CRITICAL APPRAISAL OF REFERENCES

Finally, the DNP researcher should determine whether adequate references were included to provide sufficient credibility, or if the author repeatedly cited his or her own work. The reference list should contain predominantly research published in recent years using primary sources, unless the reference is considered to be a classic in the field. In the reference list, the author should include information on the data source author (or editor in the case of an edited book), publication date of the document, as well as the title of the data source (American Psychological Association, 2010). The DNP researcher also should review any footnotes, tables, or figures included to determine the accuracy and appropriateness of information included. In particular, tables and figures should be reviewed for readability—do they require the reader to review numerous directions and footnotes in order to understand the data presented?

An integral part of the critical appraisal of the articles and other data sources being considered for inclusion in a literature review is the review of the report's treatment of informed consent, confidentiality, and the mandates of the IRB that were used if the research involved manipulation of human subjects. The following chapter discusses the ethics involved in implementing research that involves human subjects and the correct approach to applying to an IRB for a review of a proposed research protocol.

Learning Enhancement Tools

1. A DNP researcher is concerned with studying the reaction of elementary school age children to the death of a parent. Choose a format for the structure of the literature review, select the key terms to utilize during the review, and select the sources that would be used to search for appropriate articles

2. A DNP researcher is concerned with studying the organizational behavior changes that occur in nursing staff when nursing students undergo a clinical experience on the medical unit. Choose a format for the structure of the literature review, select the key terms to utilize during the review, select the sources that would be used to search for appropriate articles, and discuss how the process of critical appraisal of the data sources will be implemented.

References

American Psychological Association. (2010). *Publication manual of the American Psychological Association.* Washington, DC: Author.

Coughlin, M., Cronin, P., & Ryan, F. (2007). Step-by-step guide to critiquing research. Part 1: quantitative research. *British Journal of Nursing, 16*(11), 658–663.

F.D. Bluford Library, North Carolina State University. (2013). What is a "literature review" anyway? Retrieved from http://libguides .library.ncat.edu/literaturereview

LoBiondo-Wood, G., & Haber, J. (2009). *Nursing research: Methods, critical appraisal, and utilization.* St. Louis, MO: Elsevier.

O'Sullivan, E., & Rassel, G., & Berner, M. (2007). *Research methods for public administrators.* New York, NY: Longman.

Ryan, F., Coughlin, M., & Cronin, P. (2007). Step-by-step guide to critiquing research. Part 2: qualitative research. *British Journal of Nursing, 16*(12), 658–663.

Taylor, D., & Procter, M. (2009). *The literature review: A few tips on conducting it.* Retrieved from http://www.writing.utoronto.ca /advice/specific-types-of-writing/literature-review

Wooten, J., & Ross, V. (2005). *How to make sense of clinical research.* Retrieved from http://www.modernmedicine.com /modernmedicine/article/articleDetail.jsp?id=142654

Ethics in Clinical Research

Objectives

Upon completion of this chapter, the reader should be prepared to:

1. Describe the principle of autonomy and its relationship to the DNP researcher.
2. Describe the principle of beneficence and its relationship to the DNP researcher.
3. Describe the principle of justice and its relationship to the DNP researcher.
4. Discuss the rights of an individual who provides informed consent for participation in a research study.
5. Discuss the conditions that must be fulfilled before an institutional review board (IRB) can approve a research proposal.
6. Discuss the research categories that may qualify for an expedited review by an IRB.
7. Discuss the research categories that may qualify for an exempt review by an IRB.
8. Describe the basic sections of the average IRB application form that must be completed before a proposal can be submitted.

9. Describe how informed consent differs from confidentiality.
10. Describe the Privacy Rule and the Common Rule.
11. Discuss the importance of deidentified data.
12. Discuss the expectations of IRBs regarding identified risks to human subjects as research participants.
13. Discuss common pitfalls that can develop during the process of working with an IRB.
14. Discuss the IRB requirement of the development of a data and safety monitoring plan.

Ethical Principles

The greatest amount of attention given to ethical and legal considerations regarding research occurred immediately after World War II during the trials of war criminals. The American Medical Association was asked to develop a code of ethics for research that would provide standards for judging the crimes committed by physicians who conducted experiments on prisoners in concentration camps. This request resulted in the Nuremberg Code, which defined the terms *voluntary*, *legal capacity*, *sufficient understanding*, and *enlightened decision* (LoBiondo-Wood & Haber, 2009).

AUTONOMY

One of the main ethical principles that should be ingrained into all researchers is that of autonomy and the responsibilities it brings the researcher. Because so many research projects that doctor of nursing practice (DNP) researchers implement will utilize human subjects, it is imperative that these researchers have an understanding of the ethical principles that are important to research. **Autonomy** is the ethical principle related to informed consent. This provides a person with the right to make an informed decision about whether to participate in a research study. Potential participants must be told about any risks that could occur during the course of a research study and must be allowed to decide whether to enter the study without coercion.

BENEFICENCE

In comparison, **beneficence** is the ethical principle that guides health-care providers to act in the best interest of the research participant. It is the principle of beneficence that provides the participant with protection from harm. This can be achieved through monitoring the research participant's response during the study once informed consent is given.

JUSTICE

Finally, recruitment of research subjects is governed by the principle of **justice**. This principle affects recruitment of research subjects. It mandates that research participants be selected from multiple groups rather than only from a pool of those most likely to be coerced, such as subjects with severe physical or mental illness or those who are economically disadvantaged (American Association of Critical Care Nurses, 1999).

TOOLBOX

Think about the idea for your capstone project that you are probably already considering. Do you foresee any difficulty in maintaining the ethical principles of autonomy, beneficence, and justice with that project idea?

Informed Consent

Although autonomy, beneficence, and justice are the ethical principles that should govern the conduct of the DNP student who is engaged in research that involves human subjects, it is informed consent that ensures that these principles are observed when this type of research is implemented. **Informed consent** ultimately implies that the potential participant's ratio of risk to benefits has been clearly identified. Potential risks could consist of physical harm, pain, embarrassment, loss of privacy, and loss of time, to name only a few, whereas potential benefits could consist of participating in a treatment that could relieve a physical or psychological problem.

Informed consent is given when a person with the capacity to make decisions exercises the power to make a choice without force, fraud, deceit, or any type of coercion. Such an individual is usually an adult with decision-making capacity, although in some states a legally emancipated minor who makes decisions for himself or herself can provide informed consent. If the individual is not capable of providing informed consent, the person's family member or legal representative can provide informed consent for the person.

Rights of Participants in a Research Study

Specific guidelines regarding the informed consent process must be followed in order for federal funding to be provided to implement research projects. In addition, there are certain federal regulations that stipulate that participants in a research study have specific rights. These include:

- The right to be informed of both the nature and the purpose of the research.
- The right to receive an explanation of the procedures that will be followed and any drug or device that will be used during the research.
- The right to receive a description of any risks or discomfort that may occur during the course of the research.
- The right to receive any explanation of benefits that may be expected from the research.
- The right to receive a disclosure of any procedure, drug, or device that could be used during the research that could benefit the participant, as well as their potential risks and benefits.
- The right to receive information on forms of treatment available to the participant after the research project is concluded, if complications occur during the study.
- The right to ask questions regarding the research study or any procedure involved in it.
- The right to be told that consent to participate in the research may be withdrawn at any time, and that the participant may withdraw from the project without consequences.
- The right to receive a copy of any signed and dated written consent form that was issued during the course of the study.
- The right to decide to consent to participate or not in the research without any type of force, fraud, deceit, duress, coercion, or other influence being applied to pressure the subject (American Association of Critical Care Nurses, 1999).

The principal investigator of the research project is ultimately responsible for obtaining informed consent. However, it is the ethical responsibility of all researchers involved in the project to assure that informed consent has been obtained in an appropriate manner. Problems with informed consent can arise based on the type of research being conducted. The Code of Federal Regulations does not require written consent for surveys unless the information that is collected is recorded in a manner that allows participants to be identified and disclosure of the information could lead to criminal or civil liability for participants or damage the reputation of participants. Research that consists of field experiments or observation of participants in a covert manner presents the greatest challenge to the researcher regarding informed consent. In both of these types of studies, the researcher's need to observe participants in spontaneous behavior is not compatible with the provision of informed consent. Implementing these types of research studies could lead the primary investigator to be labeled as engaging in unethical research practices (Singleton & Straits, 2009).

 TOOLBOX

Think about the idea for your capstone project that you are probably already considering. Do you foresee any difficulty in obtaining informed consent from participants in the type of project that you are considering? If so, how will you remedy this in the project design?

Confidentiality

It is important for the DNP researcher to recognize that informed consent is not synonymous with **confidentiality**. Although **privacy** can be considered to be a person's ability to control the access of other people to information about him- or herself, confidentiality refers to protection of such information so that researchers will not disclose records that identify individuals. Regardless of the sensitivity of the information gathered during the course of a research study, the ethical investigator will guarantee the confidentiality of the data collected from human subjects. A researcher may collect anonymous information in an attempt to avoid problems with confidentiality. This means that no records are kept on the identity of subjects and data cannot be traced back to a specific person. However, some research designs do not lend themselves to confidentiality; in this case, the researcher must be capable of auditing his or her own records to ensure that information was collected accurately and reported correctly (O'Sullivan, Rassel, & Berner, 2007).

In order to ensure confidentiality, the researcher can remove subjects' names and any other identifying information as early in the research project as possible. In addition, the investigator can code subjects' identities so that such information is not divulged during any part of the research report. This is frequently done in field research, which may require more creativity in order for data to be deidentified. If other researchers or organizations request information from the primary investigator, the researcher should never release information that contains sensitive material without the research subjects' permission (Singleton & Straits, 2009).

Health Insurance Portability and Accountability Act Compliance

There are various aspects of compliance with the Health Insurance Portability and Accountability Act (HIPAA) that the DNP researcher must clearly grasp. These include an understanding of the Privacy Rule, protected health information, and release of information with prior authorization.

THE PRIVACY RULE AND THE COMMON RULE

As the DNP researcher engages in practice-oriented research, along with informed consent and confidentiality, he or she must be cognizant of the requirements of HIPAA. A researcher can gain access to medical records only through a privacy review conducted by an **institutional review board (IRB)**. The Privacy Rule was implemented as the first phase of HIPAA in 2004. It defined patient rights regarding individual health information and established protection for access to and release of a patient's medical records. HIPAA also mandates the creation of privacy boards whose sole authority is to review individual privacy rights. Privacy boards operate similar to IRBs. In comparison, an IRB derives its authority from the Federal Policy for the Protection of Human Subjects, also known as the

Common Rule. The Common Rule is similar to the Privacy Rule, although it applies only to federally funded research (Artnak & Benson, 2005).

PROTECTED HEALTH INFORMATION

If the DNP researcher opts to utilize what HIPAA refers to as **protected health information** in his or her research project, the researcher opts to use information about an individual's health status, the provision of health care, or payment for health care that can be linked to the person. The investigator should recognize that the legislation considers this type of information to fall into one of three categories:

1. No consent form is required, but the researcher must sign a restricted use agreement.
2. No consent form is required, but review by an IRB or privacy board is required.
3. Individual authorization is necessary.

There are cases when an IRB or a privacy board can allow a researcher access to protected health information without authorization. For example, if the medical record in question contains deidentified information, no individual privacy protection is required. Deidentified data means that all information that could identify an individual has been removed (Artnak & Benson, 2005).

DATA THAT CANNOT BE RELEASED WITHOUT PRIOR AUTHORIZATION

The researcher should further recognize that there are specific data elements that cannot be released during the course of a research project without prior authorization from the subject in question. These include:

- Name of the research participant
- Geographic areas smaller than a state, except for the first three digits of the ZIP code
- Dates of birth, dates of death, dates of admission, or ages greater than 89 years
- Driver's license or automobile license numbers
- Social Security numbers

- Medical records numbers
- Health plan numbers
- Account numbers
- Telephone numbers
- Fax numbers
- E-mail addresses
- License numbers, such as nurse's license or medical license
- Vehicle identification numbers
- Medical device or serial numbers
- Internet URLs
- Internet IP addresses
- Biometric information
- Any additional information that would allow the reidentification of subject information (Lavin, 2006)

TOOLBOX

Think about the idea for your capstone project that you are probably already considering. Is there any possibility that you might violate confidentiality or have difficulty complying with HIPAA mandates during the implementation of the project? If so, how will you change the project design to remedy this?

Institutional Review Boards

Ultimately, the components of informed consent are overseen by an institutional review board (IRB). This was mandated in 1991 when a federal policy for the protection of human subjects in research activities was published. This policy required that every institution that receives federal funding for research involving human participants must create an IRB and appoint its members. Federal guidelines require that an IRB be composed of at least five members, with one of the five being a person not associated with the facility. This means that a facility's IRB must review all research that involves human subjects either conducted at the facility or sponsored by the facility. Most healthcare research conducted in the United States currently is approved by an IRB because, in addition to the federal requirement for an IRB to be in place in order for funding to be awarded, many private funding agencies and most biomedical journals require an IRB to approve research that is conducted. Also, most universities and healthcare institutions require IRB approval in order to avoid liability as research is implemented (Olsen & Mahrenholz, 2000).

An institution's IRB looks for certain conditions to be fulfilled before a research proposal can be approved. These consist of:

- Minimal identified risks to human subjects.
- Equitable selection of human subjects.
- Appropriate documentation of informed consent from all participants.
- Appropriate monitoring of data to ensure safety of subjects.
- Provision for ensuring privacy of human subjects and confidentiality of data gathered (O'Sullivan et al., 2007).

EVALUATION OF A RESEARCH PROPOSAL

An IRB will usually evaluate a proposal on the basis of several areas. Because the rights of the human subjects involved are considered to be paramount, the consent form utilized will be scrutinized. The board will determine if the consent form addresses concerns such as deception of the participants, presentation of the purpose of the research, obvious or hidden costs to the subjects, benefits and risks to the participants, protection of confidentiality, the contact person if participants have questions, and what will be done with the results generated by the study. The board will also look carefully at the conditions under which subjects are excluded from and included in the research study. Approval of a project will be denied if there is an indication that the subjects believe they will receive a special benefit merely by participating, such as students who believe they will be given extra points in a class if they participate in a research project for their professor (Kamienski, 2000).

Most IRBs also have concerns regarding recruitment of participants for a research study. They usually are adamant that permission to approach a subject regarding possible participation be obtained by someone other than the researcher. This means that someone such as a coworker in the potential subject's work area could approach the person regarding the possibility of participation, and then the researcher would follow up with a conversation with the subject regarding an explanation of the research and approach the person with an invitation to participate. This area must be well planned before sending a proposal to the IRB in order to avoid a denial (Kamienski, 2000).

EXPEDITED REVIEWS BY AN IRB

A facility's IRB has the capacity to award a research proposal an **expedited review** if the risk to research subjects is considered to be at a minimal level. This shortens the length of the review process because usually only one member of the IRB will review the project to ensure protection of human subjects (Stone, 2003). Receiving an expedited review can still require a researcher to obtain informed consent, however. It should always be the goal of the DNP researcher to obtain an expedited review from an IRB. Research categories that may be eligible for an expedited review may include:

- Collection of hair and nail clippings in a manner that does not disfigure the human subject.
- Collection of excreta and external secretions including perspiration.
- Recording of information on human subjects who are at least 18 years old, using noninvasive procedures that are considered to be routine in clinical practice.
- Collecting voice recordings.
- Study of data, documents, records, pathological specimens, or diagnostic data that are already in existence (LoBiondo-Wood & Haber, 2009).

EXEMPT REVIEW BY AN IRB

Some research projects may be considered to be **exempt** from an IRB review. According to the federal guidelines generated by the Department of Health and Human Services, there are five categories that can qualify research as being exempt from IRB review:

1. Research in educational settings such as universities
2. Research involving surveys and tests in which the participant cannot be identified
3. Research involving collection of existing data if sources are either publicly available or have already been deidentified

4. Research conducted by or subject to approval by federal agencies that are designed for the good of the general public
5. Research related to the taste and quality of food

Although the DNP researcher may be reasonably certain that his or her research proposal will be exempt from a full review by an IRB, an application must still be completed and submitted; the IRB will make the final decision (Stone, 2003).

IRB APPLICATION

Regardless of the type of review the researcher is hoping for, whether a full review, expedited, or exempt, an application must still be completed and submitted, and the IRB will make the final decision. Usually the facility's application form can be downloaded from the institution's website. The researcher must bear in mind that often these forms are not formatted in a way that allows them to be saved once their blanks are filled in. Therefore, it may be more convenient for the researcher to type the proposal in a word processor and then copy and paste the information into the form. This is particularly helpful if the IRB requires changes and thus subsequent submissions of the form.

Initially the IRB application usually requires a brief statement of the study's hypothesis, research question(s), and purpose. In addition, a statement of the objectives of the research project will usually be required. Information will then be requested regarding the subjects to be utilized in the study. This will include who they are, how they will be recruited, copies of any letters or advertisements that will be used in recruitment, how many contacts will be made with each subject and the length of each contact, as well as any payment that will be given to participants. The board will be particularly interested in the inclusion of subjects from vulnerable populations, such as children, infants, prisoners, or the mentally handicapped. If the study site is a college and the study involves students whose grade could be affected by the research project, these students would be considered a vulnerable population (Kamienski, 2000).

As the application process progresses, the researcher should plan to produce copies of the informed consent to be utilized, a concise and accurate description of what the researcher will be doing to the subjects or with the subjects, and a copy of instruments that will be used in the research, including surveys, questionnaires, and any interview questions.

The researcher should also be prepared to detail the procedures that will be used to maintain confidentiality. If the researcher plans to use deception of the subjects, he or she should be prepared to describe in detail why this is necessary and how subjects will be debriefed after completion of the project. The researcher should have a contingency plan to alter the proposal if the IRB denies the proposal based on his or her use of deception. A similar plan should be in place if the researcher proposes to ask the participants questions or perform procedures that might cause participants stress or anxiety or disturb participants emotionally. Again, the IRB will be concerned by this request and will want to know why this is necessary and what the researcher intends to do to provide counseling and treatment to participants who become upset. As previously mentioned, a statement of the risk-to-benefit ratio will be needed to round out the complete proposal (Kamienski, 2000).

TOOLBOX

Think about the idea for your capstone project that you are probably already considering. Do you think that it would qualify for either an exempt or an expedited review in its current design? Why or why not?

PITFALLS OF THE IRB PROCESS

There are some common pitfalls that can sidetrack even the most seasoned researcher if not avoided when approaching the time of IRB review. For example, failure to be consistent throughout all of the documentation can derail the process. This means that the application, protocol narrative, consent forms, and any other documents must contain information with consistent details. In addition, the researcher can easily overlook the need to provide layman's language in the informed consent document, which should be written at no higher than a sixth- to eighth-grade reading level for adult participants. Because every IRB must include at least one member who is not a researcher affiliated with the sponsoring facility, the primary investigator should bear in mind that his or her protocol should be written using language that can be easily understood by non-nursing personnel. It can be considered a general standard that no IRB will approve a protocol that cannot be easily understood by its members (Colt & Mulnard, 2006).

IRB REVIEW CRITERIA

As has been previously mentioned, specific criteria must be met in order for an IRB to determine that a protocol can be approved for the recruitment and participation of human subjects. If the DNP researcher is already familiar with the criteria and how an IRB will typically interpret them, he or she can develop an IRB application that presents information that meets the board's concerns and thus avoids repetitive requests for protocol modifications. For example, clearly it is the overriding mission of an IRB to ensure that risks to subjects are minimized to the greatest extent possible. This means that questions the IRB may ask regarding risks of research and board members' expectations regarding minimizing these risks include:

- *Do the protocol's eligibility criteria adequately minimize the identified risks to subjects?* A protocol will never be approved by an IRB if the board determines there are risks to the human subjects that have not been minimized to the greatest extent possible. Such a situation would violate the overall mission of the IRB if it were allowed to persist.
- *Do the protocol's eligibility criteria adequately monitor the identified risks to subjects?* The protocol must describe explicitly the monitoring procedures the researchers have initiated in order to make certain the subjects are continually exposed to the lowest level of both risk and discomfort possible during the course of the study.
- *Are the proposed procedures justified, reasonable, and as comfortable as possible for the participants?* This also includes being as convenient for the participants as possible. For example, if a particular protocol that will involve cancer patients could produce nausea and a monitoring procedure has been developed to determine that nausea either is not being produced or is at a very minimal level, the protocol should state that the procedure would be implemented as much as possible during the patient's regularly scheduled clinic appointments. This will prevent the patient from having to schedule extra appointments, thus potentially also avoiding extra expense.

- *Are the research personnel both qualified and adequately trained to implement the study procedures?* Most IRBs now require all of the personnel who will be implementing research utilizing human subjects to undergo and document their participation in standardized training on the ethical principles of research and the regulations that pertain to such research.
- *Are the identified risks to subjects reasonable in relation to the anticipated benefits?* Many IRBs identify assessment of the risk–benefit ratio of the research study to be the most important ethical consideration of the entire project. The researcher should clearly identify if there are characteristics of the proposed subject population that will increase their risks as research participants (Pech, Cob, & Cejka, 2005).

DATA AND SAFETY MONITORING PLAN

If, in fact, a research protocol identifies that more than minimal risk to human subjects will be present during a research project, most IRBs will subsequently require the researcher to present a data and safety monitoring plan. This will be a description of how the primary investigator will monitor the research data in order to respond quickly to any adverse events or unanticipated problems that occur during the study, to ensure participant safety. A thorough description of the monitoring process should be prepared because accrual of preliminary data may indicate that the research design should be changed, information provided to subjects should be altered, or the project lacks sufficient validity and should be terminated (Pech et al., 2005).

In addition to concerns regarding the ratio of risks to benefits to the human subjects involved in the research, an IRB will also pose questions to the researcher regarding the level of confidentiality available to the participants. The researcher should be prepared with a plan to supply this information to avoid becoming sidetracked by the need to supply unanticipated data. The IRB will be concerned with determining the following:

- *Will the location of the data collection allow subjects sufficient privacy?* If information collected will be especially sensitive, the IRB will expect privacy to be provided by interviewing participants in a secured room, for example.

- *How will data be stored?* The researcher should determine where collected data will be stored and the precautions that will be implemented to prevent personnel not involved in the research study from having access to the sensitive information.
- *How will data be recorded?* The researcher should be prepared to describe the process by which data will be recorded, whether anonymously or by coded response. If the data will be coded, the researcher should be able to state where the codebook will be stored, who will have access to it, and when the identifiers for the information will be destroyed (Pech et al., 2005).

FORMULA FOR SUCCESS

Colt and Mulnard (2006) have developed a formula for success for researchers attempting to navigate through the IRB review and approval process:

- Use simplified language that is easy for anyone to understand.
- Provide rationale for the research project as well as the choice of design and the degree of risk to potential participants.
- Emphasize the multiple ways that protection of subjects is provided throughout the project.
- Provide complete and detailed information in all areas of the required documentation.
- Achieve consistency of the information provided in each section and across all documents utilized in the research study.

As previously mentioned, the institutional review board can have a great influence on the research design for a study, because the board's concerns regarding monitoring procedures can signal that the design may need to be changed somewhat or completely substituted with another design. The next chapter will discuss research designs, specifically those that are appropriate for quantitative research projects.

Learning Enhancement Tools

1. Discuss autonomy, beneficence, and justice and how these principles should relate to the conduct of a DNP researcher and his or her research participants.

2. Imagine you are the principal investigator for a research project that will study the anxiety level of nursing students who are undergoing testing for their state nursing licensure examination. Discuss all of your responsibilities regarding informed consent for this project.

3. Suppose you are developing a research proposal that will go before an institutional review board and are hoping for an expedited review. How can you format your proposal to be more likely to receive an expedited review?

4. Imagine you are developing a research proposal that will go before an institutional review board and are hoping for either an expedited or an exempt review. Discuss how the categories that will require an expedited review will differ from the categories that require an exempt review.

5. Suppose you are preparing a proposal for submission to an institutional review board. Describe the various parts that you anticipate being included in the request for information from the IRB.

6. Assume you have submitted a research proposal to an institutional review board. The IRB has concerns regarding the ratio of risks to benefits for research participants. As the researcher, describe how you would respond to the IRB's concerns and how you would keep the risk level minimal for participants.

7. Imagine that, as the primary investigator, you have submitted a proposal to an IRB. The board returns the proposal to you with the stipulation that a data and safety monitoring plan must be developed and implemented. Why would such a stipulation be given, and how can you meet the board's expectation?

References

Artnak, K., & Benson, M. (2005). Evaluating HIPAA compliance: A guide for researchers, privacy boards, and IRBs. *Nursing Outlook, 53,* 79–87.

Colt, H., & Mulnard, R. (2006). Writing an application for a human subjects institutional review board. *Chest, 130,* 1605–1607.

Kamienski, M. (2000). Tips on navigating your research proposal through the institutional review board. *Journal of Emergency Nursing, 26*(2), 178–181.

Lavin, R. (2006). HIPAA and disaster research: Preparing to conduct research. *Disaster Management & Response, 4*(2), 32–37.

LoBiondo-Wood, G., & Haber, J. (2009). *Nursing research: Methods, critical appraisal, and utilization.* St. Louis, MO: Elsevier.

Olsen, D., & Mahrenholz, D. (2000). IRB-identified ethical issues in nursing research. *Journal of Professional Nursing, 16*(3), 140–148.

O'Sullivan, E., Rassel, G., & Berner, M. (2007). *Research methods for public administrators.* New York, NY: Longman.

Pech, C., Cob, N., & Cejka, J. (2005). Understanding institutional review boards: Practical guidance to the IRB review process. *Nutrition in Clinical Practice.* Retrieved from http://ncp.sagepub.com/cgi/content/full/22/6/618

Richmond, T., & Ulrich, C. (2013). *Ethical foundations for critical care nursing research.* American Association of Critical Care Nurses: Aliso Viejo, CA.

Singleton, R., & Straits, B. (2009). *Approaches to social research.* New York, NY: Oxford University Press.

Stone, P. (2003). HIPAA in 2003 and its meaning for nurse researchers. *Applied Nursing Research, 16*(4), 291–293.

Choosing a Design for Your Capstone Project

Chapter 5: *Designing a Clinically Based Quantitative Capstone Research Project*

Chapter 6: *Designing a Clinically Based Qualitative Capstone Research Project*

Chapter 7: *Designing a Clinically Based Mixed Method Capstone Research Project*

Designing a Clinically Based Quantitative Capstone Research Project

© echo3005/ShutterStock, Inc.

Objectives

Upon completion of this chapter, the reader should be prepared to:

1. Describe the origin of quantitative research.
2. Define the categories of quantitative research.
3. Describe the advantages and limitations of using a quantitative research design.
4. Discuss the basic differences in experimental, nonexperimental, and quasi-experimental research designs.
5. Discuss the advantages and limitations of using a randomized controlled trial research design.
6. Discuss the advantages and weaknesses of using a pretest–posttest research design.
7. Discuss the advantages and weaknesses of using a nonrandomized clinical trial.
8. Describe the special challenges posed to the researcher who opts to utilize the Solomon four-group research design.
9. Discuss the advantages and limitations of using a cross-sectional survey research design.

10. Discuss the advantages and limitations of using a longitudinal study with cohorts.
11. Describe the special challenges posed to the researcher who opts to utilize a case control study as a research design.
12. Describe the various types of time series designs that are available for use as a research design.
13. Discuss threats to internal validity that can occur.
14. Describe ways to minimize threats to internal validity when developing a research design.
15. Discuss threats to external validity that can occur.
16. Describe ways to increase external validity when developing a research design.

Basic Types of Quantitative Research

A clinically based capstone research project could potentially focus either on an individual patient or on groups of patients, although quantitative research focuses on patient groups. Quantitative research is concerned with patterns that are unique to a population of patients and can be particularly useful for investigating the effectiveness of an intervention. The roots of quantitative research are in **positivism**, which maintains that there is an objective reality in the world that can be quantified in some way so that observation or measurement can occur (Seers & Critelton, 2001).

As a research classification, quantitative research consists of two broad categories: experimental studies and nonexperimental or observational studies. **Observational studies** are further delineated into:

- Cross-sectional surveys.
- Longitudinal studies using cohorts, or groups of subjects who are followed over a period of time.
- Case control studies.

Experimental studies include the following subgroups:

- Clinical trials
- Randomized controlled trials
- Pretest–posttest designs (Seers & Critelton, 2001)

A variation on the two major categories of research designs is the quasi-experimental category. Each type will be discussed according to its strengths, weaknesses, and relevance to the doctor of nursing practice (DNP) researcher.

Advantages and Limitations of Quantitative Research

Quantitative research allows the investigator to establish correlational and causal relationships between variables. When the researcher is able to analyze statistics and test a theoretically derived hypothesis using a quantitative research design, he or she can present logical outcomes that have scientific validation. When the researcher uses a quantitative research design, data can be gathered using an objective approach to observing and reporting either a phenomenon that occurs or the behavior of the research subjects. This will allow the investigator to scientifically select the instrument to be used and gather the data without becoming emotionally involved with the participants or the overall research project. Therefore, the statistical significance of the hypothesis is maintained as the primary focus of the project. In addition, the researcher is able to identify the potential risks to research subjects early in the project so that complications can be minimized before the study progresses any further (Palmer, 2009).

On the negative side, conducting quantitative research may yield a lack of subjective data about human interactions that would be necessary to answer research questions pertaining to social, internal, or holistic phenomena. When a purely quantitative research design is used, the project cannot include the establishment of human emotions, habits, perceptions, or experiences that could expose personal variables related to the research subjects that could influence the final outcome of the project. For example, patients' perceptions of treatments require a level of understanding that is more complex than a quantitative research design can produce. In addition, because the relationship between the researcher and the research subjects is detached and clinical in nature, participants may receive a negative impression of the overall project and the intent of the researcher (Palmer, 2009).

Experimental Research Designs

A design is considered to be an **experimental study** if the research subjects are randomly assigned to treatment groups and to control or comparison groups, with the comparison group receiving either no treatment or simply standard treatment.

RANDOMIZED CONTROLLED TRIALS

One example of an experimental research design is the **randomized controlled trial** mentioned in the previous section. This is considered the strongest design to provide healthcare professionals with information regarding the benefits of a specific healthcare intervention; this might be the primary reason for a DNP researcher to decide to use this as a research design. The trial is a true experiment in which research subjects are randomly selected to be in the **experimental group** and receive a new intervention or to be in the **control group** and either receive a standard intervention or no intervention at all. The two main strengths of the randomized controlled trial are:

1. The random selection of participants to be in one group or the other.
2. The longitudinal nature of the study, which means participants are followed forward in time to determine if a specific outcome occurred.

In comparison, the main disadvantages of using such a design would be:

- The cost involved in conducting a lengthy randomized controlled trial.
- The extensive follow-up period required to determine if research subjects actually experienced an outcome.
- The possibility that participants who agreed to take part in a trial may be different from those to whom the research would be applied (Roberts & Dicenso, 1999).

According to Seers and Critelton (2001), randomization and the use of a control group are essential features of this type of research design. The control group is needed for comparison purposes, and the randomization is needed to ensure that the experimental and control groups are as similar as possible, except for exposure to the intervention or treatment. Randomization also is needed to protect from selection bias because it ensures that both known and unknown factors are distributed in a uniform way among the groups. **Selection bias** is considered to be a threat to the research design's **internal validity**, meaning the ability to infer that the independent variable causes a specific change in the dependent variable (Manheim, Rich, Willnat, & Brians, 2010).

Bias can also be kept to a minimal level during a randomized controlled trial through the use of blinding. **Blinding** occurs when neither the research subject nor the person assessing the outcome of the treatment is aware of the group to which the client belongs. Under ideal circumstances, no one involved with the research project would be aware of the group assignment of the participants. A double blind trial occurs when both the research subject and the person assessing the outcome are blind to the treatment group assignment (Seers & Critelton, 2001).

The long-term implications of such requirements mean that, in order to use such a research design, a DNP student must be able to guarantee:

- Randomization can occur.
- Sufficient numbers of research participants can be used to allow for both an experimental group and a control group.
- An adequate budget is present to allow for a lengthy project requiring extensive follow-up.
- Participants are willing to be followed to determine if they experienced an outcome.
- The research subjects can be readily located.

The commitment to such a project may be greater than the student's available time or resources.

 TOOLBOX

Consider your own current work environment. Do you think that the conditions are present in that environment to guarantee that a randomized controlled trial could be successfully utilized as a research design for your capstone project? If not, try to determine which areas are not present so that you can select a more appropriate research design later in the chapter.

PRETEST–POSTTEST DESIGNS

Pretest–posttest designs look at the outcome of interest before the application of an intervention and then after an intervention. This type of

research design suffers from a fundamental weakness, making it difficult to attribute causation to the intervention when there is neither randomization nor a control group. This opens up the possibility that some
other factor has affected the outcome of the research study. However, the
DNP researcher should recognize that occasionally this research design is
the only practical method of assessing the impact of an intervention. For
example, if the researcher is assessing the respiratory status of a critically
ill patient before and after the addition of a new type of ventilator to the
treatment regimen, the pretest–posttest design would be a practical choice.
Despite its obvious weakness, the pretest–posttest design can be strengthened by using a control group that also has a pretest and a posttest, using
more than one pretest in both groups, and using multiple time points for
assessing the outcomes in both groups (Seers & Critelton, 2001).

A variation of the pretest–posttest design is the **Solomon four-group
design**. The researcher opting for this research design can examine both
the main effects of testing and the interaction of testing and the application of an intervention. The four-group design uses two groups that
receive the intervention and two groups that do not. Only one treatment
group will be administered a pretest, but all four groups will receive the
posttest. A primary advantage of this type of research design is its ability
to assess the presence of pretest sensitization; this means that the posttest
measure could be affected not only by the treatment or intervention, but
also by exposure to the pretest. However, the Solomon four-group design
has some fundamental weaknesses as well. For example, it requires a large
number of research participants. In addition, it can be difficult for the
researcher to introduce the treatment or intervention at exactly the same
time for both groups. Finally, the researcher may find it difficult to randomize subjects to only one of the four groups (McGahee & Tingen, n.d.).

SUBGROUPS OF CLINICAL TRIALS

As previously mentioned, subgroups of clinical trials can be used as a type
of experimental research design. An example of this would be a **nonrandomized clinical trial**. This type of research design would be used when
randomization is not feasible or ethical, or when there is insufficient evidence to justify the difficulty and expense of a randomized clinical trial.
This could be an option for a DNP researcher who does not have the time,
manpower, or budgetary resources to implement a randomized clinical

trial. Nonrandomized clinical trials may also be referred to as "quasi-experimental" or "nonequivalent control group" designs because the characteristics of research participants in groups that were not randomized will not be equivalent. Quasi-experimental designs will be discussed later in the chapter. This failure to ensure randomization is the primary weakness of this type of research design; therefore, an estimation of the intervention's effects can be biased if the group differences in the participant characteristics are not controlled for when the data are analyzed (Hooked on Evidence, n.d.).

Nonexperimental Research Designs

A research design is considered to be nonexperimental if there is systematic collection of data but no use of control groups or randomization of subjects and no use of statistical controls.

CROSS-SECTIONAL SURVEYS

A primary nonexperimental research design is the **cross-sectional study**. This is a study undertaken at a specific point in time. There is no follow-up of the research subjects. Data are usually collected using a questionnaire, which is increasingly being administered via the Internet. Survey responses are usually made from a prearranged list and most questions are closed-ended. Although the primary advantage of cross-sectional surveys is their ability to reach large numbers of people quickly, such a research design can be difficult for the clinically based DNP student to implement. A major disadvantage of the cross-sectional survey is that there may be missing data in the responses because respondents frequently may choose to answer only specific questions and may leave blank questions they don't understand or that require a maximal amount of effort to answer.

The response rate of the cross-sectional survey is always going to be a major concern for the DNP researcher. The higher the response rate, the more clarity is contained in the overall snapshot provided by the research design; therefore, questions must be worded to be as clear as possible. The more open questions are to interpretation, the more likely respondents are to be confused by them, and the more frequently the questions will be skipped. According to Seers and Critelton (2001), a response rate of less than 40 percent can make the responses questionable in terms of how representative they are of the target population. Such a low response rate could mean that respondents were motivated by a specific set of factors unknown to the researcher. The representativeness of a cross-sectional survey can be increased if a randomized sample is used when distributing the survey instrument. Representativeness means that the characteristics of the sample of subjects closely approximate those of the larger population of potential respondents. Ultimately, the cross-sectional survey can be an effective research design for the DNP student who has access to a specific population, such as the employees of a facility, but may be difficult to utilize with an ever-changing patient population (Seers & Critelton, 2001).

 TOOLBOX

Consider your current work environment. Do you have sufficient access to the facility's employees to allow a cross-sectional survey to be utilized as your research design for your capstone project? If not, what conditions would need to be implemented in order to allow you to have this access?

LONGITUDINAL STUDIES USING COHORTS

A **longitudinal study** is often used to focus on causative agents because it follows a group of people over time. A **cohort** is the group of research subjects the researcher follows over time. If the researcher chooses, the cohort can be sampled over multiple points in time. The DNP researcher could use this type of research design to address a question regarding potential harm to a patient in a clinical situation when it would be unethical to perform a randomized controlled trial. For example, it would be unethical to randomize research subjects who have cardiac disease to take an excessive amount of a specific medication in order to measure the impact on the subjects' cardiovascular systems. However, the researcher could certainly follow a group of cardiac patients over time to determine their compliance with their medication regimen and the changes that occurred to their cardiovascular systems over time.

The major drawback to the use of longitudinal studies using cohorts is the time and expense involved, both of which can be major concerns for the clinically based DNP researcher with a limited budget, little personnel support, and multiple deadlines. In addition, longitudinal studies suffer from **attrition**. This is the loss of research subjects that occurs during the course of the research study, making follow-up difficult (Seers & Critelton, 2001).

CASE CONTROL STUDIES

When the researcher chooses a **case control study** as the research design, research subjects are selected because they have some condition of interest. A control group made up of participants who do not have the disease or condition will be selected and typically will match the cases selected on demographic variables such as age, gender, and location. The case participants and the control participants will be questioned regarding factors that could have potentially caused the condition of interest, then the case participants and control group's exposure to each factor being studied will be compared. For example, if the researcher is examining the relationship between stress and cardiovascular disease, cases selected may be people who have experienced an acute myocardial infarction and been treated for stress with antianxiety agents. Control participants selected could be patients who are simultaneously undergoing treatment for both cardiac disease and stress. Control participants would be matched to the case participants according to age, gender, clinical diagnosis, and significant historical data.

The primary advantage to use of case control studies as a research design is that it can be quickly and easily implemented—major advantages for the DNP researcher—and also allow assessment of causation. It can be particularly useful when the condition being studied is rare, or when there is a lengthy amount of time between exposure to the potential causative conditions and the resulting outcome (Seers & Critelton, 2001). In comparison, there are several drawbacks attached to use of this research design:

- The difficulty in obtaining control subjects who are very similar to the case participants in all of the factors being investigated.
- The objection of healthy patients to participation in a research project that is disease focused (Seers & Critelton, 2001).
- Difficulty in establishing that exposure to the causative factors actually occurred before the outcome.

■ Difficulty in obtaining accurate information about exposure to the potentially causative agent that has occurred in the past, because participants' memory may be sketchy and medical records may be incomplete and inaccurate (Roberts & Dicenso, 1999).

TOOLBOX

Consider your current work environment. Do you think that sufficient conditions exist to allow a case control study to be utilized as a research design for your capstone project? If not, what would need to be changed in order for this type of design to be utilized?

Quasi-Experimental Research Designs

A variation on the previously discussed categories of research designs is the quasi-experimental category. A research design is considered to be quasi-experimental if the research subjects are not randomly assigned to groups, although there may still be a control or comparison group. Although subjects are not randomly assigned, either they can be randomly sampled or all of the relevant cases can be used. In addition, statistical controls are used instead of the random assignment of subjects. A quasi-experimental research design can be used instead of an experimental design when an experimental design is not feasible or perhaps even ethical, or when a true experiment cannot be conducted in a real-world situation. Data analysis may have to occur on the basis of archival information alone, randomization of subjects may not be an option, and there may be no pretest data available. A quasi-experimental design should also be utilized when an experimental design has become flawed due to attrition in the treatment group.

ONE-GROUP POSTTEST-ONLY DESIGN

A primary quasi-experimental research design is the one-group posttest-only design. Similar to a case study, this research design does not use a pretest baseline or a comparison group, and thus it is difficult to arrive at valid conclusions about the effects of a treatment because only posttest information is available. This type of research design is not recommended for the DNP student who wants to be able to draw conclusions about the outcome resulting from application of a specific intervention (Garson, 2009).

NONEQUIVALENT CONTROL GROUP DESIGN

This type of quasi-experimental design is used in research projects conducted in field settings. It looks very similar to a true experiment except for a lack of random assignment to groups. The essential problem with the nonequivalent control group design is the difficulty the researcher can have in assuming that the experimental and comparison groups are similar when the study is initiated. The design also requires the researcher to contend with multiple threats to the internal validity of the study. This means there will be competing explanations for the results that are obtained. Such threats to internal validity will include:

- *Selection*—This results from the way in which research subjects were chosen for the project, particularly if precautions were not utilized to achieve a **representative sample**.
- *History*—A specific event occurring either inside or outside the experimental setting has an effect on the dependent variable.
- *Maturation*—The natural developmental changes, such as the aging process, that would occur to research subjects over the course of time and are unrelated to the research project being conducted.
- *Testing*—The effect of taking a pretest on the subject's posttest score. Taking a pretest may improve the research subject's score on the posttest, and thus the result of the differences between posttest and pretest scores may not be an outcome of the application of an intervention but may instead be the result of the experience gained through the testing process.
- *Instrumentation*—This threat to internal validity occurs when there are changes in the way variables are measured or the techniques used for observation that will cause changes in the measurements that are obtained.
- *Mortality*—The loss of study subjects from the time of administration of the pretest to the time of administration of the posttest. If the subjects who remain in the study are vastly different from

the subjects who opt to remove themselves from the project, the results obtained will most likely be affected (LoBiondo-Wood & Haber, 2009).

The DNP researcher who opts to use this research design must be prepared to minimize the threats to internal validity to the greatest extent possible. This may be difficult if the researcher does not have the budgetary resources for training all data collectors to minimize the threat of instrumentation or if an insufficient number of subjects are available to minimize the threat of mortality as subjects leave the study.

 TOOLBOX

Consider your current work environment. If you opted to utilize a non-equivalent control group design as a research design for your capstone project, how would you cope with the threats to internal validity that are known to exist with this type of research design?

TIME SERIES

The **time series** research design involves the collection of data over an extended period of time and the introduction of an experimental treatment during the data collection process. A primary advantage of the time series is that the extended time perspective greatly increases the likelihood that changes that occur can be attributed to the introduction of the treatment or intervention that is being implemented (Polit & Beck, 2006). There are multiple variations on this research design:

- *Simple interrupted time series design*—This is a one-group pretest–posttest design that utilizes multiple pretests and posttests. Trends noted in multiple pretests can be compared to trends noted in multiple posttests to determine whether postintervention improvement is the result of a maturation effect that would have led to improvement anyway. This could be a possible research design for the DNP researcher who has access to a group of research subjects in a clinical setting for an extended period. Because there is no control group, however, the researcher cannot assess other threats to internal validity such as history. As with the nonequivalent control group design, other threats to internal validity that may occur include selection bias, instrumentation bias, and testing (Garson, 2009).

- *Interrupted time series with a nonequivalent no-treatment comparison group*—This is a two-group pretest–posttest design using an untreated control group, but with the addition of multiple pretests and posttests. A comparison group is used, so even though randomization does not occur, the same threats to validity can occur but they usually can be more easily disproved. The main challenge with this research design is the need to show that the two groups used were equal on all of the variables that were important to causation prior to the introduction of treatment. This may be difficult for the researcher who has little knowledge of the status of the research subjects prior to initiation of the treatment intervention (Garson, 2009).

- *Interrupted time series with multiple replications*—This interrupted time series has the treatment intervention and removal of the treatment occurring multiple times according to a schedule; the design is strengthened when the researcher times these interventions and removals randomly. The difficulty associated with this design is its assumption that the researcher is dealing with the effect of an intervention that dissipates before the next intervention is applied without a cumulative effect. This would not be an effective research design to use when the researcher is working with, for example, the effects of some pain medications or psychiatric drugs that may be cumulative over time (Garson, 2009).

- *Interrupted time series with switching replications*—This research design uses two groups, each serving as either the treatment or comparison group on an alternating basis. This is accomplished through multiple applications of the treatment intervention and removal of the treatment. Although this design requires a high level of control over the research subjects by the researcher, it is a strong design that can rule out threats to validity. The main difficulty encountered with use of this research design is that it is ineffective when the treatment intervention has been introduced gradually or when the effect of the treatment intervention does not dissipate easily. This means that this design probably would not be effective when a research project involves the effects of chemotherapy because these effects would not dissipate easily and are typically administered in a cycle of treatments (Garson, 2009).

TOOLBOX

Consider your current work environment. Do you think that it lends itself to use of a time series research design if you opted to utilize it as the setting for your capstone project? Why or why not?

EXTERNAL VALIDITY

The importance of internal validity and threats that must be minimized already has been discussed. However, **external validity** must also be considered. This pertains to the generalizability of the results obtained. A study will have little external validity if it is so specific to a certain population that its results cannot be applicable to anyone else. Like internal validity, there are specific threats to external validity that also must be minimized by the researcher to the greatest extent possible. These include:

- *Pretest sensitization*—Posttest scores of pretested subjects may not be representative of the unpretested population of subjects if the subjects are pretest sensitized to the effects of the intervention or treatment being applied.
- *Interaction of selection and experimental treatment*—If the process of selection has been biased, a test group that responds to the independent variable in ways not typical of the larger population of subjects may be produced.
- *Reactive effects of experimental arrangements*—This occurs when the conditions of the experiment are not representative of real-world situations.
- *Multiple-treatment interference*—If multiple treatments are applied simultaneously, changes that are different from what would occur if one treatment were used alone may occur.
- *Irrelevant responsiveness of measures*—The measures being used may include irrelevant components that indicate change has occurred when in fact it has not.

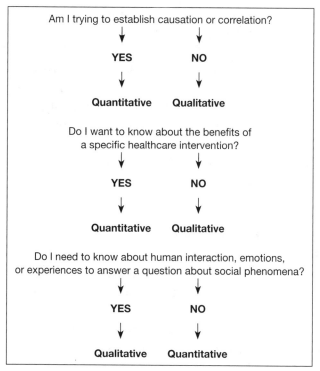

FIGURE 5-1 Decision tree to determine if a quantitative research design is appropriate.

■ *Irrelevant replicability of treatments*—Researchers may fail to include the part of the intervention or treatment actually responsible for creating change each time the research subjects are exposed to it (Manheim et al., 2005).

As the DNP student continues to decide on a research design for the research project, he or she must investigate qualitative research designs as well as quantitative designs. The following chapter will review the qualitative designs.

Learning Enhancement Tools

1. Describe the ideal conditions under which a DNP researcher could utilize a randomized controlled trial as a research design.
2. Describe the ideal conditions under which a DNP researcher could utilize a nonrandomized clinical trial as a research design.

3. Describe the ideal conditions under which a DNP researcher could utilize a pretest–posttest research design.
4. Develop a set of criteria you would use in critiquing an experimental research design used in a research project. Describe why you selected each criterion and how you would implement each one.
5. Suppose you are a DNP researcher who is considering using a cross-sectional survey as a research design for a project involving administrators' training in disaster preparedness. You are employed in a 425-bed acute care hospital that is affiliated with a large university. Describe what you can do to make the survey as representative as possible.
6. Describe the ideal conditions under which a DNP researcher could utilize a longitudinal research design using a cohort.
7. Develop a set of criteria you would use in critiquing a nonexperimental observational research design that is used in a research project. Describe why you selected each criterion and how you would implement each one.
8. Outline a plan for a research study that would effectively fit use of a case control study as a research design.
9. Develop a set of criteria you would use in critiquing a quasi-experimental research design used in a research project. Describe why you selected each criterion and how you would implement each one.
10. Outline a plan for a research study that would effectively fit the use of one-group posttest only as a research design.
11. Outline a plan for a research study that would effectively fit use of nonequivalent control group as a research design.
12. Imagine you are planning to use a quasi-experimental research design for your research project. Explain how you can reduce the threats to internal validity as you implement the design.
13. Describe the ideal conditions under which a DNP researcher could utilize a time series research design.
14. Describe the circumstances under which a DNP researcher would choose to utilize the following research designs:
    a. Simple interrupted time series design
    b. Interrupted time series with a nonequivalent no-treatment comparison group

    c. Interrupted time series with multiple replications

    d. Interrupted time series with switching replications

15. Suppose you are planning to use a quasi-experimental research design for your research project. Explain how you can reduce the threats to external validity as you implement the design.

Resources

Bordens, K., & Abbott, B. (2008). *Research design and methods: A process approach.* New York, NY: McGraw-Hill.

Creswell, J. (2008). *Research design: Qualitative, quantitative, and mixed methods approaches.* Thousand Oaks, CA: Sage Publications.

Endacott, R. (2007). Clinical research 1: Research questions and design. *Accident and Emergency Nursing, 15*(2), 106–109.

Fontana, J. (2004). A methodology for critical science in nursing. *Advances in Nursing Science, 27*(2), 93–101.

Halcomb, E., & Andrew, S. (2005). Triangulation as a method for contemporary nursing research. *Nurse Researcher, 13*(2), 71–82.

Hopwood, N. (2004). Research design and methods of data collection and analysis: Researching students' conceptions in a multiple method case study. *Journal of Geography in Higher Education, 28*(2), 347–353.

Leedy, P., & Ormrod, J. (2009). *Practical research: Planning and design.* Upper Saddle River, NJ: Prentice-Hall.

Russell, C. (2005). Interpreting research in nephrology nursing: Evaluating quantitative research reports. *Nephrology Nursing Journal, 32*(1), 61–64.

Sandelowski, M. (2000). Focus on research methods: Combining qualitative and quantitative sampling, data collection, and analysis techniques in mixed-method studies. *Research in Nursing & Health, 23,* 246–255.

Shadish, W., Cook, T., & Campbell, D. (2002). *Experimental and quasi-experimental designs for generalized causal inference.* Boston, MA: Houghton-Mifflin.

Verschuren, P. (2001). Case study as a research strategy: Some ambiguities and opportunities. *International Journal Social Research Methodology, 6*(2), 121–139.

References

Garson, D. (2009). *Research design.* Retrieved from http://faculty.chass
.ncsu.edu/garson/PA765/design.htm

Hooked on Evidence. (n.d.). *Hooked on evidence study design type definitions.* Retrieved from www.hookedonevidence.com/formsubmit
/popups/designtypedef.cfm

LoBiondo-Wood, G., & Haber, J. (2009). *Nursing research: Methods, critical appraisal, and utilization.* St. Louis, MO: Mosby.

Manheim, J., Rich, R., Willnat, L., & Brians, C. (2005). *Empirical political
analysis: Research methods in political science.* New York, NY: Addison Wesley Longman.

McGahee, T., & Tingen, M. (n.d.). The use of the Solomon four-group
design in nursing research. *Southern Online Journal of Nursing
Research, 9*(1), 1–7. Retrieved from ww.resourcenter.net/images/snrs
/files/sojnr_articles2/Vol09Num01Art14.html

Palmer, J. (2009). Nursing research: Understanding the basics. *Plastic Surgical Nursing, 29*(2), 115–121.

Polit, D., & Beck, C. (2006). *Essentials of nursing research: Methods,
appraisals, applications.* Philadelphia, PA: Lippincott.

Roberts, J., & Dicenso, A. (1999). Identifying the best research design
to fit the question. Part 1: Quantitative design. *Evidence-Based
Nursing, 2,* 4–6.

Seers, K., & Critelton, N. (2001). Quantitative research: Designs relevant
to nursing and healthcare. *Nursing Times, 6*(1), 487–500.

CHAPTER 6

Designing a Clinically Based Qualitative Capstone Research Project

© echo3005/ShutterStock, Inc.

Objectives

Upon completion of this chapter, the reader should be prepared to:

1. Discuss the principles that function as the basis of qualitative research.
2. Describe the advantages and limitations of using a qualitative research design.
3. Discuss the specific challenges faced by the researcher who is engaged in qualitative research involving sensitive issues.
4. Discuss the differences between qualitative and quantitative research.
5. Discuss the use of ethnography as a qualitative research design.
6. Differentiate between an etic perspective and an emic perspective.
7. Discuss the use of phenomenology as a qualitative research design.
8. Differentiate between descriptive and interpretive phenomenology.
9. Discuss the use of grounded theory as a qualitative research design.
10. Describe the characteristics of a core variable.

11. Discuss the use of life history as a qualitative research design.
12. Differentiate between an interview guide and a life history grid.
13. Discuss the use of ethnomethodology as a qualitative research design.
14. Describe the key features of an ethnomethodological research design.
15. Delineate the limitations known to be associated with an ethnomethodological research design.

Basic Types of Qualitative Research

A clinically based capstone project can use a qualitative research design when the DNP researcher is concerned mainly with the process being implemented rather than the outcomes being achieved or products being utilized. The qualitative researcher is concerned with how research subjects make sense of their lives, experiences, and structures in their own world and the meaning that these experiences and structures have for them. This indicates that qualitative research frequently is descriptive because the researcher is concerned with the process, meaning, and understanding that can be gained. Hoepfl (1997) broadly defines qualitative research as any type of research that uses a means other than statistical procedures or some method of quantification to generate findings.

In qualitative research, the researcher is the primary instrument for data collection as well as data analysis. Data collection frequently occurs through fieldwork, which means the researcher goes on-site to the research subjects' location to observe and record behavior in its natural setting. In addition, data is frequently recorded using field notes. These are free-flowing descriptions of research subjects, activities, and setting that can also include sketches or maps. Recognizing that writing extensive field notes can be very difficult during participant observations, some researchers advocate writing brief notes to serve as a memory aid after the conclusion of the observation while full field notes are being constructed (Hoepfl, 1997). A valuable source of information for the qualitative researcher can be document analysis. This can include letters, diaries, and newspaper articles in addition to the standard reports and official records. Some researchers have used journal entries and memos to supplement interviews with research participants (Hoepfl, 1997).

Regardless of the format of the research design selected, the researcher engaged in qualitative research is most often interested in inductive research. This means the researcher builds hypotheses and theories from details derived from the collection of data from the research subjects. The researcher will be interested in the generation of new hypotheses rather than testing hypotheses (Siegle, n.d.).

The basic difference between qualitative and quantitative research can be best described in terms of their philosophical bases. Qualitative research is based on principles of phenomenology, which acknowledges the individual qualities of each research subject while exploring human responses and the influence of society on each person's perception of reality. In comparison, quantitative research is based on the principles of positivism. Knowing that quantitative research is the best approach to use in order to establish the existence of a cause-and-effect relationship between variables, it is logical that positivism seeks to conduct research that is both objective and measurable so that a direction for a hypothesis will emerge. Therefore, it becomes clear that qualitative research can be a logical choice when the researcher is interested in issues other than a cause-and-effect relationship between variables (Palmer, 2009). The researcher engaged in quantitative research is concerned with the following:

- What knowledge exists about a problem that will allow a hypothesis to be formulated and then tested?
- What concepts are available for testing the hypothesis?
- How can the concepts be operationalized or measured?
- What scientific theory can explain the data as they currently exist?
- How can the results be interpreted and then reported to be of interest to the nursing community initially and then to stakeholders for health care in general? Are there implications that could be of interest to stakeholders in other fields as well? Do the results have global implications?

In contrast, the researcher engaged in qualitative research is primarily concerned with the following:

- What do research subjects know about their culture that can be discovered by the researcher?
- What concepts do research subjects use to classify their experiences?

- How do these subjects define the concepts they use to classify their experiences? Where do the subjects derive the information they use to formulate their definitions of the concepts?
- Is there a folk theory that subjects are using to explain their experiences? What is the basis of the folk theory once it is identified?
- How can the researcher translate the subjects' cultural knowledge into a cultural description that will be of interest to the nursing community initially and then to stakeholders for health care in general? Is there an aspect of the cultural description that will be of interest to stakeholders in other fields as well? Does the cultural description have global implications? (Siegle, 2009)

Key (1997) summarized the differences between qualitative and quantitative research. Whereas the quantitative approach has as its philosophical basis in phenomenology, which emphasizes the meaning that experiences have for individuals, the qualitative approach is based in positivism, which places emphasis on the idea that truth is only found in scientific knowledge. The goals of the DNP student who chooses a qualitative approach to the capstone project will be to achieve understanding through discovery, frequently of the lived experience of a small group of individuals, and to describe the understanding that has been achieved. The goals of the DNP student who chooses a quantitative approach to the capstone project will be to achieve a prediction of a phenomena so that it could be described, explained, and ultimately controlled. The qualitative approach is frequently selected because it is a flexible one, occurring in a natural setting and using a small sample that does not have to be randomized. In contrast the quantitative approach is structured, occurring in an artificial setting and using a randomized sample of participants that is representative of the larger population. When data collection occurs in a capstone project having a qualitative basis, the student researcher serves as the data collection instrument through interviews and observations; in contrast, data collection in a project having a quantitative basis occurs through the use of scales, tests, or instruments. Ultimately, the DNP student chooses a qualitative approach to the capstone project because the intent is to utilize inductive reasoning with the researcher being the mode of analysis. The DNP student would choose a quantitative approach if the intent is to utilize deductive reasoning with statistical methods being the mode of analysis of the collected data.

Advantages and Limitations of Qualitative Research

A primary advantage of qualitative research stems from its subjective nature. The data gathered is unique to the individual research subject's perspective, so the subject is given the opportunity to express feelings and perceptions in an environment that is nonjudgmental. Qualitative research allows a connection to be established between phenomena being studied and research subjects' perceptions of those phenomena. Another advantage of qualitative research is its flexibility. It allows the DNP researcher to be prepared to adjust the study in response to obstacles that arise during the study and to alter the established course of the project so that new research questions can be developed and other methods for data collection can be established as needed. Qualitative research can also provide a realistic description of how a research subject relates to his or her environment as well as to the interventions being implemented in the study. This means that a research question regarding the reason why a patient is not responding as expected to treatment could be solved through qualitative research. It can use subjective information and observations of research participants to describe the natural setting of the variables being studied, and thus may produce more comprehensive information than could be generated through quantitative research. Qualitative research also lends itself particularly well to academia because questions regarding how students respond to a specific teaching strategy can be resolved using a qualitative research design (Palmer, 2009).

Although qualitative research can be a rich source of untapped data for the DNP researcher, its potential limitations must be considered as well. It has sometimes been viewed in a negative light because of its reliance on subjective data and the difficulty involved in channeling perceptions or emotions into measurable data. The very subjective data that can describe the **context** of the variables being considered can make it difficult to prevent researcher-induced bias. Results may be questioned in terms of validity and credibility. The primary limitation attached to this type of research design is the potential lack of logical reasoning and statistical analysis required by a scientific field such as health care. A qualitative study places a great deal of reliance on the knowledge and reliability of the researcher and the relationship that he or she establishes with research subjects during the course of the project. If the researcher becomes too emotionally involved with research subjects, a threat to the research may develop as subjects begin to feel vulnerable during interviews. This means that some types of qualitative research designs may require greater scrutiny by an institutional review board than the researcher originally anticipated in order to prevent the research subjects from feeling that their privacy is being overly invaded (Palmer, 2009). In addition, the DNP researcher who opts to use a qualitative research design will find that there are few guidelines regarding when to conclude the data collection process. This may lead to overextension of the sampling procedure to such an extent that the boundaries of the research project are expanded inappropriately (Hoepfl, 1997).

Even greater challenges can emerge for the qualitative researcher who opts to engage in research that involves sensitive issues. Dickson-Swift, James, Kippen, and Liamputtong (2007) found specific issues arise for the researcher who selects a particularly sensitive topic:

- The researcher must recognize that he or she is actually entering the life of the research subject; when this process occurs at a time of crisis and involves extensive interviews, the researcher must be able to show both discretion and respect for the subject's willingness to disclose extremely personal information.
- The researcher must be able to develop rapport with the research subject from the first encounter; participant disclosure will be increased if there is a strong rapport between the researcher and the participant.
- Researcher self-disclosure may occur to facilitate disclosure by the research subject, but this may cause the researcher to feel vulnerable.
- The researcher may feel the need for reciprocity, or the desire to give something back to the subject to acknowledge what the person has given to the researcher. This can lead to the development of a social relationship between the researcher and the research subject.
- A researcher who is hearing many life stories of traumatized research subjects may begin to feel desensitized and distant from his or her own feelings.

- The researcher may begin to develop emotional attachments to research subjects and thus may continue to think about research subjects after completing data collection.
- The researcher who performs data collection in a setting such as subjects' homes may feel physically vulnerable if the setting causes him or her to feel unsafe or emotionally vulnerable when the setting leads to a great amount of self-disclosure.
- The researcher may ultimately feel guilt related to collecting sensitive data and may wrestle with questions regarding exploitation of research subjects.

The researcher who chooses to select a sensitive topic must be prepared before initiating the study to address these challenges to avoid spending valuable time struggling with a project that is not viable.

Qualitative Research Designs

There are various qualitative research designs that the DNP researcher can select from when formulating the capstone project. These include ethnography, phenomenology, grounded theory, life history, and ethnomethodology. Motivational interviewing, which isn't a specific research design, is also relevant to qualitative research.

ETHNOGRAPHY

When a researcher selects **ethnography** as the research design for a study, he or she is primarily concerned with the need to learn about a culture from the people who actually are immersed in it every day. The term *culture* can be used to mean not only a population of people with common ethnicity, but also a society, a community, or an organization. Ethnography entails intensive involvement with the participants being studied through immersion in their world via fieldwork. The researcher uses participant observation and in-depth interviews to discover the meanings that participants have for their knowledge, behaviors, and activities (Ploeg, 1999). Informants are interviewed multiple times, and they are asked to identify other informants who would be useful to the researcher and are representative of the community being studied. This is referred to as **chain sampling**. This would occur, for example, when the informant being interviewed by the DNP researcher in an area of hospital administration suggests the researcher speaks with members of another subdivision of the same department who are involved in similar activities. It is most typical for the researcher who uses ethnography as a research design to live in the culture being studied for an extensive period of time, so the DNP researcher could easily study the employees of the hospital where he or she is employed.

If the research is primarily concerned with how members of the culture being studied perceive their own world, this is referred to as an **emic perspective**. This would be used, for example, when the research centers around nurses employed in a specific area of a hospital and their perception of their own unit. If the research is more concerned with the way nonmembers perceive and interpret the behaviors of members of the culture, this is an **etic perspective** (Garson, 2008). This would be appropriate when the research focuses on nonnurses employed by the hospital or even volunteers associated with the hospital on a frequent basis and their perception of the behaviors of the nurses in a specific area of the hospital. The context of the culture is particularly important in ethnography, whether social, political, or economic. This means that this design easily could be utilized by a DNP researcher who is interested in studying hospital employees, whether nurses or administrative employees (Ploeg, 1999).

PHENOMENOLOGY

The researcher who decides to use a phenomenological approach to a study is primarily interested in accurately describing the lived experiences of the research subjects rather than formulating theories or models of the phenomenon being studied. In-depth interviews are most frequently used as the primary means of data collection (Ploeg, 1999). The role of the researcher is often that of a facilitator to encourage the respondent to talk freely. This means the only interview questions are those that promote clarification of an area or further exploration of an issue. Data analysis occurs through interpretation of the interview material as meaningful information is identified and categorized into themes (Balls, 2009).

A phenomenological research design may be approached from two perspectives: descriptive phenomenology or interpretive phenomenology. **Descriptive phenomenology** uses a concept known as **bracketing** to maintain researcher objectivity. This consists of setting aside the researcher's knowledge of the experience being investigated and approaching the data without preconceived ideas about the phenomenon being studied (Balls, 2009). Some researchers who advocate the descriptive phenomenological approach opt to not conduct a detailed literature review before beginning the study and to not format specific research questions other than the desire to describe participants' lived experiences as they relate to the topic of the project. The descriptive approach also proposes that there are aspects to any participant's lived experience that are common to anyone who has that experience. These aspects are referred to as **universal essences** (Lopez & Willis, 2004). The descriptive approach could be used by a DNP researcher interested in describing the lived experiences of parents whose children are hospitalized with a chronic illness.

In comparison, **interpretive phenomenology** proposes that the researcher cannot eliminate preconceptions about a phenomenon and, in fact, it is those experiences that are used to interpret the experiences of other people (Balls, 2009). The interpretative approach proposes that a person's reality is influenced by the world in which he or she lives to such an extent that his or her choices are confined by the specific conditions of his or her daily existence. The DNP researcher who uses an interpretative phenomenological approach would interpret the narratives of participants to determine the historical, social, and political forces that are shaping their experiences. This approach does not prohibit the use of a conceptual framework, and in fact allows a theoretical approach to be used to add focus and to assist in decisions about sampling, subjects, and research questions. If the researcher opts to utilize a framework, he or she has a responsibility to show that the framework did not bias the participants' narratives and to demonstrate how the framework was used in data interpretation and in the generation of findings. The DNP researcher could use the interpretative approach to study the lived experiences of nurse managers in a hospital that is undergoing a buyout by another corporation. The interpretative approach would investigate the historical, social, and political forces that are influencing the managers' experiences (Lopez & Willis, 2004).

 TOOLBOX

Consider your current work environment. Do you think that a phenomenological research design could be used effectively in this environment? If not, what would need to be changed in order to accommodate such a design?

GROUNDED THEORY

The researcher who opts to use grounded theory is interested in utilizing theory that is derived from everyday experiences. The researcher attempts to explain a specific social situation by identifying the guiding principle underlying it (Byrne, 2001). Rather than developing a theory and then seeking out evidence to support that theory, the researcher using grounded theory as a research design gathers data and then develops an explanatory theory derived from the data (Walker & Myrick, 2006). Research topics that would lend themselves well to use of grounded theory by a DNP researcher would be interaction between client and nurse, the process of discharge planning, interaction between physician and nurse, or the management styles utilized by nurse managers.

The sources of data acquired through grounded theory will include any resource that provides information about the social interaction being investigated. The grounded theory underlying the social interaction being investigated will be determined by the researcher through the **constant comparative method**, which means that data will be analyzed concurrently throughout the process of data collection as the researcher searches for a **core variable** that will be the foundation for formulation of the grounded theory. The core variable that is sought by the researcher typically:

- Recurs on a frequent basis.
- Links various data.
- Has greater implications for development of formal theory.
- Develops detail in the research.
- Includes people from various backgrounds (Byrne, 2001).

The researcher using a grounded theory design begins to analyze the data through a process known as coding, initially examining the data line by line and then comparing and contrasting the data to create categories. These categories are used to develop the theory, which emerges as the researcher implements **data reduction**. Data reduction occurs as information relevant to the topic is filtered and information that is not relevant to the topic is discarded. Data will be collected using the process of **data saturation**—data are collected until no additional new information is located (Byrne, 2001). Grounded theory as a research design lends itself well to being used by a researcher who functions in a quality assurance–type area and is already familiar with the root-cause-analysis investigative process.

TOOLBOX

Consider your current work environment. Do you think that a grounded theory research design could be used effectively in this environment? If not, what would need to be changed in order to accommodate such a design?

LIFE HISTORY

The researcher who opts to utilize life history as a research design is interested in exploring, discovering, and understanding the lives of participants, with research subjects actively reconstructing their lives as they tell their stories. The researcher is able to explore a variety of the participants' experiences and relationships and examine changes over time as lifelong data are collected. The researcher who uses the life history design views research subjects as collaborative partners. Each participant will be guided through his or her life history by the researcher and encouraged to reflect on memories and insights into behaviors. The life history approach is intended to provide an understanding of how past events and relationships influence current phenomena and how people instill meaning into their lives. As the design is implemented, context is determined. This is the subject's worldview that influences how his or her life is lived and interpreted and allows the subject to assign meaning to his or her life events, thoughts, experiences, and relationships. Context is crucial as the researcher attempts to understand how the subject views an event in his or her life or a specific experience (Haglund, 2004).

Some researchers advocate use of an interview guide as well as a life history grid when utilizing the life history research design. The **interview guide** can be particularly useful in obtaining institutional review board approval because it ensures the interviewer will ask all participants similar questions. The interview guide for the life history design should move in chronological order, including contexts that are particularly important to the participants, and should include both open-ended questions and follow-up questions. Multiple 1-hour interviews should be scheduled with participants, with the first interview scheduled when the research subject initially gives consent and the second interview scheduled immediately after the first interview. This will allow the researcher to begin the interview with questions that are the least personal and reserve more sensitive questions for subsequent interviews. The **life history grid** is important as a tool for the researcher because it adds details during the analysis so that life patterns can be diagrammed. It allows the researcher to organize the participant's life events, correlate events in the life history, and summarize the written record. The grid can be used to identify patterns of experiences to understand the stories that research subjects have narrated about their lives. If the researcher opts to complete the grid during the course of the interviews, it may serve to engage the participant in the research process (Haglund, 2004).

The life history research design could be used effectively by the researcher who is interested in exploring and understanding the lives of nurses who served in World War II, for example. This type of design, because of its inclusion of contextual data, participants' interpretations, as well as emotional responses, may provide a depth of understanding that would be difficult to match with other, less effective designs (Haglund, 2004).

 TOOLBOX

Consider your current work environment. Do you think that a life history research design could be used effectively in this environment? If not, what would need to be changed in order to accommodate such a design?

ETHNOMETHODOLOGY

The researcher who utilizes ethnomethodology as a research design is concerned with how members of a social group (such as a specific area of a hospital, for example) perceive, define, and ultimately classify the ways in which they perform their daily activities (such as patient care duties) and the meaning the members assign to these activities. Ethnomethodology is used to show how group members produce order within their own ranks so that cultural activities are interpreted and understood. A DNP researcher could use this research design to study the practices that are culturally unique to nursing, such as the giving of reports from nurse to nurse or the pinning ceremony that is implemented at the successful graduation from a nursing program (Harper, 2008).

The researcher who opts to use ethnomethodology as a research design believes that social order is made up of patterns of behavior and interactions that can be chaotic; however, members produce order from this chaos mentally by interpreting rules to guide their social actions.

This belief can be considered in light of the socialization of a new nurse in nursing practice, within which the nurse learns accepted and expected attitudes. As the nurse's practice becomes more routine, the attitudes influencing the practice will become so incorporated into the nurse's psyche that he or she will no longer have to interpret the underlying reasons for specific aspects of practice (Harper, 2008).

Ethnomethodological ethnography has specific unique features that must be considered by the researcher who is considering using it as a research design:

- *Taken for granted assumptions*—The routine activities undertaken by the members of a group, including the expectations of what should happen in the course of a normal day.
- *Common-sense knowledge and procedures*—The knowledge used by the group members to make sense of their world; for a DNP researcher, this could consist of the body of knowledge that all nurses share.
- *Typification*—The way group members classify objects or experiences; this could include the terminology nurses use to classify the acuity levels of their patients.
- *Accounting*—All of the activities group members use to make sense of their world; for the DNP researcher, this would consist of how nurses use their taken-for-granted assumptions, common-sense knowledge, and experience to make decisions.
- *Indexicality*—This means that actions and verbal statements depend on the context of the situation for their meaning.
- *Reflexivity*—The relationship between a description of how an event occurred and the circumstances of an event; for the DNP researcher, this could consist of a nurse describing the behaviors associated with different levels of anxiety and also describing patients who exhibited these behaviors.

In addition to these key features that must be considered by the researcher who decides to use ethnomethodological ethnography as a research design, certain limitations also are associated with such a design. For example, the design does not address the external constraints imposed upon research subjects that will limit their choices, both in action and in thought patterns. This type of design will not be effective for a researcher who needs to explain the cause of research subjects' behaviors, primarily because the design's intention is to describe the interpretive practices used by subjects rather than the causes of action. However, for the DNP researcher interested in exploring how nurses rationalize their decisions relating to daily nursing activities that are so routine that they require no thought, it can be a very effective design for a research project (Harper, 2008).

 TOOLBOX

Consider your current work environment. Do you think that ethnomethodology could be utilized as a research design in this environment? If not, what would need to be changed in order to accommodate such a design?

MOTIVATIONAL INTERVIEWING

Although motivational interviewing is not a specific research design itself, a discussion of it is included here due to its relevance to qualitative research. In recent years, motivational interviewing has been gaining more acceptance as a technique that could be utilized as part of a qualitative research design. Motivational interviewing is an approach to behavioral change in patients that emphasizes collaboration between the nurse and the patient. It emphasizes the use of open-ended questions, reflective listening, confirmation, summarizing, and empathy (Cronk et al., 2012).

The technique has been found to be particularly effective in assisting patients to understand the need for lifestyle changes that will lead to positive changes in their physical and mental health. Considered a form of patient empowerment, motivational interviewing can help a patient gain control over self-destructive lifestyle habits and become an active participant in health promotion (Brobeck, Berdgh, Odencrants, & Hildingh, 2011). A trademark of the technique is the response of the nurse to the patient as a competent individual rather than simply as someone in need of rescue from inappropriate lifestyle choices (Miller & Moyers, 2007).

Miller and Moyers have indicated that there are eight elements that are particularly important in learning to utilize motivational interviewing:

1. Openness to the healthcare professional's collaboration with the patient so that his or her autonomy is respected; there is genuine interest expressed in the patient's viewpoint and life experiences

2. Development of a supportive and facilitative atmosphere so that patients have less fear expressing their ambivalence regarding their ability to make needed lifestyle changes
3. Ability to identify language used by the patient that indicates a commitment to moving in the direction of behavioral change as well as sustaining positive changes that have already been made
4. Ability to strengthen and reinforce change-oriented language used by the patient so that the commitment to change is deepened
5. Ability to respond to resistance to change indicated by the patient in such a way as to reflect what is indicated and show respect for the patient's thoughts and feelings while not reinforcing the resistance
6. Recognizing the patient's readiness to negotiate a plan for change
7. Ability to increase and strengthen the patient's commitment to change
8. Blending motivational interviewing with other approaches to continue to assist the patient with health promotion through the development of healthy lifestyle choices and practices

Motivational interviewing has proven itself to be a highly beneficial technique that can be effectively incorporated into a qualitative research design. DNP students who opt to utilize it as the basis for a study may find it beneficial to undergo training on its use in order to derive the maximum benefit from such utilization.

 TOOLBOX

Consider your current work environment. Do you think that the patient population served by your facility would benefit from use of motivational interviewing? If not, what would need to be changed in order to accommodate use of this technique?

Selecting a Qualitative Research Design

Hoepfl (1997) has described a basic process for selecting the most appropriate qualitative research design for a study. The researcher who is attempting to decide on a design should systematically:

- Decide on a focus for the study; this will allow the researcher to establish boundaries and decide on types of data to include and exclude as data collection occurs.

- Determine whether the qualitative research paradigm characteristics fit with the overall goals of the research; this will allow the researcher to determine early in the research process if in fact a qualitative design meets the needs of the research project.
- Decide where data will be collected and whom the data will be collected from, incorporating factors such as confidentiality issues.
- Determine how data collection will proceed; for example, the first phase of data collection may consist of open-ended participant observation, while the next phase might consist of more focused interviews.
- Decide on instrumentation that will be needed beyond simply using the researcher as the human instrument; this will help the researcher decide if additional time needs to be incorporated into the project to allow for the design of an instrument.
- Decide how detailed and specific research questions will be and how accurately and detailed the data will be recorded.
- Decide on procedures for data analysis.
- Address the logistics of data collection; interviews will need to be scheduled, personnel for data collection may need to be recruited, and a budget will need to be planned.
- Plan how the issues of reliability and validity will be addressed.

As the DNP student continues to decide on a research design for the research project, mixed framework research designs must be investigated in addition to the quantitative and qualitative designs. Mixed framework designs are research designs that incorporate elements of both of the previously discussed categories of research. Another chapter will review the mixed framework designs.

Learning Enhancement Tools

1. Describe the ideal conditions under which a DNP researcher could utilize ethnography as a research design.
   a. Describe a study that has an ethnographic research design and an emic perspective.
   b. Describe a study that has an ethnographic research design and an etic perspective.

2. Describe the ideal conditions under which a DNP researcher could utilize a phenomenological research design.
   a. Describe a study that has a phenomenological research design and a descriptive perspective.
   b. Describe a study that has a phenomenological research design and an interpretative perspective.
3. Describe the ideal conditions under which a DNP researcher could utilize grounded theory as a research design.
   a. Describe an outline for a research study that would use grounded theory as a research design and would require the researcher to implement both data saturation and data reduction.
   b. Describe an outline for a research study that would use grounded theory as a research design. Discuss how the researcher would implement the constant comparative method and how the core variable would be derived.
4. Describe the ideal conditions under which a DNP researcher could utilize life history as a research design.
   a. Describe an outline for a research project using life history as a research design. Formulate an interview guide for the project.
   b. Describe an outline for a research project using life history as a research design. Formulate a life history guide for the project.
5. Describe the ideal conditions under which a DNP researcher could utilize ethnomethodology as a research design.
6. Discuss how the DNP researcher using an ethnomethodological research design could incorporate all of the key features of such a design into a research project.
7. Explain how the DNP researcher who is interested in using an ethnomethodological research design can plan to circumnavigate the limitations that are known to be associated with such a design.
8. Imagine that you are a DNP researcher who has chosen to perform qualitative research with rape victims who arrive at your hospital's emergency department. Discuss specific ways in which you can cope with the challenges posed by performing research on such a sensitive topic while consistently remaining cognizant of the needs of your research subjects.

Resources

Alexander, B. (2005). Performance ethnography: The reenacting and inciting of culture. In N. K. Denzin & Y. S. Lincoln (Eds.), *The Sage handbook of qualitative research* (3rd ed., pp. 411–441). Thousand Oaks, CA: Sage.

Annells, M. (2007). What's common with qualitative nursing research these days? *Journal of Clinical Nursing, 16*(2), 223–224.

Balls, P. (2009, August 13). Phenomenology in nursing research: Methodology, interviewing and transcribing. *Nursing Times, 105* (32–33), 30–33.

Birch, M., & Miller, T. (2000). Inviting intimacy: The interview as therapeutic opportunity. *International Journal of Social Research Methodology, 3*, 189–202.

Crist, J., & Tanner, A. (2003). Interpretation/analysis in hermeneutic interpretive phenomenology. *Nursing Research, 52*(3), 202–205.

Dickson-Swift, V., James, E., Kippen, S., & Liamputtong, P. (2006). Blurring boundaries in qualitative health research on sensitive topics. *Qualitative Health Research, 16*, 853–871.

Hubbard, G., Backett-Milburn, K., & Kemmer, D. (2001). Working with emotions: Issues for the researcher in fieldwork and teamwork. *International Journal of Social Research Methodology, 4*, 119–137.

Johnson, B., & Clarke, J. (2003). Collecting sensitive data: The impact on researchers. *Qualitative Health Research, 13*, 421–434.

LeVasseur, J. (2003). The problem of bracketing in phenomenology. *Qualitative Health Research, 13*, 408–420.

Madison, D. (2011). *Critical ethnography: Method, ethics, and performance.* Thousand Oaks, CA: Sage Publications.

Rager, K. (2005). Self-care and the qualitative researcher: When collecting data can break your heart. *Educational Researcher, 34*, 23–27.

Smith, C., & Gallo, A. (2007). Applications of performance ethnography in nursing. *Qualitative Health Research, 17*, 521–527.

Sque, M. (2000). Researching the bereaved: An investigator's experience. *Nursing Ethics, 7*, 23–33.

Stubblefield, C., & Murray, R. (2002). A phenomenological framework for psychiatric nursing research. *Archives of Psychiatric Nursing, 16*(4), 149–155.

References

Balls, P. (2009, August 13). Phenomenology in nursing research: Methodology, interviewing and transcribing. *Nursing Times, 105*(32–33), 30–33.

Brobeck, E., Bergh, H., Odencrants, S., & Hildingh, C. (2011). Primary healthcare nurses' experiences with motivational interviewing in health promotion practice. *Journal of Clinical Nursing,* 20, 3322–3330.

Byrne, M. (2001, June). Grounded theory as a qualitative research methodology. *AORN Journal, 73*(6), 1155–1156.

Cronk, N., Russell, C., Knowles, N., Matteson, M., Peace, L., & Ponferrada, L. (2012). Acceptability of motivational interviewing among hemodialysis clinic staff: A pilot study. *Nephrology Nursing Journal, 39*(5), 385–391.

Dickson-Swift, V., James, E., Kippen, S., & Liamputtong, P. (2007). Doing sensitive research: What challenges do qualitative researchers face? *Qualitative Research, 7,* 327–353.

Garson, D. (2008). *Ethnographic research.* Available at www.statisticalassociates.com

Haglund, K. (2004). Conducting life history research with adolescents. *Qualitative Health Research, 14,* 1309–1319.

Harper, P. (2008). Ethnomethodological ethnography and its application in nursing. *Journal of Research in Nursing, 13,* 311–322.

Hoepfl, M. (1997). Choosing qualitative research: A primer for technology education researchers. *Journal of Technology Education, 9*(1). Retrieved from http://scholar.lib.vt.edu/ejournals/JTE/v9n1/hoepfl.html

Key, J. (1997). *Research design in occupational education.* Retrieved from http://www.okstate.edu/ag/agedcm4h/academic/aged5980a/5980/newpage110.htm

Lopez, K., & Willis, D. (2004). Descriptive versus interpretive phenomenology: Their contributions to nursing knowledge. *Qualitative Health Research, 14,* 726–735.

Miller, W., & Moyers, T. (2007). Eight stages in learning motivational interviewing. Journal of Teaching in the Addictions, (5), 3–17.

Palmer, J. (2009). Nursing research: Understanding the basics. *Plastic Surgical Nursing, 29*(2), 115–121.

Ploeg, J. (1999). Identifying the best research design to fit the question. Part 2: Qualitative designs. *Evidence Based Nursing, 2,* 36–37.

Siegle, D. (2009). Assumptions of qualitative designs. Retrieved from http://www.gifted.uconn.edu/siegle/research/Qualitative/qualquan.htm

Walker, D., & Myrick, F. (2006). Grounded theory: An exploration of process and procedure. *Qualitative Health Research, 16,* 547–559.

CHAPTER 7

Designing a Clinically Based Mixed Method Capstone Research Project

Objectives

Upon completion of this chapter, the reader should be prepared to:

1. Describe the underlying premise of a mixed method research design.
2. Discuss the principles that function as the basis of a mixed method research design.
3. Describe the advantages and limitations of using a mixed method research design.
4. Discuss the importance of triangulation and complementarity in deciding to implement a mixed research design.
5. Describe the two primary types of mixed method research subtypes.
6. Discuss the types of across-stage mixed method research designs.
7. Discuss the various classifications of mixed method research designs.
8. Describe the specific types of mixed research designs.
9. Describe how timing plays a part in selecting the type of mixed research design to be implemented.

10. Describe how weighting plays a part in selecting the type of mixed research design to be implemented.
11. Describe how mixing plays a part in selecting the type of mixed research design to be implemented.
12. Discuss how concurrent timing is used in a mixed research design.
13. Discuss how sequential timing is used in a mixed research design.
14. Describe what occurs during the stages of the mixed research process.
15. Discuss the specific skills that a researcher will need in order to implement a mixed research study.

Introduction to Mixed Method Research

The doctor of nursing practice (DNP) researcher who chooses to use a mixed method approach to his or her research design is interested in essentially combining the qualitative and quantitative methods. When the strengths of the two methods are combined, the researcher can achieve a broader perspective than would have been possible using only one type of research method. However, use of a mixed method approach entails the researcher having a thorough understanding of the fine points of both quantitative and qualitative research to avoid generating and ultimately reporting inaccurate findings (Palmer, 2009).

Researchers who promote the mixed method approach to research base their ideas on the compatibility thesis as well as pragmatism. The **compatibility thesis** is essentially the idea that the quantitative and qualitative research methods can be compatible and can be used together in a research study. **Pragmatism** adherents believe that a researcher should use any approach or combination of approaches that will function the best in a real-world situation, regardless of assumptions of paradigms or philosophies. Out of these ideas can come the fundamental principle of mixed research, which is that the research should use a combination of research methods that have complementary strengths but without overlapping weaknesses (University of South Alabama, n.d.).

Advantages and Limitations of Mixed Method Research

As with use of qualitative and quantitative research alone, mixed method research has specific advantages and limitations that must be considered as the researcher plans the study. The advantages and limitations, as might be expected, are very similar to those that were reviewed in the chapters on quantitative and qualitative research. The limitations should be addressed specifically in the early stages of the planning process so as to minimize their effect on the study.

Advantages of mixed method research can include:

- The use of pictures and narrative to add meaning to numbers.
- The mixed method can be used to study large numbers of people.
- The mixed method may have higher credibility than use of quantitative research or qualitative research alone.
- The mixed method may generate statistically significant results.
- Data analysis could be performed with statistical software.
- The mixed method can generate numerical data.
- The mixed method may be able to show a cause-and-effect relationship.
- The mixed method can be used to study a small number of cases in depth.
- The mixed method can be used to describe complex phenomena.
- The mixed methods can be used to test a grounded theory.
- The mixed method can answer a broader and more complex range of research questions because the researcher is not confined to use of a single approach to the research.
- Strengths of the additional research method can compensate for the weaknesses of the other method.
- The mixed method can provide stronger evidence for a conclusion.
- The mixed method can reveal insights that would not have been evident when using only one research method.
- The mixed method can increase the generalizability of the results to a larger population.

Limitations of using a mixed method approach to research can include:

- The mixed method may require a research team.
- The mixed method will require the researcher to have a thorough understanding of the intricacies of each method in order to successfully combine them.

- The mixed method will require the researcher to accurately interpret conflicting results that are generated.
- The mixed method can be more time consuming than using quantitative research or qualitative research alone, requiring the use of additional personnel, and more expensive, requiring a more expansive budget and potentially additional time spent in fund-raising activities (University of South Alabama, n.d.).

Deciding to Utilize a Mixed Method Approach

The DNP researcher who is considering the use of a mixed method approach should determine if the purpose of the research is congruent with the potential benefits of combining the research approaches. For example, the desire for triangulation is a frequently used reason for initiating mixed method research. **Triangulation** means the researcher uses the different methods in order to achieve corroboration of results achieved from the different approaches. This can increase the validity of the study. **Complementarity** is another excellent reason for using the mixed method approach. This means the researcher is striving to enhance, illustrate, or clarify the results achieved through use of input from both quantitative and qualitative designs. This can also increase the validity of the research and can further increase the interpretability of the results generated. Other purposes for choosing a mixed method approach can be the desire to extend the range of the inquiry used in the study as well as the desire to use results achieved so that one method strengthens the other method. This can mean that the researcher is able to include sampling that would not have been possible without using mixed methods (University of South Alabama, n.d.).

Mixed Research Approaches

There are two major types of mixed research—mixed model research and mixed method research. **Mixed model research** is used when quantitative and qualitative approaches are either mixed within the research process or across the various stages of the process. Mixed model research that occurs within the research stages could consist of using a questionnaire for data collection that includes both open-ended and closed-ended questions. Mixed model research that occurs across the research stages could consist of data collection through open-ended interviews, with the results of those interviews then quantified. There are six research designs that are across-stage mixed model designs:

1. Qualitative research objectives that lead to collection of qualitative data, which initiate the researcher performing quantitative analysis
2. Qualitative research objectives that lead to collection of quantitative data, which initiate the researcher performing qualitative analysis
3. Qualitative research objectives that lead to collection of quantitative data, which initiate the researcher performing quantitative analysis
4. Quantitative research objectives that lead to collection of qualitative data, which initiate the researcher performing qualitative analysis
5. Quantitative research objectives that lead to collection of qualitative data, which initiate the researcher performing quantitative analysis
6. Quantitative research objectives that lead to collection of quantitative data, which initiate the researcher performing qualitative analysis

In comparison, **mixed method research** occurs when both a qualitative phase and a quantitative phase are included in the same research study. Mixed method research designs are classified according to time order and paradigm emphasis. This means that the designs are classified according to the researcher's desire to conduct phases concurrently, at roughly the same time, or sequentially so that one occurs before the other. Also, the designs are classified according to the researcher's need to use either a dominant status design, with either a qualitative or quantitative design being the primary focus of the research, or an equal status design that has essentially an equal focus on both quantitative and qualitative aspects of the design. What does knowledge of these research approaches mean to the DNP researcher? It means that unless the researcher is positive that he or she has a fluent understanding of the inner workings of both qualitative and quantitative research, the mixed research approach should not be utilized (University of South Alabama, n.d.).

Specific Mixed Research Designs

Once the DNP researcher decides that a mixed approach to the research would best serve the needs of the study and that he or she has sufficient knowledge to implement such an approach, a specific mixed design must be selected (**Table 7-1**). The most common approach to mixing methods is the triangulation design (Creswell & Plano Clark, 2010).

TRIANGULATION DESIGN

In congruence with the definition of triangulation earlier in the chapter, this design is used to obtain different data that are still complementary on the same topic of research. This can be an effective design to use when a researcher wants to compare and contrast quantitative statistical results with qualitative findings or to further validate or clarify quantitative numerical results with qualitative data. Implementation of the design occurs when the researcher implements the quantitative and qualitative methods at the same time and with both methods carrying equal weight in the study. The design involves the collection and analysis of quantitative and qualitative data during the same time frame yet during separate collection procedures for increased understanding of the research problem. The two data sets will then be merged; this can be done by transforming data from qualitative to quantitative and vice versa to facilitate the combining of the data sets during data analysis (Creswell & Plano Clark, 2010).

Because the triangulation design seems to have a common-sense appeal, it is frequently a wise choice for novice researchers who are new to mixed research. It is also an excellent design if a team of researchers is available, because quantitative and qualitative data can be collected and analyzed separately. However, the aspects of this design that make it so appealing also make it very challenging. Because all data collection occurs during the same time frame, the design may require a great deal of effort and expertise, necessitating the use of a team of researchers. This translates into a study that will be both lengthy and expensive. This may not be an appropriate design for the researcher who recognizes that a team will not be available. Furthermore, the researcher must decide before

TABLE 7-1   Comparison of the Major Mixed Methods Designs

Type of Design	Variations	Timing	Weighting of Methods	Mixing
Triangulation	Convergence Data transformation Validation of quantitative data Multilevel	Concurrent, with quantitative and qualitative data collection occurring at the same time	Both methods usually considered to be equal in importance	Data merged during the interpretation or analysis phase
Embedded	Embedded/experimental Embedded/correlational	Concurrent and sequential	Unequally weighted	Embed one type of data within a larger design using the other type of data
Explanatory	Follow-up explanations Participant selection	Sequential: quantitative, then qualitative	Usually quantitative weighted more significantly	Connect data between the two phases
Exploratory	Instrument development Taxonomy development	Sequential: qualitative, then quantitative	Usually qualitative weighted more significantly	Connect data between the two phases

Source: Data from Creswell, J., & Plano Clark, V. (2010). Designing and conducting mixed methods research. Thousand Oaks, CA: Sage.

implementation of the design how discrepancies in the quantitative and qualitative results will be addressed (Creswell & Plano Clark, 2010).

 TOOLBOX

Imagine that you have opted to utilize triangulation as part of your mixed method research design. Consider your current work environment. Who among the employees of your current facility would you opt to utilize as part of the team required to implement this type of design?

EMBEDDED DESIGN

The embedded design is used when one data set provides a secondary yet supportive role in a study that is based primarily on the other major research method. It is used when the researcher needs to include qualitative or quantitative data to answer a research question that is included within a study that is primarily quantitative or qualitative. It is particularly useful when there is a need to include a qualitative section within a quantitative design. The hallmark of the embedded design is the inclusion of one type of data within a methodology that is framed by the other type of data. Although both types of data are included, one type always plays a secondary role within the design (Creswell & Plano Clark, 2010).

A primary advantage of this design is that it can be used when the researcher does not have enough time or resources to commit to extensively researching both quantitative and qualitative data collection because one data type will be viewed as being supplementary. Also, because the primary focus of the design is traditionally quantitative, agencies tend to be more willing to provide funding for such a design than other types of research. The two research methods will be used to answer different

 TOOLBOX

Suppose you have opted to use a cross-sectional survey as a quantitative research design to obtain data regarding the job satisfaction of first-year registered nurse graduates. How could you include a qualitative section as part of this study so that it could function as an embedded design?

research questions, so the researcher can keep the two sets of results generated separate in the research report and may even opt to report them in separate reports. There is no need to merge the two different data sets in order to answer the same research question, such as is required with the triangulation design (Creswell & Plano Clark, 2010).

EXPLANATORY DESIGN

The explanatory design consists of two phases, with the basic premise being that qualitative data will assist in explaining initial quantitative results. This type of design is well suited for a study in which the researcher needs to explain nonsignificant results, unexpected results, or statistical outliers that did not fall into the mainstream pattern. This design begins with the collection and analysis of quantitative data, followed by collection and analysis of qualitative data. The qualitative phase of the design is formulated to follow from the results of the quantitative phase. Typically, greater emphasis is placed on the quantitative phase (Creswell & Plano Clark, 2010).

The explanatory design has two variations: the follow-up explanations model and the participant selection model. The follow-up explanations model is used when the researcher needs qualitative data to help explain quantitative results. The researcher will identify specific quantitative findings that need additional explanation and will then collect qualitative data from research subjects who can most successfully explain these findings. The participant selection model is used when a researcher needs quantitative information to identify research subjects to participate in a follow-up qualitative study. This model will also primarily emphasize the qualitative phase (Creswell & Plano Clark, 2010).

The explanatory design may be a wise choice for the DNP researcher who does not have access to a team to assist in the research process. It is straightforward to implement because the two methods are conducted in separate phases and only one type of data is collected at a time; therefore, one researcher can implement the design. The final report also may be easier for readers to follow because it can be written in two phases. However, the explanatory design requires an extensive amount of time to implement because of its two-phase format, with the qualitative phase being the most lengthy. Another challenge for the researcher can be the need to decide whether the same individuals should be used for both phases of the design, whether subjects from the same sample should be used for both phases, and also whether subjects should be drawn from the same population of potential participants for the phases. A significant drawback can be the difficulty in obtaining approval from an institutional review board for this design because the researcher will not be able to specify how subjects will be selected for the second phase of the research until the initial findings are obtained (Creswell & Plano Clark, 2010).

 TOOLBOX

Suppose you are interested in implementing a cross-sectional survey of oncology nurses who have worked in that area of nursing for at least 10 years. As follow-up to the survey, you want to implement a phenomenological phase to the research in which you obtain information on the lived experiences of RNs who have worked as oncology nurses and have also experienced cancer themselves. How would you approach your facility's institutional review board in order to obtain approval to implement this design?

EXPLORATORY DESIGN

The researcher who chooses the exploratory design has the premise that the results of the qualitative method can help develop the quantitative method. Further development or exploration can be needed because measures or instruments are not available, variables are unknown, or no guiding framework is utilized. This design can be particularly effective when the researcher is exploring a phenomenon because it begins qualitatively and also is well suited to the development and testing of an instrument or the identification of important variables to study quantitatively. The exploratory design has two phases that start with qualitative data to initiate exploration of a phenomenon and then progress to a second phase that uses quantitative data. Researchers build on the results of the qualitative phases by developing an instrument, identifying variables, or stating proposed reasons for testing based on an emergent theory. These developments will forge a connection between the initial qualitative phase and the quantitative component of the research. The qualitative phase usually is given greater emphasis with the exploratory design (Creswell & Plano Clark, 2010).

There are two major variations of the exploratory design: the instrument development model and the taxonomy development model. The instrument development model is used to develop and implement a quantitative instrument based on qualitative findings. The researcher will first explore the research topic qualitatively, using only a few participants. The qualitative findings will serve as a guide for the development of a quantitative survey instrument. The researcher will then implement and validate the instrument quantitatively. Researchers who choose this variation of the exploratory design tend to emphasize the quantitative component.

In comparison, the taxonomy development model is used when an initial qualitative phase is conducted to identify important variables, develop a classification system, or develop a theory, and then a second phase consisting of quantitative tests is carried out to study the results in more detail. The initial qualitative phase will produce specific categories that then can be used to direct the research question and data collection in the second quantitative phase (Creswell & Plano Clark, 2010).

Because it uses separate phases, this design is usually straightforward to implement as well as report; however, the researcher should recognize that the use of two phases requires additional time to implement. Also, the researcher may have difficulty specifying the procedures of the quantitative phase when applying for initial institutional review board approval. A decision will be required regarding the use of the same individuals for participation in both the qualitative and quantitative phases of the research (Creswell & Plano Clark, 2010).

 TOOLBOX

Suppose you have decided to implement the instrument development model as part of an exploratory research design. Your topic is the stress level experienced by spouses or partners of cancer patients during the first 90 days after diagnosis. How could you explore this topic qualitatively with a few participants in order to guide the development of a quantitative survey instrument?

Selecting a Type of Mixed Research Design

Researchers should consider some key factors when selecting a mixed research design for a research project. These include timing, weighting, and mixing. Timing refers to the order in which the researchers use the data within a study. In a mixed research design, timing is classified as concurrent or sequential. **Concurrent timing** means the researcher implements both quantitative and qualitative methods during a single phase of the research study. **Sequential timing** occurs when the researcher implements the methods in two distinct phases, using one type of data before using the other data type (Creswell & Plano Clark, 2010).

Weighting refers to the emphasis of the two methods used in the study. This means the researcher decides whether the quantitative or qualitative component will have equal priority or if one component will have a greater priority than the other. Weighting is greatly influenced by practical considerations. Because it requires more time, money, and personnel to implement a study that equally weights the two methods, a researcher with limited resources may choose to prioritize one method over the other and dedicate less of his or her budget and time to the secondary method (Creswell & Plano Clark, 2010).

In addition to timing and weighting, the decision of how to mix the quantitative and qualitative methods will also be a concern when choosing a mixed method design. The two data sets can be merged, one set can be embedded within the other, or the two sets can be connected. The data sets can be merged by analyzing them separately in a results section and then merging the two sets of results together during the discussion phase, or by transforming one data type into the other type. The data sets can be connected when analysis of one type of data leads to the need for the other type of data (Creswell & Plano Clark, 2010).

Stages of the Mixed Research Process

A specific sequence of steps should be followed to implement a mixed research approach. They can be followed in a different order as the needs of the researcher change or as problems that must be addressed arise. The steps are:

1. Determine the appropriateness of the use of a mixed design.
2. Decide if the purpose of the research is congruent with the rationale for using a mixed design.
3. Select the mixed model or mixed method research design.

4. Collect the data. Primary data collection methods consist of tests, questionnaires, interviews, focus groups, observation, and already existing data. Data collection is discussed in detail elsewhere in this text.

5. Analyze the data, bearing in mind that qualitative data can be converted into quantitative data and vice versa. Data analysis in mixed research consists of:

   - *Data reduction*—Reduces the volume of qualitative and quantitative data. This can be accomplished through memoing, for example, for qualitative data, and descriptive statistics such as averages and percentages for quantitative data.
   - *Data display*—Describes quantitative and qualitative data pictorially. This can be done using charts, graphs, and tables.
   - *Data transformation*—Allows quantitative data to be converted into narrative data that can be analyzed qualitatively and qualitative data to be expressed quantitatively using numerical coding and then statistics.
   - *Data correlation*—Involves the correlation of quantitative and qualitative data for clarity.
   - *Data consolidation*—Combines quantitative and qualitative data to create new sets of data.
   - *Data comparison*—Involves the comparison of data from both the qualitative and quantitative sources.
   - *Data integration*—Allows both quantitative and qualitative data to be integrated into a cohesive data set or to become two separate but equally important parts of an entire data set (Johnson & Onwuegbuzie, 2004).

6. Validate the data. Data validation should occur throughout the research project. The study has internal validity if the design provides a logical basis to show that the independent variable does or does not cause a specific change in the dependent variable. External validity is present if the results can be generalized to the larger population (Manhiem, Rich, Willnat, & Brians, 2010).

7. Interpret the data. Data interpretation should begin with the collection of the first piece of datum and should continue throughout the study. Use reflexivity and negative-case sampling throughout data interpretation. **Reflexivity** means the researcher uses self-awareness and critical self-reflection to better understand his or her

personal biases and the way these may affect the research process and conclusions. **Negative-case sampling** means the researcher attempts to locate and scrutinize cases that do not confirm his or her expectations and the tentative explanations that have been proposed (University of South Alabama, n.d.).

8. Write the research report. The writing process can actually begin during data collection. The report should reflect that mixing occurred during the research process (University of South Alabama, n.d.).

The researcher who is considering implementing a mixed research study should first gain experience with both quantitative and qualitative research before attempting to implement mixed research. The researcher should be able to craft quantitative hypotheses, select the method of data collection most appropriate for this method, understand how to use statistical analysis, and verify that the instrument used provides both reliability and validity—the results generated can be generalized to the larger population, and scores received from participants are consistent over time. In addition, the researcher must be able to develop qualitative research questions, must be familiar with how to use interviews, and must understand how to code text and develop themes based on the codes. The researcher who is considering implementing mixed research should determine if there is adequate time to collect and analyze two different types of data. Furthermore, adequate resources and personnel must be available for the collection and analysis of both quantitative and qualitative data. Once the DNP researcher has decided which type of research design will be most effective for the research project, other issues pertaining to organizing the study must be addressed (Creswell & Plano Clark, 2010). The following chapter will discuss issues pertaining to obtaining a sample of research subjects, while subsequent chapters will address data collection and data analysis.

Learning Enhancement Tools

1. Imagine that you are a DNP researcher who is considering using a mixed method approach to design a research study on addressing the needs of hospice patients who speak English as a second language. How can you most effectively use the principle of

complementarity to design a study using a mixed method approach to the research?

2. Describe an original approach to mixed model research that mixes the quantitative and qualitative approaches within the stages of the research process.

3. Describe an original approach to mixed model research that mixes the quantitative and qualitative approaches across the various stages of the research process.

4. Describe a possible research study for an across-stage mixed model research project using one of the following research designs:

   a. Qualitative research objectives, collection of qualitative data, performing quantitative analysis. Describe what should occur in the stages of the mixed research process for such a design, including how data analysis should occur.

   b. Qualitative research objectives, collection of quantitative data, performing qualitative analysis. Describe what should occur in the stages of the mixed research process for such a design, including how data analysis should occur.

   c. Qualitative research objectives, collection of quantitative data, performing quantitative analysis. Describe what should occur in the stages of the mixed research process for such a design, including how data analysis should occur.

   d. Quantitative research objectives, collection of qualitative data, performing qualitative analysis. Describe what should occur in the stages of the mixed research process for such a design, including how data analysis should occur.

   e. Quantitative research objectives, collection of qualitative data, performing quantitative analysis. Describe what should occur in the stages of the mixed research process for such a design, including how data analysis should occur.

   f. Quantitative research objectives, collection of quantitative data, performing qualitative analysis. Describe what should occur in the stages of the mixed research process for such a design, including how data analysis should occur.

5. Describe a possible research study that could be developed using a triangulation mixed research design. Discuss how, as the lead DNP researcher for this project, you would plan to circumnavigate the challenges associated with this design.

6. Describe a possible research study that could be developed using an embedded mixed research design. Discuss how, as the lead DNP researcher for this project, you would plan to circumnavigate the challenges associated with this design.

7. Describe a possible research study that could be developed using an explanatory mixed research design. Discuss how, as the lead DNP researcher for this project, you would plan to circumnavigate the challenges associated with this design.

8. Describe a possible research study that could be developed using the variation of the explanatory mixed research design known as the follow-up explanations model. Discuss how, as the lead DNP researcher for this project, you would plan to circumnavigate the challenges associated with this design.

9. Describe a possible research study that could be developed using the variation of the explanatory mixed research design known as the participant selection model. Discuss how, as the lead DNP researcher for this project, you would plan to circumnavigate the challenges associated with this design.

10. Describe a possible research study that could be developed using an exploratory mixed research design. Discuss how, as the lead DNP researcher for this project, you would plan to circumnavigate the challenges associated with this design.

11. Discuss the various factors that must be considered in opting for a mixed method research design. Draw a decision tree illustrating the researcher's progress through these factors.

12. Compare and contrast the four major types of mixed method research designs.

13. Describe a possible research study that could be developed using the variation of the exploratory mixed research design known as the instrument development model. Discuss how, as the lead DNP researcher for this project, you would plan to circumnavigate the challenges associated with this design.

14. Describe a possible research study that could be developed using the variation of the exploratory mixed research design known as the taxonomy development model. Discuss how, as the lead DNP researcher for this project, you would plan to circumnavigate the challenges associated with this design.

Resources

Adcock, R., & Collier, D. (2001). Measurement validity: A shared standard for qualitative and quantitative research. *American Political Science Review, 95*(3), 529–546.

Bartlett, J., Kotrlik, J., & Higgins, C. (2001). Organizational research: Determining appropriate sample size in survey research. *Information Technology, Learning, and Performance Journal, 19*(1), 43–50.

Creswell, J. (2008). *Research design: Qualitative, quantitative, and mixed methods approaches.* Thousand Oaks, CA: Sage.

Manheim, J., Rich, R., Willnat, L., & Brians, C. (2010). *Empirical political analysis: Research methods in political science.* New York, NY: Addison Wesley Longman.

Mason, J. (2006). Mixing methods in a qualitatively driven way. *Qualitative Research, 6*(1), 9–25.

Onwuegbuzie, A., & Johnson, R. (2006). The validity issue in mixed research. *Research in the Schools, 13*(1), 48–63.

Onwuegbuzie, A., & Leech, N. (2007). On becoming a pragmatic researcher: The importance of combining quantitative and qualitative research methodologies. *International Journal of Social Research Methodology: Theory & Practice, 8*(5), 375–387.

Onwuegbuzie, A., & Teddlie, C. (2010). *Handbook of mixed methods in social and behavioral research.* Thousand Oaks, CA: Sage.

Sandelowski, M., Volls, C., & Barraso, J. (2006). Defining and designing mixed research synthesis studies. *Research in the Schools, 13*(1), 29–40.

Tashakkori, A., & Teddlie, C. (2003). (Eds.). *The handbook of mixed methods in the social and behavioral sciences.* Thousand Oaks, CA: Sage.

References

Creswell, J., & Plano Clark, V. (2010). *Designing and conducting mixed methods research.* Thousand Oaks, CA: Sage.

Johnson, R., & Onwuegbuzie, A. (2004). Mixed methods research: A research paradigm whose time has come. *Educational Researcher, 33,* 14–26.

Manheim, J., Rich, R., & Willnat, L., & Brians, C. (2010). *Empirical political analysis: Research methods in political science.* New York, NY: Addison Wesley Longman.

Palmer, J. (2009). Nursing research: Understanding the basics. *Plastic Surgical Nursing, 29*(2), 115–121.

University of South Alabama. (n.d.). *Mixed research: Mixed method and mixed model research.* Retrieved from www.southalabama.edu/coe /bset/johnson/lectures/lec14.htm

UNIT **III**

Implementing Your Capstone Project

Chapter 8: Sampling

Chapter 9: Data Collection

Chapter 10: Issues Related to Survey Data Collection

Chapter 11: Data Analysis

Chapter 12: Writing the Research Report for Potential
Publication

Sampling

Objectives

Upon completion of this chapter, the reader should be prepared to:

1. Describe the importance of obtaining a representative sample.
2. Describe the importance of simple random sampling and discuss ways to implement this type of sampling.
3. Describe the importance of stratified random sampling and discuss ways to implement this type of sampling.
4. Discuss the difference between proportional and disproportional stratified sampling.
5. Describe the importance of cluster random sampling and discuss ways to implement this type of sampling.
6. Discuss the difference between one-stage and two-stage cluster sampling.
7. Describe the importance of convenience sampling and discuss the most effective way to implement this type of sampling.
8. Describe the risk of bias and degree of representativeness associated with convenience sampling.
9. Describe the importance of quota sampling and discuss the most effective way to implement this type of sampling.

10. Describe the importance of purposive sampling and discuss the most effective way to implement this type of sampling.
11. Describe the importance of snowball sampling and discuss the most effective way to implement this type of sampling.
12. Discuss the difference between random selection and random assignment.
13. Describe the procedure for determining the sample size when random sampling is utilized.
14. Describe the primary characteristics of maximum variation sampling.
15. Describe the primary characteristics of homogeneous sample selection.
16. Describe the primary characteristics of extreme case sampling.
17. Describe the primary characteristics of typical case sampling.
18. Describe the primary characteristics of critical case sampling.
19. Describe the primary characteristics of negative case sampling.
20. Describe the primary characteristics of opportunistic sampling.
21. Describe the primary characteristics of mixed purposeful sampling.
22. Describe sampling strategies for recruiting participants for a sample for qualitative research.

Introduction to the Process of Sampling

The procedure used to obtain the sample of research subjects for participation in a research study is of such vital importance that even a minor error on the part of the researcher can prevent him or her from generating accurate data and a credible report. The researcher's goal in sampling is to obtain a **representative sample**—this means the sample is similar to the **population** from which it was drawn in all areas except that it contains fewer people than the population (University of South Alabama, n.d.).

Quantitative Sampling Designs

Sampling in quantitative research is either random sampling or nonrandom sampling. Random sampling is particularly important because it will generate representative samples, whereas nonrandom sampling will not.

TYPES OF RANDOM SAMPLING

A researcher who intends to utilize quantitative research should be familiar with several types of random sampling:

- *Simple random sampling*—This is the most basic type of random sampling. It allows everyone in the group from which the sample is being drawn to have an equal chance of being selected for the final sample. Simple random sampling can be implemented in its most basic form by putting all of the names of potential research participants from the population into a receptacle and then drawing the needed number of names at random. A computer program also can be used for simple random sampling. This is known as a random number generator that assigns each person in the population a number. The program will then provide the researcher with a list of randomly selected numbers within a range that the researcher provides. After receiving the random numbers, the researcher identifies the people with those assigned numbers and contacts them to determine their willingness to participate in the research study (University of South Alabama, n.d.).

- *Systematic sampling*—Systematic sampling uses what is known as a **sampling interval**. This is the population size divided by the desired sample size. A number will be randomly selected between 1 and the sampling interval. This will determine which research subjects will be selected for the sample out of the sampling frame. The **sampling frame** is a list of all the potential participants who make up the population. For example, if the sampling interval is 20 and the randomly selected number between 1 and 20 was 7, then the researcher reviews the numbered list of potential participants and selects subjects 7, 14, 21, and 28. A potential problem that can occur with sampling is periodicity, which means a cyclical pattern emerges in the sampling frame, usually because several ordered lists have been attached together. This can be avoided by reorganizing the multiple lists into one general list (University of South Alabama, n.d.).

- *Stratified random sampling*—This type of sampling occurs when the researcher initially selects a stratification variable. This can be anything that is used to classify the sampling frame, such as gender or race. If race is used as the stratification variable, the researcher will then select a random sample from each race in the sampling frame. The various sets of subjects will be put together and the final sample is then generated. There are two types of stratified random sampling:

1. *Proportional stratified sampling*—This occurs when the researcher makes certain that the subsamples that are selected (such as those based on race or gender) are in proportion to their sizes in the population.

2. *Disproportional stratified sampling*—This occurs when the researcher is not concerned with ensuring that the subsamples selected are in proportion to their sizes in the population (University of South Alabama, n.d.).

■ *Cluster random sampling*—This type of sampling is utilized when clusters or groups of potential participants, rather than individual subjects, are included only if the clusters are approximately equal in size. If the clusters are known to be unequal in size, probability should be considered to be proportional to the size of the group utilized. This will allow a representative sample to be produced. There are two types of cluster random sampling:

1. *One-stage cluster sampling*—To utilize this type of sampling, the researcher initially selects a random sample of the clusters or groups. The researcher then includes in the final sample all of the individual names included in the chosen clusters.

2. *Two-stage cluster sampling*—To utilize this type of sampling, the researcher selects a random sample of the clusters or groups, just as would be done in one-stage cluster sampling. The second stage involves taking a random sample of potential subjects from each of the clusters that was selected in the first phase (University of South Alabama, n.d.).

 TOOLBOX

Consider your potential topic for your capstone project. Is there a random sampling method that could be effectively utilized with it? Take into account the need to move your project successfully through the facility's institutional review board approval process.

TYPES OF NONRANDOM SAMPLING

In comparison to random sampling, there are four primary types of nonrandom sampling techniques that can be utilized with quantitative research:

1. *Convenience sampling*—This type of sampling is utilized when the researcher selects people who are most easily located or who are most available for participation in the research study. The major advantage for this type of sampling is the ease with which the researcher can locate research subjects; the major disadvantage is the risk of researcher bias is greater than in any other type of sampling. Because the researcher will obtain information only from people who volunteer to participate, the factors motivating people to volunteer should be determined. People who opted to participate may not constitute a representative sample in relation to the overall population. This is considered to be the weakest form of sampling in relation to generalizability to the greater population (LoBiondo-Wood & Haber, 2009).

2. *Quota sampling*—This is a variation on convenience sampling. It involves setting quotas and then using convenience sampling to select participants to fill the quotas. This allows the researcher to use the knowledge available about the population to build some representativeness into the sample being selected. However, researcher bias will still be an issue for this type of sampling, as previously discussed with convenience sampling (LoBiondo-Wood & Haber, 2009).

3. *Purposive sampling*—With this type of sampling, the researcher specifies the characteristics of the population of interest and then locates individuals who match those characteristics. The researcher typically chooses subjects who are considered to be typical of the population. Purposive sampling is particularly effective when:
   - The population being studied is very unusual, such as a group of patients with a rare disease.
   - There is a newly developed instrument that requires pretesting.
   - There is a scale or test that needs to be validated, and the researcher needs to collect exploratory data regarding a very specific population.

- The researcher wants to describe the lived experience of a phenomenon, such as patients who have been victims of domestic violence.

    A significant limitation of this type of sampling is that the researcher must assume that errors of overrepresenting or underrepresenting segments of the population will somehow resolve themselves. However, this is not a valid assumption (LoBiondo-Wood & Haber, 2009).

4. ***Snowball sampling***—Each subject being used in the research study is asked to identify other potential research subjects who have the characteristics being studied. This technique is particularly effective with a population that is difficult to find and therefore has no sampling frame (University of South Alabama, n.d.). However, it also risks a breach of confidentiality as research subjects identify other individuals with characteristics of interest to the researcher.

Convenience sampling, quota sampling, and purposive sampling would all be wise choices for the doctor of nursing practice (DNP) researcher who has access to a continuous source of patients.

LoBiondo-Wood and Haber (2009) have developed a summary of the various types of sampling separated according to their respective risk of bias and degree of representativeness. This is included in **Table 8-1**.

 TOOLBOX

Consider your potential topic for your capstone project. Is there a nonrandom sampling method that could be effectively utilized with it? Take into account the need to move your project successfully through the facility's institutional review board approval process. If a nonrandom method would be more effective than a random sampling method, provide rationale for your answer.

TABLE 8-1 Sampling Types Separated According to Risk of Bias and Degree of Representativeness

Type of Sampling Strategy	Risk of Bias	Degree of Representativeness
Nonprobability sampling		
Convenience	Greatest of any sampling strategy	Questionable representativeness because sample is self-selecting
Quota	Can have unknown sources of bias that will affect the external validity of the research study	Representativeness can be built in through knowledge of the population of interest
Purposive	The greater the heterogeneity of the population, the greater the bias; conscious bias on the part of the researcher can be present	Representativeness is limited, as is the ability to generalize to a larger population due to the sample being hand selected
Probability sampling		
Simple random	Low risk of bias	Maximum level of representativeness; as sample size increases, possibility of nonrepresentativeness decreases
Stratified random	Low risk of bias	High degree of representativeness
Cluster	Greater risk of sampling errors than simple or stratified random sampling	Less representative than simple random or stratified random sampling
Systematic	Easy to inadvertently introduce bias due to lack of randomization	Because bias can occur as a result of coincidental nonrandomness, tends to be less representative than other types of probability sampling

Source: Data from LoBiondo-Wood, G., & Haber, J. (2009). *Nursing research: Methods, critical appraisal, and utilization.* St. Louis, MO: Mosby.

Random Selection and Random Assignment

In implementing sampling designs, it is important to recognize the difference between random selection and random assignment. Random selection means that the researcher uses an equal probability selection method to select a sample from a population using a random sampling technique. Each element of the population has an equal chance of being included in the sample. The sample that is produced as a result of this procedure will be a mirror image of the overall population (LoBiondo-Wood & Haber, 2009).

In comparison, random assignment occurs when the researcher already has a sample of research subjects that is then randomly divided into two or more groups. Usually the groups will be mirror images of each other and will be roughly equivalent on all variables (University of South Alabama, n.d.). The ultimate purpose of random assignment is the distribution of research participants into either the experimental group or the control group of the research project on a random basis, with each research subject having an equal probability of being assigned to any group. Random assignment is important because it assumes that any important variables will be equally distributed between the groups, and thus variation will be kept to a minimum (LoBiondo-Wood & Haber, 2009).

Determining Sample Size

Once the researcher has decided which type of quantitative sampling is most appropriate for the research study, practical issues related to the sampling process must be handled. Such issues include deciding the size sample to collect based on the type of research being implemented. Clearly the researcher should attempt to get as large a sample as possible for the study in order to make it as representative of the overall population as possible. However, if the population is inclusive of 100 individuals or fewer, the researcher should not select a sample, but should instead include the entire population (Brians, Manheim, Rich, & Willnat, 2010).

Brians and colleagues (2010) have identified several factors that can help a researcher determine how large a sample will be needed for a research project. One such factor is **homogeneity**. This is the degree to which individuals who compose a population resemble one another in regards to the characteristics being studied in a research project. The more homogeneous the individuals in a population, the smaller the sample required to be representative of that population. In addition, the more variables being studied by the researcher, the larger the sample will need to be. This is a requirement because the more questions asked in the research project, the more likely the researcher will be to find differences among the subjects. Furthermore, the degree of accuracy required by the researcher is also a consideration. Because the sample estimates the characteristics of the population, this estimate is always going to contain a margin of error. The researcher must determine how much sampling error can be tolerated. The greater the degree of accuracy desired, the larger the sample must be. In addition, always plan to utilize a larger sample when:

- The population is heterogeneous, meaning it differs in multiple characteristics.
- The goal is to break down the data into multiple categories.
- The researcher expects that a weak relationship will be shown between variables.
- A less efficient sampling technique is used.
- A low response rate is expected (University of South Alabama, n.d.).

Web-based sample size calculators are available to provide the researcher with a specific sample number. Usually, such a tool will calculate the size sample needed for the project based on the size population utilized and the confidence interval desired. The **confidence interval** is the extent to which the sample mean deviates from the population parameter (Singleton & Straits, 2009). The sample size calculator will tell the researcher that *x* number of research subjects should be sampled in order to have a 95 percent level of confidence, plus or minus 5 percent.

 TOOLBOX

Consider how large a sample of participants you would need for the type of capstone project that you are considering. Should that number increase or decrease based on the anticipated homogeneity of your population?

The researcher should bear in mind that in order to ensure a small confidence interval, such as plus or minus 2 percent, a large sample size will be required (Neuendorf, 2002).

Qualitative Sampling Designs

As previously mentioned, sampling for qualitative research tends to be purposive in nature so that cases that will yield relevant data will be selected. The sample usually originates from a theory that either is in the process of being tested or is growing progressively. In addition, the sample usually evolves as the study progresses, data are analyzed, and new insight is revealed. The process of sampling will continue until virtually no new information is being revealed. The researcher who will be utilizing sampling for qualitative research should be cognizant of the kinds of research subjects to be included in the sample, the optimum time to contact potential research participants, and the kinds of situations that will be studied. The researcher may encounter difficulty in recruiting participants for a sample when the topic being studied is particularly sensitive, when the potential participants are not offered any type of incentive, or when there are no existing relationships that may be used to assist in recruitment. To circumvent these potential problems, the researcher can:

- Attempt to partner with a group that is already affiliated with the type of people who would be most desirous as participants.
- Contact potential participants through informal networks of colleagues.
- Recruit participants for sample from existing organizations, using contact people to assist in gaining admittance to agencies.
- Recruit from lists of professionals, such as nurse practitioners.
- Send follow-up invitations to arrange interviews and set meeting times that do not conflict with the participants' other obligations (MacDougall & Fudge, 2001).

As previously mentioned, sampling in qualitative research is usually purposive in nature. Specific purposive sampling techniques can be used. These include:

- *Maximum variation sampling*—The researcher selects a wide range of cases from which to compose the sample.
- *Homogeneous sample selection*—The researcher selects a small but homogeneous set of cases with the intent of studying them closely.
- *Extreme case sampling*—The researcher chooses cases that represent extremes on a specific variable.
- *Typical-case sampling*—The researcher selects cases that seem to be average for the variable being studied.
- *Critical-case sampling*—The researcher selects cases that are considered to be very important in relation to the variable being studied.
- *Negative-case sampling*—The researcher selects cases that are opposite to the generalizations being made about a variable to confirm that he or she is not selectively finding cases to support his or her personal theory.
- *Opportunistic sampling*—The researcher selects useful cases as the opportunity presents itself.
- *Mixed purposeful sampling*—The researcher combines the sampling strategies previously mentioned into a more complex design that is based on the researcher's specific needs (University of South Alabama, n.d.).

 TOOLBOX

Do you think that one of the qualitative (purposive) sampling techniques could be used effectively with your capstone project? If so, which one do you think would be most appropriate? Defend your answer. If you don't think that one of the techniques would work well, be prepared to defend that position as well.

Qualitative Sampling Strategy

MacDougall and Fudge (2001) have described a multistage process for recruiting participants for a sample used in a qualitative research project. The stages consist of:

1. *Prepare*—The researcher should describe the desired sample by preparing a list of geographic locations that will be utilized as well as the characteristics that will be sought in potential participants.

   a. Comprehensive lists of sources of information regarding potential subjects should be obtained. Contact should be made with people who are familiar with communities of potential participants. MacDougall and Fudge (2001) categorize these as key contacts or champions, with **key contacts** being people who can suggest possible groups or participants who might take part in the study, and **champions** being people who are interested in the research and will either assist in recruiting participants or allow the researcher to use the champion's credibility in the community to recruit.

   b. The researcher should also contact colleagues to seek out recent related research projects to determine how they involved groups or potential participants in their projects. This is important so that the current recruitment strategies of the project in progress can build on existing relationships. As the researcher begins to build lists of groups, key contacts, and champions that should provide participants with desired characteristics for the sample, alternative possibilities should also be developed, particularly if potential participants will be difficult to reach or if the topic being researched is particularly sensitive.

2. *Contact*—In this stage, the researcher should personally seek endorsement from key contacts with communities who may develop into champions, providing written information about the research project and stressing the valuable insights that potential participants can provide not only for the research project, but also for the community as a whole.

   a. If the researcher discovers that the key contact will not develop into a champion but instead has assumed the role of a gatekeeper who is making it difficult to make contact with potential participants, the researcher should begin to tactfully withdraw contact and move on to another key contact. This prevents time being wasted in negotiations that will not lead to the desired goal of contact with participants but will only produce awkward entanglements.

b. The researcher preferably should arrange to meet individual participants in the presence of the key contact or champion. The participants should be given a description of the research, opportunities for questions, and an information sheet written specifically for them. At this point, consent forms that have been approved by the institutional review board should be in place, a time and place for interviews to be conducted should be announced, and the researcher should have arranged a way to effectively, yet ethically, obtain addresses of potential participants to maintain communication with them as the research project progresses.

c. The researcher should plan to communicate with potential participants after announcing the meeting time and place and then again approximately 2 weeks before the meeting, asking for a confirmation of plans to attend. At this point, a plan should also be in place to allow for continued communication with key contacts, champions, or participants who show particular enthusiasm regarding the project and would like to be kept abreast of progress being made and actions that have resulted from the research.

3. *Follow-up*—This phase ensures that relationships will be maintained with the research participants even after the research is concluded. A plan should be in place to continue involvement with useful agencies that will be interested in learning about actions that have resulted from the prepare and contact phases.

a. The researcher should ensure that participants are given feedback on the themes that were discussed in the focus group or the interviews. Also, participants should be given the opportunity to give the researcher feedback on their experience during the research process. If appropriate, the contributions of the key contacts and champions should be acknowledged in some manner.

b. If there are public events associated with the research, the researcher should ensure that key contacts and champions are invited and their contributions acknowledged.

c. The researcher should ensure that time has been allotted for participation in actions that are a direct result of the research project (MacDougall & Fudge, 2001).

TOOLBOX

What is your strategy for recruiting participants for your capstone project?

Once the researcher has developed the research problem, completed the literature review, completed the necessary requirements of an institutional review board, selected a design for the research project, and developed a plan for how sampling will proceed, the researcher is prepared to proceed with data collection. The following chapter will discuss how the researcher can decide on the most appropriate data collection method to utilize based on the type of research study being pursued.

Learning Enhancement Tools

1. Imagine you are a DNP researcher who is trying to decide whether to utilize simple random sampling or systematic sampling in your research study. Describe how each type of sampling can be implemented and the advantages or limitations of each type.
2. Discuss the differences between proportional and disproportional stratified sampling. Describe how each type would be utilized in a research study.
3. Discuss the differences between one-stage and two-stage cluster sampling. Describe how each type would be utilized in a research study.
4. Outline a plan for a research study that would utilize convenience sampling. Describe the advantages and limitations of this type of sampling.
5. Outline a plan for a research study that would utilize quota sampling. Describe the advantages and limitations of this type of sampling.
6. Outline a plan for a research study that would utilize purposive sampling. Describe the advantages and limitations of this type of sampling.

7. Outline a plan for a research study that would utilize snowball sampling. Describe the advantages and limitations of this type of sampling.

8. Suppose you are a DNP researcher who is preparing to conduct qualitative research using in-depth interviews with nurse managers who have had experience with nurse employees engaging in substance abuse. Describe your plan for recruitment strategies to generate a sample of participants for this study.

9. Suppose you are a DNP researcher who is preparing to conduct qualitative research using in-depth interviews with nurse managers who have had experience with nurse employees receiving discipline of their nursing license by the state board of nursing. You are interested in using mixed purposeful sampling in this research project. Discuss in detail how you could implement this technique, describing specifically the sampling strategies that you will select to incorporate into the final sampling plan.

10. Imagine you are a DNP researcher who is preparing to conduct qualitative research using in-depth interviews with nurse managers who have had experience with nurse employees receiving discipline of their nursing license by the state board of nursing. You are developing a plan for recruiting participants for a qualitative sample. Describe in detail the strategies you will use in recruiting subjects during the preparation phase of the recruitment process.

11. Imagine you are a DNP researcher who is preparing to conduct qualitative research using in-depth interviews with nurse managers who have had experience with nurse employees receiving discipline of their nursing license by the state board of nursing. You are developing a plan for recruiting participants for a qualitative sample. Describe in detail the strategies you will use in recruiting subjects during the contact phase of the recruitment process.

12. Suppose you are a DNP researcher who is preparing to conduct qualitative research using in-depth interviews with nurse managers who have had experience with nurse employees receiving discipline of their nursing license by the state board of nursing. You are developing a plan for recruiting participants for a qualitative sample. Describe in detail the strategies you will use in recruiting subjects during the follow-up phase of the recruitment process.

13. Suppose you are a DNP researcher who is making the final decision regarding a sampling strategy for your research project. Describe how you will decide on a nonprobability sampling strategy based on risk of bias and desired level of representativeness.
14. Imagine you are a DNP researcher who is making the final decision regarding a sampling strategy for your research project. Describe how you will decide on a probability sampling strategy based on risk of bias and desired level of representativeness.

Resources

Bernardo, J. M. (1997). Statistical inference as a decision problem: The choice of sample size. *The Statistician, 46,* 151–153.

Campbell, M., Thomson, S., Ramsay, C., MacLennan, G., & Grimshaw, J. (2004). Sample size calculator for cluster randomized trials. *Computers in Biology and Medicine, 34*(2), 113–125.

Connelly, L. (2003). Balancing the number and size of sites: An economic approach to the optimal design of cluster samples. *Controlled Clinical Trials, 24*(5), 544–559.

Cosby, R., Howard, M., Kaczorowski, J., Willan, A. R., & Sellor, J. (2003). Randomizing patients by family practice: Sample size estimation, intracluster correlation and data analysis. *Family Practice, 20*(1), 77–82.

Hayes, R., & Bennett, S. (1999). Simple sample size calculation for cluster-randomized trials. *International Journal of Epidemiology, 28*(2), 319–326.

Lake, S., Kammann, E., Klar, N., & Betensky, R. (2002). Sample size re-estimation in cluster randomization trials. *Statistics in Medicine, 21*(10), 1337–1350.

Lee, S., & Zelen, M. (2000). Clinical trials and sample size considerations: Another perspective. *Statistical Science, 15,* 95–103.

Lindley, D. (1997). The choice of sample size. *The Statistician, 46,* 129–138.

Talbot, L. (Ed.). (1995). Populations and samples. *Principles and practice of nursing research.* St. Louis, MO: Mosby.

Turner, R., Prevost, A., & Thompson, S. (2004). Allowing for imprecision of the intracluster correlation coefficient in the design of cluster randomized trials. *Statistics in Medicine, 23*(8), 1195–1214.

Wears, R. (2002). Advanced statistics: Statistical methods for analyzing cluster and cluster-randomized data. *Academic Emergency Medicine, 9*(4), 330–341.

References

Brians, C., Manheim, J., Rich, R., & Willnat, L. (2010). *Empirical political analysis: Research methods in political science.* New York, NY: Addison Wesley Longman.

LoBiondo-Wood, G., & Haber, J. (2009). *Nursing research: Methods and critical appraisal for evidence-based practice.* St. Louis, MO: Mosby.

MacDougall, C., & Fudge, E. (2001). Planning and recruiting the sample for focus groups and in-depth interviews. *Qualitative Health Research, 11,* 117–126.

Neuendorf, K. (2002). *The content analysis guidebook.* Thousand Oaks, CA: Sage Publications.

Singleton, R., & Straits, B. (2009). *Approaches to social research.* New York, NY: Oxford University Press.

University of South Alabama. (n.d.). *Sampling.* Retrieved December 28, 2009, from www.southalabama.edu/coe/bset/johnson/lectures/lec7.htm

CHAPTER 9

Data Collection

Objectives

Upon completion of this chapter, the reader should be prepared to:

1. Describe the steps involved in instrument development.
2. Discuss the advantages and disadvantages of the use of physiological measurements as a data collection method.
3. Discuss the advantages and disadvantages of the use of participant observation as a data collection method.
4. Describe the different types of participant observation.
5. Discuss the advantages and disadvantages of the use of the e-mail interview as a data collection method.
6. Discuss the advantages and disadvantages of the use of existing records as a data collection method.
7. Describe content analysis as a data collection method.
8. Describe the steps in the typical process of content analysis as a research process and data collection technique.
9. Describe the disadvantages of the traditional mail survey and the telephone survey.
10. Discuss how a researcher could utilize the focus group as a data collection method.

11. Describe the differences between structured and unstructured observational methods.
12. Identify special issues that are unique to data collection occurring in mixed method research.
13. Describe how the programmatic research approach will affect data collection.
14. Discuss the different types of questions that can be utilized in most questionnaires.

Introduction to the Process of Data Collection

For the doctor of nursing practice (DNP) researcher, the process of data collection should flow naturally from the progress that has already been made on the project, although selecting the appropriate method and the specific instrument to utilize can be time-consuming. The method of data collection must be appropriate to the problem being researched, the hypothesis that has been formulated, the research setting, and the population of interest. For example, if the researcher is interested in observing the behavioral changes exhibited in patients suffering from Alzheimer's disease, it would be inappropriate to use a lengthy questionnaire that would require the patient to concentrate for long periods to answer questions (LoBiondo-Wood & Haber, 2002).

The process of data collection actually has its origin in the literature review, because it is then that the researcher begins to define variables and determine how they will be **operationalized**, or measured. This provides the germ of an instrument that will be useful in measuring the defined variables. The researcher can even construct his or her own instrument, although this can be a time-consuming process that can overwhelm the novice researcher. Instrument development can be a tedious process because of its multiple steps. It requires:

- Defining the concept to be measured.
- Developing the items to be included on the instrument.
- Assessing the items for **content validity**—determining whether the instrument and its items are representative of the content the researcher intends to measure.
- Developing instructions for the research participants.
- Developing a pretest for the items.

- **Pilot testing** the items—this serves as a pretest to the major survey.
- Estimating **reliability**—determining the instrument is consistent and will give the same results if the research is replicated.
- Ensuring **validity**—ensuring the instrument measures what it was intended to measure.

The DNP researcher who is involved in a time-limited capstone project should avoid constructing an original instrument and instead utilize an existing instrument, if one exists with proven validity and reliability (LoBiondo-Wood & Haber, 2002).

 TOOLBOX

Do you think that an instrument will be needed for your capstone project? If so, try to locate an existing instrument on the Internet that you could utilize. Be able to defend your choice in terms of validity and reliability.

Types of Data Collection Methods

There are five general types of data collection methods, some of which can be used with both qualitative and quantitative research. These consist of physiological measurements, observational methods, interviews, questionnaires, and records or other types of existing data. The advantages and disadvantages of each type will be discussed, along with the most relevant uses of each as a data collection method.

A brief discussion of programmatic research is required here; this is an approach to nursing research that is discussed in this chapter because of its profound effect on the data collection process. Programmatic research is usually considered to be research conducted on a large scale by teams of researchers. It is designed to be a lengthy endeavor and is usually research that is considered to be for the public good. Data collection will occur on a team-wide basis with multiple researchers all collecting data simultaneously. Generally, a large amount of funding is required for such a project, and this amount of funding will not be awarded without evidence of prior completion of multiple extensive projects. Because of the multiple researchers involved and the resources required for such an effort, a plan will need to be in place to sustain the research with adequate resources, both financial and personnel related, and to guide the research so data collection can occur over a lengthy period of time as needed. Collaboration will be required not only among multiple researchers, but also among multiple agencies. Because data collection occurs simultaneously with multiple researchers in the same research project, strict oversight is required to ensure that the same procedures and protocols are being used by all to avoid bias as well as problems with reliability and validity. Although a DNP researcher would certainly function well as a researcher in such a project, it is not recommended that a DNP clinician spearhead such an extensive and lengthy project (University of Ballarat Institute for Regional and Rural Research, 2004).

PHYSIOLOGICAL MEASUREMENTS

Physiological measurements can consist of the data nurses collect about their patients on an everyday basis, such as temperature, pulse, respiration, and blood pressure, in addition to body weight, results of laboratory tests, and radiological examinations. Physiological data collection usually is objective, precise, and sensitive. Unless a technical malfunction of the equipment occurs, two readings of the same piece of equipment taken by two different nurses simultaneously will usually generate the same result. The instrument used will usually detect small changes in the variable being studied, such as variations of one tenth of a degree in body temperature. Also, a patient usually cannot distort his or her physiological information to any great degree without actually ingesting a toxifying substance. However, the instruments used in physiological data collection can usually be obtained only in a hospital because of their cost and occasionally due to the training required to utilize them. In addition, some instruments used in physiological data collection are so sensitive that environmental changes can affect them (LoBiondo-Wood & Haber, 2002).

The researcher must bear in mind that physiological measurements in DNP research will be multifaceted, composed of:

- The true value of what is being measured, such as 140/90 as a blood pressure reading.
- The degree to which the measure varies, such as being lower in the morning and higher in the evening, in the case of blood pressure.

- The accuracy of the instrument with which the variable is being measured, such as a sphygmomanometer.
- The position of the patient, as in blood pressure fluctuating depending on whether the patient is lying or standing.
- The skill of the person obtaining the measurement.

This is another situation in which both reliability and validity will be critical issues. For example, if the patient's pulse is measured every 5 minutes by the same nurse using the same technique, it is expected that similar results would be obtained. This would be reliability. When multiple readings of a measurement are assessed from the same person, it is known as **intrarater reliability**. If multiple readings of a measurement are assessed from several nurses, it is known as **interrater reliability**. The validity that the researcher must be concerned with in such a case is **criterion-related validity**. This requires the comparison of the measure in question with the best existing measure of the variable (Ciliska, Cullum, & Dicenco, 1999).

 TOOLBOX

Do you anticipate using physiological measurements as part of data collection in your capstone project? If so, how would you achieve interrater reliability for these measurements?

OBSERVATIONAL METHODS

Observational methods include participant observation, which Key (1997) described as the researcher keeping detailed records of what is occurring with the subjects being studied, while occasionally reviewing records as a social scientist and constantly monitoring both the observations and records for any intrusion of personal bias. There are five types of participant observation:

1. *External participation*—This is the lowest degree of involvement by the researcher, with the observation being done usually via television or videotape.
2. *Passive participation*—The researcher is present at the scene with the subject in the role of spectator but does not attempt to interact with the subject or participate in the scene with him or her.

3. *Balanced participation*—The researcher walks a tenuous tightrope between being a participant and a spectator. The researcher is not a full participant in all of the research subject's activities.

4. *Active participation*—The researcher generally does what the majority of the participants in the research setting are doing. Active engagement by the researcher will occur as he or she learns the rules of the research setting.

5. *Total participation*—This is the highest level of involvement for the researcher and means that the researcher becomes a natural participant. This type of observation generally is used when the researcher chooses to study something in which he or she already functions as a natural participant (Key, 1997).

Participant observation is an effective data collection method when the researcher is interested in gathering information about a research subject's physical symptoms, verbal communication, nonverbal behavior, performance of specific skills, or environment. It is important to note that participant observation is considered to be an unstructured observational method. This means the researcher has a high degree of contact with the research population being studied, tries to collect information within the structures that are meaningful to the research subjects, and tries not to allow his or her own ideas and values to become injected into the situation being studied. The most common forms of record-keeping in this type of data collection are logs and field notes. Logs are considered to be a record of both events and conversations that will be maintained on a daily basis, while field notes can certainly include a log but tend to be more analytical. Field notes will not merely list a record of what has occurred but will also give the researcher's interpretation of the events (Polit & Hungler, 2000).

In comparison, structured observational methods involve the development of a system for categorizing, recording, and encoding the observations. Also, record-keeping forms will be prepared in advance and will usually be quite elaborate. Because of the in-depth categorizing that is required and the extensive record-keeping forms utilized, it is not recommended that the novice DNP researcher utilize a structured observational method when an unstructured observational method is a viable alternative (Polit & Hungler, 2000).

According to Hoepfl (1997), observation can provide the researcher with a deeper understanding than an interview alone because it provides information about the context in which events occur. Thus, observation can give the researcher knowledge regarding areas that participants are not aware of or that they have chosen not to discuss. It is especially valuable for its ability to allow the researcher a complete understanding of a particularly complex situation. Proponents of this method of data collection believe that more structured methods may be too constricting to provide an accurate account of human behavior and its intricate nature.

Critics of participant observation point out that observer bias and influence from the observer are particular problems with this method. The researcher may have difficulty in maintaining objectivity as observations are recorded and may record inaccurate events due to memory errors. In addition, the researcher may experience difficulty in entering a group intended for study and being accepted as a fellow member. Emotional involvement on the part of the researcher tends to occur as the researcher begins to participate in the activities of the group. This means that participant observation may be ineffective as a data collection method for the DNP researcher who is studying a research population of employees in a facility where he or she has just been hired, because the researcher will be struggling with the dynamics of organizational behavior in becoming incorporated into the group (Polit & Hungler, 2000).

 TOOLBOX

Do you think that participant observation would be an effective method of data collection for your capstone project? If so, which type would you choose and why?

INTERVIEWS AND QUESTIONNAIRES

Interviews used in research studies typically can be structured in a few different ways:

- *Structured interviews*—These can consist of a fixed series of questions that cannot be altered or a fixed series of questions that contain prompts to the interviewer so he or she can obtain more detailed answers from the subject.

- *Semistructured interviews*—These usually consist of a series of issues the interviewer wants to discuss; they can be addressed in any order.
- *Unstructured interviews*—These are completely open-ended interviews without a structured set of questions.

As technology has progressed, the e-mail interview has become a frequent data collection tool for researchers. It has several advantages that can make this a recommended tool for the DNP researcher. For example, the e-mail interview is a wise choice for the researcher with a particularly slim budget, because it allows multiple interviews to be conducted simultaneously and requires no travel expenses, no additional equipment to be obtained, and no additional personnel to be hired and trained. In addition, the e-mail interview allows research subjects to be interviewed at an unlimited distance, so participants could literally be obtained globally. Such an interview also provides the research subject with time for reflection, because there is no time constraint and the participant may feel that he or she can formulate an e-mail response more freely than he or she could verbalize a face-to-face response to questions (Hunt & McHale, 2007).

There are some potential disadvantages to the e-mail interview that the DNP researcher should be prepared to accommodate. For example, it will be difficult to obtain a representative sample, because potential respondents who do not have Internet access will be excluded. Also, the researcher will not be able to be certain that he is interviewing the person he thinks he is interviewing. This can open both validity and ethical issues.

The respondent may lose enthusiasm for the interview if it becomes too lengthy or complicated and may decide either to not complete the interview or to withdraw from the interview. This can leave the researcher with a partially completed interview that may not be usable for data analysis or with the ethical issue of not knowing whether the person has withdrawn or is simply taking a lengthy time for completion. Finally, an e-mail interview eliminates the possibility of the researcher being able to interpret the nonverbal cues of the respondent, such as facial expressions or hand movements (Hunt & McHale, 2007).

There are guidelines that can assist the DNP researcher who opts to use the e-mail interview as a data collection tool in circumventing these disadvantages. These suggestions include:

- Alert participants regarding the number of questions they will be asked as part of the entire interview process.
- Encourage the participant to ask questions before the interview begins.
- Have clear-cut procedures that will address informed consent, the right to withdraw from the interview procedure, and how to ensure that the person completing the interview is truly the research participant.
- Set time limits for how long the interview can be reviewed by the participant before a response must be submitted.
- Plan to close the time period when the interview is open for completion with a statement thanking the participant for participating and asking for the participant's comments and feedback (Hunt & McHale, 2007).

While the e-mail interview is increasing greatly in popularity, the use of the traditional mail survey is decreasing in popularity with researchers because of its expense, the extensive amount of time required to prepare the mail-outs and accumulate residential addresses, and the frequently low return rate of the surveys. Telephone surveys, however, are still in use. Random digit dialing can be used to generate a sample of all area telephone numbers. The drawback of this type of survey is primarily related to the poor response received from respondents after the first few questions. As respondents begin to tire of answering the questions, they may begin to give unreliable answers or simply hang up on the interviewer. In addition, this type of survey will become more difficult to implement as more people rely on cell phones as their primary telephones and no longer have listings in residential telephone books (O'Sullivan & Rassel, 1999).

As previously mentioned, the design of a new instrument is never recommended when an existing one with proven validity and reliability that has already been pilot tested is available. However, the DNP researcher should be able to discern what type of question will best collect the data he or she is focusing on. There are five main types of questions that will typically be used on most questionnaires:

1. *Structured interviews*—This type can easily be used to measure the general attitude of the interviewee, is easy to understand, and is quickly completed. Researchers can also add a text box

for respondents to put a response to any of the questions in their own words. Instructions should be included, particularly if the researcher wants respondents to give free text responses to specific questions. The researcher should recognize, however, that free text responses will require additional time and effort on the part of the researcher to code and analyze.

2. *Rating scales*—This type of question can describe the interviewee's attitude on either a five- or seven-point scale and also can differentiate between positive and negative. It can be used with interviewees who are capable of understanding linear scales and the meaning of numerical values.

3. *Visual analogue scales*—This type of question can precisely measure an interviewee's attitude. The data will need to be transformed to allow for statistical analysis. This question type can be used with interviewees who understand linear scales and who also have no difficulties with their vision.

4. *Structured interviews*—This type of question is similar to a numerical rating scale. It is easier to utilize than other question types for interviewees who are visually challenged, those with low literacy levels, and children.

5. *Open-ended items*—This type of question requires analysis with qualitative methods. Although it is well suited to creative participants, it may make a negative impression on interviewees who have difficulty putting thoughts and feelings on paper in detail (Boynton & Greenhalgh, 2004).

If the researcher is not vigilant, he or she can run into various pitfalls associated with the wording of questionnaires. For example, if the researcher presents a question that uses the word *frequently*, the implication is that there is a frequency involved. A more appropriately worded question would avoid the word *frequently*, and instead would present a rating scale that is frequency-based with options such as hourly, once daily, once every 3 days, once weekly, and so on. Another example of a potential wording pitfall would be the use of the word *regularly*. This implies that a pattern of activity is present. This can mean different things to different people, with one patient thinking that *regularly* attending cardiac rehabilitation means three times weekly without variation, while another patient might believe that *regularly* means once weekly with an additional time attended if convenient (Boynton & Greenhalgh, 2004).

 TOOLBOX

Do you think that a survey could be used effectively as part of data collection for your capstone project? If so, what type of questions would you include? Could you implement an e-mail survey? Why or why not?

FOCUS GROUPS

The focus group is a form of in-person interviewing that can be used to obtain in-depth information from a group of participants on a specific group of topics. The group interaction is the hallmark of the focus group. Such an interview technique consists of the preparation phase, the formation of the groups, the interviewing of the participants, and finally the analysis and reporting of the results. The researchers should decide on the purpose of the study and what information is needed and then compose no more than 10 open-ended questions to pose to the focus group participants. It is important to ensure that all of the participants have the opportunity to discuss each question and respond as desired. The focus group can consist of as few as 4 members but usually no more than 15 people. The participants should be people who have never met prior to arriving at the site for the group interaction; however, the participants should be similar enough to prevent the majority of the group time from being taken up with attempting to find common ground among the group members. The similarity between group members can be that they are all nurses, for example, or all cancer patients (O'Sullivan & Rassel, 1999).

The researcher organizing a focus group will need to arrange for a moderator for the group as well as someone to serve as a transcriber and possibly an additional person to set up recording equipment. Videotaping of the participants will entail distribution of an informed consent form. The moderator is vital to the progression of the group because it is his or her duty to lead the group from question to question and prevent participants from getting stagnated in complicated questions or conversation that has no bearing on the group's topic of discussion. Once the focus group has concluded, the moderator and observers will assemble to discuss the conversational progression of the participants and to record their impression of each of the participants and their individual contributions to the group as well as to the overall interview (O'Sullivan & Rassel, 1999).

A unique feature of the focus group is the topic guide, which is a list of the topics that will be covered. It is most effectively designed as an outline of issues with probing questions listed under each issue and should be jointly designed with the research team and the moderator. A cue to the degree of detail required in the topic guide will be the degree of experience of the moderator. A less experienced moderator may require a more detailed topic guide with very specific questions written under each issue (Debus, n.d.).

How can an inexperienced researcher know that a focus group might be a more effective means of data collection than an individual interview? According to Debus (n.d.), the researcher should consider using a focus group when:

- Group interaction is likely to produce new thoughts that would not emerge otherwise.
- The subject matter is not so sensitive that participants will hesitate to discuss it in a group.
- The topic is such that participants can voice their thoughts in 10 minutes or less.
- The interviewer is not likely to become fatigued.
- The volume of material is not extensive.
- A single subject matter is being examined.
- It will be helpful for key decision makers to observe firsthand consumer information.
- Target respondents can be easily assembled in one location.
- A quick turnaround is required.
- The researcher has a limited budget.

 TOOLBOX

Could you utilize focus groups as part of data collection for your capstone project? If so, what would you use as your topic guide? Would you choose to be the moderator or would you use an outside moderator?

RECORDS OR EXISTING DATA

Records or currently existing data can be used when available data are examined in a new way in order to answer specific research questions. This can be an excellent data collection method for the DNP researcher because of the savings in terms of time. It allows for the examination of trends over the course of time. The researcher also avoids the time involved in approaching potential research subjects to ask for their participation in the research project (LoBiondo-Wood & Haber, 2002).

As might be expected, there are disadvantages attached to the use of existing records as a data collection method. Some facilities may be reluctant to allow researchers access to their records, particularly when there is a concern regarding protected health information. Also, if the researcher is allowed access to records, he or she will be reviewing only those records that have survived over the course of time. If these are not representative of the larger population being studied, then the researcher may face the problem of bias as he or she makes an educated guess regarding the records' accuracy (LoBiondo-Wood & Haber, 2002).

A variation on the theme of data collection occurring on an organizational scope is the organizational assessment. This allows the researcher to explore the existence of significant elements present in the entity, such as the mission and vision statements and the documented profile of the organization's workforce. The following checklist contains examples of significant areas that might be included in an organizational assessment, although this list may vary based on the organization's structural composition.

Conducting an Organizational Assessment

1. ___ Stated purpose of the organization
2. ___ Stated vision of the organization
3. ___ Stated mission statement of the organization
4. ___ Stated values of the organization
5. ___ Major services provided by the organization
6. ___ Major facilities included as part of the organization
7. ___ Technologies utilized by the organization
8. ___ Profile of the organization's workforce:
   a. ___ Educational levels of employees at various levels
   b. ___ Key requirements for employment at various levels
   c. ___ Workforce diversity of employees at various levels

9. ___ Legal and regulatory environment of the organization
10. ___ Applicable occupational health and safety regulations
11. ___ Accreditation, certification, or registration requirements of the organization
12. ___ Relevant health care and other industry standards
13. ___ Environmental and financial regulations applicable to the organization
14. ___ Organizational structure and governance system identified
15. ___ Identified stakeholder groups at each level of the organization
16. ___ Identified suppliers, partners, collaborators, or distributors utilized
17. ___ Relative size and growth rate in relation to competitors
18. ___ Identified areas of innovation and collaboration
19. ___ Identified areas of strategic planning
20. ___ Identified challenges to long-term sustainability

Source: Data from Baldrige Performance Excellence Program (2011). Self-assessment and action planning: Using the Baldrige Organizational Profile for Health Care. Downloaded June 3, 2013 from http://patapsco.nist.gov/eBaldrige/HealthCare_Profile.cfm.

 TOOLBOX

What could be the advantages in terms of approaching an institutional review board for a DNP student who opts to perform a secondary data review?

CONTENT ANALYSIS

Content analysis can be a variation on the use of existing data. It is, in its simplest form, the quantitative analysis of message characteristics. It allows the researcher to describe these messages in the media, such as television programs; in documentary data; or in other communications in an objective, systematic, and quantitative manner (LoBiondo-Wood & Haber, 2002). Neuendorf (2002) has described the progression of the typical content analysis research process:

1. *Theory and rationale*—The researcher must decide what content will be described and why it is specifically of interest to the

researcher. He or she must develop a literature review to generate either researcher questions or hypotheses.

2. *Conceptualizations*—The researcher decides which variables will be used in the study and how they will be defined.

3. *Operationalizations*—The researcher decides how variables will be measured as well as the unit of data collection. The unit of data collection can be individual words, characters, themes, time periods, or interactions.

4. *Codebook*—The researcher develops a codebook for the coding of variables.

5. *Sampling*—The researcher decides how to randomly sample a subset of the content. This could occur by time period, by issue, by page, by channel, or another similar subset.

6. *Training and pilot reliability*—The researcher should schedule a training session for the personnel serving as coders so that consensus can be developed on the coding of the variables. Reliability of the variables should be determined, so if the study were to be replicated under the same conditions, essentially the same results would be achieved.

7. *Coding*—Intercoder reliability should be established to ensure that all coding is being done consistently.

8. *Tabulation and reporting*—Results can be reported in various ways, with trends over time being a common method of reporting results.

Although content analysis can seem deceptively simple to the novice researcher, it has the disadvantage of requiring the researcher to rely on previously recorded documents or messages. Thus, the accuracy of the existing data can be questionable, and bias may be present.

 TOOLBOX

Imagine you are considering using content analysis in your capstone project in order to analyze the current messages delivered by the media regarding nurses. What points do you think would be of greatest interest to include in the analysis?

Data Collection in Mixed Method Research

Data collection that occurs in mixed method research has its own particular issues that researchers must be prepared to address. For example, data collection in a research project of this design will occur either concurrently or sequentially. Concurrent data collection occurs when quantitative and qualitative data collection occurs at approximately the same time. Sequential data collection occurs when quantitative or qualitative data are collected first and the results that are achieved are used to provide information for the other form (quantitative or qualitative). Sequential data collection is accomplished with the idea that there will be a connection between the two different forms of data. Either the first or the second data collection can be considered the greater priority, depending on the research problem and the emphasis the researcher desires (Creswell & Plano Clark, 2010).

An additional concern that is unique to mixed method research involves the need to approach institutional review boards. Creswell and Plano Clark (2010) have noted that in an IRB proposal using the concurrent approach, both the quantitative and qualitative forms of data collection can be described at the beginning of the project, whereas in a proposal using the sequential approach, only the initial phase of data collection can be described definitively. This will likely lead to the IRB requiring the researcher to complete an addendum when the second stage data collection procedures have been solidified.

As previously mentioned, the DNP researcher can choose among various approaches to data collection. Although interviews and questionnaires have been discussed in some detail, data collection through survey research has enough unique features to warrant a chapter of its own. The subsequent chapter will discuss data collection through the process of survey research.

Learning Enhancement Tools

1. Imagine you are a DNP researcher who is conducting research on emotional changes in adolescents who have experienced the death of a sibling. You have decided to develop a new instrument for this study. Describe in detail the process you will go through as you develop the new instrument.

2. Describe a detailed outline for a study you could implement as a DNP researcher that could utilize physiological measurements as a data collection method.

3. Describe a detailed outline for a study you could implement as a DNP researcher that could utilize participant observation as a data collection method.

4. Describe a detailed outline for a study you could implement as a DNP researcher that could utilize the e-mail interview as a data collection method.

5. Describe a detailed outline for a study you could implement as a DNP researcher that could utilize existing records as a data collection method.

6. Describe a detailed outline for a study you could implement as a DNP researcher that could utilize content analysis as a data collection method.

7. As a DNP researcher, you have decided to use content analysis as a data collection method to study current television shows that depict nurses. Describe in detail the various steps you would use to proceed through content analysis for this research project.

8. Describe a detailed outline for a study you could implement as a DNP researcher that could utilize a focus group as a data collection method.

9. Suppose you are a DNP researcher and are interested in using an observational data collection method as part of a research project using family members of cancer patients as the research population. Describe how you make the decision of whether to use a structured or unstructured observational method for data collection.

10. Describe a plan that would allow data collection to occur in a research project that has a mixed method design.

11. Imagine you are a DNP researcher who is participating in a research project that is using programmatic research as the research design. Describe how use of this type of research will affect data collection for a researcher.

12. Suppose you are a DNP researcher who is planning to design a questionnaire on the attitude of nursing staff on a particular floor toward nursing students who were performing clinical rotation on that floor. Describe in detail which types of questions would be best to include in a questionnaire on this topic and also state how many questions of each type you would include.

Resources

Buchanan, T., & Schmidt, J. (1999). Using the Internet for psychological research: Personality testing on the World Wide Web. *British Journal of Psychology, 90*, 125–144.

Burke, J., O'Campo, P., Peak, G., Gielen, A., McDonnell, K., & Trochim, W. (2005). An introduction to concept mapping as a participatory public health research method. *Qualitative Health Research, 15*, 1392–1410.

Drewnowski, A. (2001). Diet image: A new perspective on the food-frequency questionnaire. *Nutrition Review, 59*, 370–372.

Emden, C., & Borbasi, S. (2000). Programmatic research: A desirable (or despotic) nursing strategy for the future. *Collegian, 7*(1), 32–37.

Garratt, A., Schmidt, L., Mackintosh, A., & Fitzpatrick, R. (2002). Quality of life measurement: Bibliographic study of patient assessed health outcome measures. *British Medical Journal, 324*, 1417.

Gilbody, S., House, A., & Sheldon, T. (2001). Routinely administered questionnaires for depression and anxiety: Systematic review. *British Medical Journal, 322*, 406–409.

Gosling, S., Vazire, S., Srivastava, S., & John, O. (2004). Should we trust Web-based studies? A comparative analysis of six preconceptions about Internet questionnaires. *American Psychologist, 59*(2), 93–104.

Groger, L., Mayberry, P., & Straker, J. (1999). What we didn't learn because of who would not talk to us. *Qualitative Health Research, 9*, 829–835.

Harris, K., & Graham, S. (1999). Programmatic intervention research: Illustration from the evolution of self-regulated strategy development. *Learning Disability Quarterly, 22*(4), 251–262.

Houtkoop-Steenstra, H. (2000). *Interaction and the standardised survey interview: The living questionnaire.* Cambridge, UK: Cambridge University Press.

Koo, M., & Skinner, H. (2005). Challenges of Internet recruitment: A case study with disappointing results. *Journal of Medical Internet Research, 7*(1). Retrieved from www.jmir.org/2005/1/e6

Lohr, K. (2002). Assessing health status and quality of life instruments: Attributes and review criteria. *Quality of Life Research, 11*, 193–205.

Meyen, E., Aust, R., & Gauch, J. (2002). E-learning: A programmatic research construct for the future. *Journal of Special Education Technology, 17*(3), 37–46.

Minnick, A., & Leipzig, R. (2000). Beyond interviewing skills: Twelve steps for training interviewers. *Outcomes Management for Nursing Practice, 4*(4), 182–186.

Ross, M., Mansson, S., Daneback, K., Cooper, A., & Tikkanen, R. (2005). Biases in Internet sexual health samples: Comparison of an Internet sexuality survey and a national sexual health survey in Sweden. *Social Science and Medicine, 61*(1), 245–252.

Roster, C., Rogers, R., Albaum, G., & Klein, D. (2004). A comparison of response characteristic from Web and telephone surveys. *International Journal of Market Research, 46*(3), 359–373.

Schaeffer, N. (2003). Hardly ever or constantly? Group comparisons using vague quantifiers. *Public Opinion Quarterly, 55*, 395–423.

Trochim, W., Milstein, B., Wood, B., Jackson, S., & Pressler, V. (2004). Setting objectives for community and systems change: An application of concept mapping for planning a statewide health improvement initiative. *Health Promotion Practice, 5*(1), 8–19.

Widerszal-Bazyl, M., & CieSlak, R. (2000). Monitoring psychosocial stress at work: Development of the psychosocial working conditions questionnaire. *International Journal of Occupational Safety Ergonomics*, special issue, 59–70.

Yampolskaya, S., Nesman, T., Hernandex, M., & Koch, D. (2004). Using concept mapping to develop a logic model and articulate a program theory: A case example. *American Journal of Evaluation, 25*, 191–207.

Yuille, J., Marxsen, D., & Cooper, B. (1999). Training investigative interviewers: Adherence to the spirit, as well as the letter. *International Journal of Law and Psychiatry, 22*(3/4), 323–336.

References

Baldrige Performance Excellence Program. (2011). *Self-assessment and action planning: Using the Baldrige Organizational Profile for Health Care.* Retrieved from http://patapsco.nist.gov/eBaldrige/Business_Profile.cfm

Boynton, P., & Greenhalgh, T. (2004). Hands-on guide to questionnaire research: Selecting, designing, and developing your questionnaire. *British Medical Journal, 328*, 1312–1315.

Ciliska, D., Cullum, N., & Dicenso, A. (1999). The fundamentals of quantitative measurement. *Evidence Based Nursing, 2,* 100–101.

Creswell, J., & Plano Clark, V. (2007). *Designing and conducting mixed methods research.* Thousand Oaks, CA: Sage.

Debus, M. (n.d.). *The handbook for excellence in focus group research.* Washington, DC: Academy for Educational Development Healthcom. Retrieved January 21, 2010, from www.globalhealthcommunication.org/tools/60

Hoepfl, M. (1997). *Choosing qualitative research: A primer for technology education researchers.* Retrieved from http://scholar.lib.vt.edu/ejournals/JTE/v9n1/hoepfl.html

Hunt, N., & McHale, S. (2007). A practical guide to the e-mail interview. *Qualitative Health Research, 17*(10), 1415–1421.

Key, J. (1997). *Research design in occupational education.* Retrieved from http://www.okstate.edu/ag/agedcm4h/academic/aged5980a/5980/newpage2.htm

LoBiondo-Wood, G., & Haber, J. (2002). *Nursing research: Methods, critical appraisal, and utilization.* St. Louis, MO: Mosby.

Neuendorf, K. (2002). *The content analysis guidebook.* Thousand Oaks, CA: Sage Publications.

O'Sullivan, E., & Rassel, G. (1999). *Research methods for public administrators.* New York, NY: Longman.

Polit, D., & Hungler, B. (2000). *Essentials of nursing research: Methods and applications.* Philadelphia, PA: Lippincott.

CHAPTER 10

Issues Related to Survey Data Collection

© echo3005/ShutterStock, Inc.

Objectives

Upon completion of this chapter, the reader should be prepared to:

1. Describe the different types of information that can be obtained through use of a survey as a data collection method.
2. Describe the various stages of planning the development of a survey for data collection.
3. Discuss the process of recruiting the sample for survey research.
4. Discuss the process of planning the content of a survey instrument.
5. Describe how sampling can occur when survey research is being implemented.
6. Discuss the various cross-sectional survey designs that can be selected for implementation.
7. Discuss the various longitudinal survey designs that can be selected for implementation.

Introduction to Survey Data Collection

The DNP researcher who opts to utilize survey research as a method of data collection chooses to do so because he or she wants to make inferences about the larger population. Survey research can produce data that are based on real-world observations. It is more likely than some other research approaches to produce data that are based on a representative sample and that can be generalized to a population. Because surveys can produce a large amount of data in a short period of time at a relatively low cost, a set time span can usually be set for the research project. This can be useful in preparing proposals for institutional review boards (Kelley, Clark, Brown, & Sitzia, 2003). Usually the researcher can obtain five different types of information from the respondents who complete surveys:

1. Facts, such as demographics and personal history
2. Perceptions, which are statements about what the respondents think they know about the world
3. Opinions, which are statements of the respondents' judgments about events that have occurred or specific objects
4. Attitudes, which are the respondents' basic orientation toward ideas, objects, or events and can be the basis for respondents' opinions
5. Behavioral reports, which are statements of how respondents choose to act in specific situations (Brians, Manheim, Rich, & Willnat, 2010)

Once the researcher has decided to utilize survey research as the method of data collection, he or she should begin planning the development of the survey by progressing through specific stages. According to Brians and colleagues (2010), these consist of:

1. *Conceptualizing*—The researcher decides on the purpose of the survey research, develops the hypotheses, specifies the concepts to be utilized, and decides how the concepts will be operationalized (measured) using the survey questions.
2. *Survey design*—The researcher establishes the procedures he or she will utilize in implementing the survey and decides on the nature of the sample that will be used. Kaye and Johnson (1999) recommend that the design of a Web-based survey should allow it to be

as short as possible so that respondents can complete it quickly and not have to scroll through the survey frequently, use as few graphics as possible so that a Web-based survey can be downloaded rapidly, and use drop-down boxes to save space. In addition, the researcher who is using a Web-based survey should check the survey using a variety of browsers to locate any browser-related design problems.

3. *Instrumentation*—The questions are drafted for the survey and the instrument itself is formatted.

4. *Planning*—The budget is planned, the materials that will be needed are delineated, and personnel that will be needed to assist are either requested, as in the case of graduate teaching assistants, for example, or are recruited from the researcher's company. Kaye and Johnson (1999) recommend that as part of the planning process, the survey should be publicized by listing it with as many major search engines as possible; researchers should offer an incentive for completing the survey, such as continuing education hours; and they should determine the most effective sites for publicizing the survey by asking respondents how they found out about the survey.

5. *Sampling*—The researcher chooses the people to be interviewed. Kaye and Johnson (1999) recommend that respondents can be located by linking the survey to key online sites; announcements should be posted on discussion groups that will be used by the targeted population; and the intended audience should be specified in the introduction to the survey because virtually anyone could potentially complete the survey. Once a sample is selected, the chosen respondents can be e-mailed a request to complete the survey, along with a specific number for identification that will maintain anonymity and a password for accessing the survey on a website.

6. *Training/briefing*—The interviewers or other personnel are prepared so they can administer the survey in a uniform fashion to all participants. The greater the number of interviewers, the longer this will take to complete.

7. *Pretesting*—The survey instrument is administered to a small group of participants who are similar to the larger sample to be utilized. This ensures that the instructions given to participants can be easily understood and that the survey items will produce the type of response desired by the researcher.

8. *Surveying*—The survey is administered to members of the sample population. Kaye and Johnson (1999) recommend including a verification page with a thank-you response to the respondent so he or she is not left wondering whether the submitted survey was actually transmitted successfully.

9. *Monitoring*—The researcher reviews records of contacts and refusals and discusses administration of instruments with research personnel to verify that the correct people are contacted as potential respondents.

10. *Verifying*—Follow-up contacts are used to make certain interviews are actually performed or surveys are actually returned, whether by e-mail or by postal service mail.

11. *Coding*—The data collected at this point are converted into numerical terms to allow for analysis.

12. *Processing*—The data are further organized for analysis.

13. *Analyzing*—The data are analyzed using statistical tools so conclusions can be derived regarding their content and the implications for the greater community.

14. *Reporting*—Findings are summarized into research reports for dissemination into the healthcare community and related stakeholders and possible publication.

As part of the follow-up to the administration, processing, and analysis of survey research, the researcher should closely examine the response rate to the survey. The researcher should determine:

- How many people were sent the survey if it was a hard-copy mail-out survey?
- What was the method of distribution, and was this a new method of distribution for this type of research? Was this type of research traditionally distributed using a hard copy mail-out method but was distributed for the first time using a Web-based survey?
- How many surveys were returned? Of the number returned, how many were completed and therefore usable? Can a reason for the incomplete surveys be determined? Is there a specific question that seemed to confuse respondents?
- If different populations were used, was there a different response rate in various populations? Did certain populations seem to understand the questions differently?

- What specific things were used by the researcher to try to increase the response rate, such as incentives and publicity? Did the incentives seem to be ineffective or poorly chosen for the target population?
- If the response rate seems to be an extreme case, either extremely high or extremely low, can the aberration be explained? (Baruch & Holtam, 2008)

 TOOLBOX

Suppose you are planning to survey nurses on a local hospital's oncology floor regarding their stress level when caring for dying patients. Do you think that you will obtain information on facts, perceptions, opinions, attitudes, or behavioral reports? Explain why you believe that the survey will yield the information that you selected.

Recruiting the Sample for Survey Research

In the process of recruiting the sample for survey research, the researcher frequently has to negotiate access to the potential respondents by going through purposive sampling. The **gatekeepers** are the authority figures who control the researcher's access to the research participants. These can be, for example, nursing school deans if faculty will be surveyed or nurse managers if the survey will involve nurses. The researcher must be prepared to show the gatekeepers that the research is worthwhile and will not negatively affect them or the participants. Also, the researcher must be able to show the gatekeepers that the research has credibility and that he or she has personal credibility (Lindsay, 2005).

Once access to potential participants has been negotiated with the gatekeepers, the researcher must convince the research subjects that the proposed project will benefit them in some way. The subjects will be more likely to agree to participate if they believe the research will provide them with new skills or knowledge they did not have prior to participating. The researcher must be prepared to let the potential participants know the survey will not take long to complete, confidentiality will be maintained, and some type of incentive will be offered for participation. This can be a monetary payment or an hour of continuing education time for nurses (Lindsay, 2005).

An important point in recruiting potential research subjects that is frequently overlooked is timing. When initially negotiating access through the gatekeepers and later recruiting the subjects, the researcher must be flexible enough to present the benefits of completing the survey at a time that is most convenient for the gatekeepers and later for the subjects. This may involve talking with a nurse manager at 4:00 p.m., with night-shift nurses at midnight, and then with day-shift nurses at 7:00 a.m. (Lindsay, 2005).

TOOLBOX

Assume you are planning to survey nurses on a local hospital's oncology floor regarding their stress level when caring for dying patients. Who would be the gatekeepers in this case, and how would you negotiate access to them?

Planning the Content of a Survey Instrument

In planning the format of the questionnaire that will be used in survey research, the researcher should recognize the importance of making the questions clear and easy to read. The use of all capital letters should be avoided. Questions should be numbered and grouped together according to subject. Instructions should be provided at the beginning of the instrument and, if necessary, at the beginning of each new group of questions. In addition, questions that actually consist of two or more subquestions should be avoided. An example of this would be, "How satisfied are you with your current nursing position and with your nurse manager?" Closed-ended questions, such as multiple choice questions, are answered rapidly by respondents and easy for the researcher to code as well as analyze. Open-ended questions, in which the respondent composes his or her reply rather than choosing one from a selection, can be used in survey instruments as well. Open-ended questions take longer for the research subjects to answer but can provide a rich source of information that would not be available with closed-ended questions. However, they can be very time-consuming for the researcher to code and difficult to analyze, because the researcher will need to decide how to treat partially answered questions and skipped questions, as well as answers that don't seem to be applicable to the question (Kelley et al., 2003). Examples of a survey instrument that uses both open-ended and closed-ended questions may be found in **Figure 10-1**.

The following questions relate to your reasons for participating in nursing classes. Different people have different reasons for participating in such a class, and we want to know how true each of these reasons is for you. There are three groups of items, and those in each group pertain to the sentence that begins that group. Please indicate how true each reason is for you using the following scale:

1	2	3	4	5	6	7
not at all true		somewhat true				very true

A. I actively participate in my nursing classes:

1. Because I feel like it's a good way to improve my skills and my understanding of patients.

2. Because others would think badly of me if I didn't.

3. Because learning the content well is an important part of becoming a nurse.

4. Because I would feel bad about myself if I didn't study these concepts.

B. I follow my instructor's suggestions:

5. Because I will get a good grade if I do what he/she suggests.

6. Because I believe my instructor's suggestions will help me nurse effectively.

7. Because I want others to think that I am a good nurse.

8. Because it's easier to do what I'm told than to think about it.

9. Because it's important to me to do well at this.

10. Because I would probably feel guilty if I didn't comply with my instructor's suggestions.

C. The reason that I will continue to broaden my nursing knowledge is:

11. Because it's exciting to try new ways to work interpersonally with my patients.

12. Because I would feel proud if I did continue to improve at nursing.

13. Because it's a challenge to really understand what the patient is experiencing.

14. Because it's interesting to use the nursing process to try to identify what needs the patient has.

DEMOGRAPHIC DATA COLLECTION FORM

Student Classification

☐ Junior   ☐ Senior   ☐ RN-to-BSN

Sex: Age:

Ethnicity

☐ Caucasian   ☐ Hispanic   ☐ African-American   ☐ Asian   ☐ Other

Marital Status	**Dependent Children**	**No. of Dependent Children**
☐ Single ☐ Married ☐ Divorced ☐ Widowed	☐ 2-parent family ☐ 1-parent family ☐ No children	

FIGURE 10-1   Self-Regulation Questionnaire (*Continued*)

Previous Healthcare Experience ☐ Yes ☐ No	Current GPA 4.00 to 3.5 2.99 to 2.50 3.49 to 3.0 2.49 to 2.00	
Number of Hours Spent Independently on School Work per Week:		
< 5 6 to 10 11 to 15	16 to 20 21 to 25 26 to 30	> 30
Number of Hours Spent in Collaboration on School Work per Week:		
< 5 6 to 10 11 to 15	16 to 20 21 to 25 26 to 30	> 30
Hours Employed per Week:		
0 1 to 10	11 to 20 21 to 30	31 to 40
PLANNING THE CONTENT OF A SURVEY INSTRUMENT		
Years Since Previous Degree:		
1 to 3 years 4 to 5 years 6 to 10 years	11 to 15 years > 15 years No previous degree	
Previous Degree GPA:		
4.00 to 3.50 3.49 to 3.00	2.99 to 2.50 2.49 to 2.00	

INSTRUMENTATION

The Learning Self-Regulation Questionnaire (LSRQ), originally designed by Williams and Deci (1996) to assess academic self-regulation in a medical school course, was used in this study following minor modification to reflect studies in the field of nursing. This tool has been used in various forms in multiple research studies (Black & Deci, 2000; Ryan & Connell, 1989; Williams & Deci, 1996). Permission to use and modify the LSRQ for this research was obtained from Deci (personal communication, November 10, 2007).

The LSRQ is a 14-item questionnaire that assesses academic self-regulation on two scales, controlled regulation and autonomous regulation. Three primary questions (A, B, and C) were presented with multiple response choices (1–14) to which the respondent indicated the likelihood of that choice using a Likert-type response with answer choices ranging from 1, indicating "not at all true," to 7, indicating "very true." Participant responses were tallied for two subscales: autonomous regulation and controlled regulation. The autonomous regulation subscale score was determined by averaging the answers to the following questions: 1, 3, 6, 9, 11, 13, and 14. The controlled regulation subscale score required the averaging of responses to questions 2, 4, 5, 7, 8, 10, and 12.

FIGURE 10-1 Self-Regulation Questionnaire (*Continued*)

Instrument validity refers to the strength of the survey tool to measure what is intended to be measured (Polit & Hungler, 1999). The instrument validity of the LSRQ was ensured through the review of previous published studies that used this research tool and reported good internal consistency and construct validity for this research instrument. The original instrument was used by Ryan and Connell (1989) to assess learning autonomy in children and was later modified twice by Williams and Deci (1996) to reflect curriculum content used with college students. Williams and Deci reported strong validity for both modified versions of this tool. In addition, Black and Deci (2000) reported construct validity for the LSRQ. This instrument was slightly modified to reflect nursing curriculum similar to the modifications in previous studies.

Reliability refers to the consistency of a measurement tool in measuring a particular attribute (Polit & Beck, 2006). When determining instrument reliability, the instrument should be examined for stability and internal consistency. Stability of an instrument examining a psychosocial construct such as academic self-regulation or learning style preference is questionable. The LSRQ is similar to the VARK questionnaire, which helps students determine their preference for receiving, giving, and processing information. While test-retest reliability procedures support instrument stability, test-retest methods are not reliable when assessing stability of the instrument due to multiple factors, which may impact participant responses such as attitude and mood differences and experience that may have occurred between the two measurements (Polit & Beck).

Internal consistency, the reliability of the LSRQ subscales to measure the expected characteristics, autonomous regulation and controlled regulation, is supported by reviewing the reported Cronbach's alpha reliabilities for the instrument from previous studies. Previous studies report the alpha reliabilities ranging from 0.75 to 0.80 for autonomous regulation subscale and from 0.67 to 0.75 for controlled regulation subscale (Black & Deci, 2000; Williams & Deci, 1996).

Since this questionnaire was modified to reflect nursing curricula and questions were generalized to learning efforts related to all nursing courses, not just one specific course, additional factorial analysis was required. The reliability of survey tools utilizing a Likert scale format producing interval and ratio measures can be determined by performing a Cronbach's alpha test of internal consistency (LoBiondo-Wood & Haber, 2006). The desired score of 0.70 or greater on a scale of 0 to 1.0 demonstrates survey tool reliability. The reliability of the modified LSRQ was verified with a reported Cronbach's alpha on the autonomous regulation subscale and the controlled regulation subscale were 0.768 and 0.725, respectively.

The DDCT was used to collect the following data: (a) student classification (nominal scale as TBNS or NTBNS); (b) sex (nominal scale); (c) age (interval scale); ethnicity; (d) marital status (single, married, divorced, widowed); (e) family unit (two-parent family, single-parent family, or no children); (f) number of dependent children; (g) previous healthcare experience; (h) current GPA; (i) number of hours spent independently on school work per week; (j) number of hours spent in collaboration on school work per week; (k) hours employed per week; and (l) years since previous degree (if any); and (m) previous degree GPA.

PROCEDURES

Permission to utilize and modify the original LSRQ was obtained. The dean of the Auburn University Montgomery School of Nursing granted the researcher permission to conduct the research. The Auburn University Montgomery Institutional Review Board granted

FIGURE 10-1   Self-Regulation Questionnaire (*Continued*)

approval of the research study, and the Auburn University Institutional Review Board also approved the research study, as the principal investigator was conducting the research to satisfy degree requirements as a graduate student at Auburn University. The researcher contacted faculty within the School of Nursing to coordinate collection dates.

RECRUITING SCRIPT

Introduction: Hi, my name is Michelle Schutt. I am a doctoral student at Auburn University, and I am conducting a study for my dissertation in partial fulfillment for the education doctorate from Auburn University.

Invitation to Participate: You were selected as a potential participant for a research study entitled "Examination of Learning Self-Regulation Variances in Nursing Students" because you are presently enrolled at the Auburn Montgomery School of Nursing. All of you are invited to participate in this study that will evaluate learning self-regulation. I will study the differences in learning self-regulation across different groups of nursing students.

Agreement to Participate: If you agree to participate, I will need you to read the information letter. Your completion of the survey conveys consent to participate in this research. The information letter states that participants will anonymously complete a two-sided document, with one side being a short demographic tool and the opposite side being a short survey, and return the survey in a sealed envelope. There will be no future requirements of the participants.

Anticipated Risks: The risks associated with this study are minimal but could include a breach in confidentiality, social discomforts, or feelings of coercion to participate. Should you need to discuss your feelings about participating in this research, you can speak with me, your advisor, or someone at the Auburn Montgomery Counseling Center. Contact information for the Auburn Montgomery Counseling Center is attached to the informed consent form.

Confidentiality of Data: All information obtained about you will remain confidential in a locked filing cabinet in Room 315 Moore Hall. The only other individuals who will review the data will be professors in the Auburn University educational doctoral program assisting with data analysis. No identification will be provided on the forms to link the response to an individual student.

How the Study Will Help: Your participation will greatly benefit future nursing students and will support efforts to improve teaching effectiveness in the Auburn Montgomery School of Nursing, other schools of nursing, and education as a whole.

Decision to Participate or Not and Withdrawal of Consent: Your decision whether or not to participate will not prejudice your future relations with Auburn University, Auburn Montgomery, or the Auburn Montgomery School of Nursing.

If you decide to participate, you are free to withdraw your consent and to discontinue participation at any time without penalty. If you decide to withdraw from the study prior to completing the requested demographic tool and survey, please simply do not return these collection tools. Once these tools are collected, your specific response tool will not be retrievable as it will not have your name or an identifying code on it.

If you have questions concerning the study, presently or in the future, I will be happy to answer/address those concerns. You can contact me by e-mail at mschutt1@aum.edu or by phone at (334) 328-4293.

FIGURE 10-1 Self-Regulation Questionnaire (*Continued*)

IRB REQUIRED ALTERNATIVE RECRUITING SCRIPT

NOTE: This script will be used for obtaining informed consent and data collection for two groups of participants: (1) Junior participants during April 2008 and (2) RN-to-BSN participants during May 2008.

Introduction: Hi, my name is Dr. Debbie Faulk. I am here on behalf of Michelle Schutt, a doctoral student at Auburn University, and I am conducting a study for my dissertation in partial fulfillment for the education doctorate from Auburn University.

Invitation to Participate: You were selected as a potential participant for a research study entitled "Examination of Learning Self-Regulation Variances in Nursing Students" because you are presently enrolled at the Auburn Montgomery School of Nursing. All of you are invited to participate in this study that will evaluate learning self-regulation. I will study the differences in learning self-regulation across different groups of nursing students.

Agreement to Participate: If you agree to participate, I will need you to sign an informed consent form. The form states that you agree to the following: Participants will anonymously complete a two-sided document, with one side being a short demographic tool and the opposite side being a short survey. There will be no future requirements of the participants.

Anticipated Risks: The risks associated with this study are minimal but could include a breach in confidentiality, social discomforts, or feelings of coercion to participate. Should you need to discuss your feelings about participating in this research, you can speak with me, your advisor, or someone at the Auburn Montgomery Counseling Center. Contact information for the Auburn Montgomery Counseling Center is attached to the informed consent form.

Confidentiality of Data: All information obtained about you will remain confidential in a locked filing cabinet in my office in Room 318 Moore Hall until course grades have been entered in Webster in May (August), at which time I will surrender the data collection tools to Mrs. Schutt. The only other individuals who will review the data will be professors in the Auburn University educational doctoral program assisting with data analysis. No identification will be provided on the forms to link the response to an individual student.

How the Study Will Help: Your participation will greatly benefit future nursing students and will support efforts to improve teaching effectiveness in the Auburn Montgomery School of Nursing, other schools of nursing, and education as a whole.

Decision to Participate or Not and Withdrawal of Consent: Your decision whether or not to participate will not prejudice your future relations with Auburn University, Auburn Montgomery, or the Auburn Montgomery School of Nursing.

If you decide to participate, you are free to withdraw your consent and to discontinue participation at any time without penalty. If you decide to withdraw from the study prior to completing the requested demographic tool and survey, please simply do not return these collection tools. Once these tools are collected, your specific response tool will not be retrievable as it will not have your name or an identifying code on it. If you have questions concerning the study, presently or in the future, I will be happy to answer/address those concerns. You can contact me by e-mail at mschutt1@aum.edu or by phone at (334) 328-4293.

Source: Courtesy of Michelle A. Schutt, EdD, RN.

FIGURE 10-1   Self-Regulation Questionnaire (*Continued*)

When possible, a pilot test of the survey instrument should be conducted. This will allow the researcher to identify questions that are poorly worded or difficult to understand. The researcher should determine whether the majority of respondents seem to understand the questions in the same way. When the researcher uses closed-ended questions, pilot testing should demonstrate whether enough answer options are offered for each question, and whether questions are routinely missed or skipped by respondents. The procedures used in the pilot test should be the same as those that are intended to be used in the administration of the primary survey instrument. This will demonstrate whether procedures used in administration are the source of nonresponses (Kelley et al., 2003).

No matter how the format of the survey instrument is structured, each survey should be accompanied by a cover letter that tells the prospective participant the purpose of the research study, the name and contact information of the researcher, how the information will be used, any potential benefits or harm the research subject can expect, and what will happen to the information he or she provides. An informed consent form should be attached, as well as a detailed discussion of the safeguards that will be used to guarantee either the anonymity of the research subjects or the confidentiality of the information that they will provide (Kelley et al., 2003). This can be implemented as easily with an electronic version as with a paper version.

 TOOLBOX

Imagine you are planning to survey nurses on a local hospital's oncology floor regarding their stress level when caring for dying patients. Develop the cover letter that will accompany the survey.

Sampling During Survey Research

Random sampling is usually the type of sampling utilized when questionnaires are being used to collect data. This allows the results to be generalized to a larger population, with the results then being subjected to statistical analysis. There are various types of random sampling, each of which can be utilized in survey research. They include:

- *Simple random sampling*—Each person in the population is chosen by chance and is as likely to be selected as anyone else is.

- *Systematic sampling*—Subjects to be included in the sample are selected at specific intervals within the population; for example, every seventh person.
- *Stratified random sampling*—A specific group is selected from the larger population and a random sample is then chosen from that group. This would be used when the DNP researcher decides to survey nursing students at a college as the greater population and then selects to random sample only the junior class from the larger population.
- *Cluster sampling*—This technique is frequently used in nationwide research projects because it randomly assigns research subjects to groups within a much larger population, and then research subjects within the assigned groups are surveyed (Kelley et al., 2003).

Alternatively, nonrandom sampling can be used when the survey instruments are more informal, such as with interviews and focus groups. Just as it sounds, nonrandom sampling targets subjects within a population. There are three main types of nonrandom sampling that can be used in some way with a survey instrument:

1. *Purposive sampling*—A specific population is selected, and only its members are surveyed; an example would be selecting sophomore nursing students as the population and then surveying only those students who are age 30 or older.
2. *Convenience sampling*—The sample is composed of those individuals who are the easiest to recruit; an example would be sending an e-mail to potential subjects in a specific population and asking them to respond if they would like to be surveyed about a particular topic. Only the respondents would be sent the survey instrument.
3. *Snowballing*—The sample actually develops as the survey progresses because as one person completes the survey, he or she is asked to recommend other potential research subjects who can be asked to participate (Kelley et al., 2003).

The decision of which type of sampling to utilize will largely depend on the degree of sampling error the researcher can tolerate. **Sampling error** is considered to be the possibility that the sample selected is not completely representative of its population of origin. The researcher will never be successful in completely eliminating sampling error, but he or she should recognize that random sampling will always give a better approximation of the population's characteristics than nonrandom sampling (Kelley et al., 2003).

The sample size will depend on the aim of the research project, the statistical analysis the researcher plans, and the resources of the researcher, both personnel and financial. If less formal surveys are planned, such as using focus groups or interviews, the sample size chosen can safely be smaller than the size needed for a more formalized survey. Although the larger the sample size, the more representative it will be of the larger population; for some populations, it will be difficult to obtain a large number of responses. The researcher should ensure that the nonresponse rate is calculated along with all statistics related to the response rate because there are always implications related to the nonresponse rate. The researcher should determine if a specific section of the population was neglected regarding recruitment and therefore produced a large number of nonresponders (Kelley et al., 2003).

TOOLBOX

What type of sampling would you utilize in order to survey oncology nurses regarding their stress levels experienced when caring for dying patients?

Designs in Survey Research

Designs in survey research are usually either cross-sectional or longitudinal in nature. **Cross-sectional designs** gather information about a target population at a specific point in time and essentially produce a snapshot about the respondents. **Longitudinal designs** require the researcher to ask the same questions of respondents at two or more points in time. The researcher's choice of survey design is based on the purpose of the research. For example, a cross-sectional survey design can be either a contextual design or a social network design. A **contextual design** would sample cases within specific groups to accurately describe characteristics of the groups' contexts. This could be used, for example, if a researcher is interested in determining whether the increased patient satisfaction with the nursing care provided in the hospitals in a specific area of the state can be explained by the contextual resources available in that area. A **social network design** would be used if the researcher is interested in gaining information on the relationships among individuals and organizations and the processes that link them. Because the researcher will be interested in gaining information on the relationships that are present, this can be a time-consuming technique and will require the surveying of every person in the target population being studied (Singleton & Straits, 2009). This may prove difficult for the DNP researcher to implement because of the time constraints present with a capstone project.

In comparison, a longitudinal design can be a **trend study** if each survey collects data on the same variables with a new sample of the same target population so the researcher is able to observe changes in the population overall. If the researcher decides to study, over time, a specific group of individuals who typically experience the same significant event within a specific period of time, the research project becomes a **cohort study**. In addition, if the researcher opts to study how specific individuals are changing over time, the design will be that of a **panel study** because the respondents will be surveyed repeatedly (Singleton & Straits, 2009).

After the researcher has decided to use survey research as the method of data collection and has constructed the survey instrument, recruited the sample, and decided on a survey design to utilize in the implementation of the survey itself, the remaining step after implementation is the analysis of the collected data. The subsequent chapter will discuss analysis of the data that are collected, regardless of the type of research project implemented.

 TOOLBOX

How could a survey of oncology nurses regarding their stress levels experienced while caring for dying patients be developed into a cohort study? How could it be utilized as a panel study?

Learning Enhancement Tools

1. Suppose you are a DNP researcher who is planning to utilize survey research to collect data on patients' satisfaction with the discharge process from the hospital. You are employed in a 450-bed

teaching hospital that is affiliated with a large university that has a nursing school. Describe how you will progress through the process of implementing survey research.

2. Imagine you are a DNP researcher who is planning to utilize survey research to collect data on the students' satisfaction with the facilities used for clinical rotation. You are employed by a school of nursing in a large university that is affiliated with a 450-bed teaching hospital. Describe how you will progress through the process of implementing survey research.

3. Suppose you are a DNP researcher who is planning to utilize survey research to collect data on the grieving process of siblings of victims of violent crimes. Describe in detail how the planning process of the survey would vary depending on whether a traditional mail-based survey is used or a Web-based survey is used.

4. Suppose you are a DNP researcher who utilized a Web-based survey to collect data on the grieving process of siblings of victims of violent crimes. The response rate was extremely low. Describe the process the researcher should use to analyze the response rate to this survey, particularly because it is unusually low.

5. Suppose you are a DNP researcher who is interested in using survey research to study nurses' attitudes toward their colleagues on the neurology floor who become involved in substance abuse. Describe the process you would use in presenting the idea of the survey research to the hospital vice president for nursing, the day shift and night shift house supervisors, and the neurology floor's nurse manager.

6. Imagine you are a DNP researcher who is interested in using survey research to study nurses' attitudes toward their colleagues who become involved in substance abuse. Discuss in detail the process you will use to design the survey instrument for this particular research project.

7. Imagine you are a DNP researcher who is interested in using survey research as the primary method of data collection for your research project. Develop a detailed scenario in which you would utilize a survey instrument and the type of sampling selected is:
   a. Simple random sampling
   b. Systematic sampling
   c. Stratified sampling
   d. Cluster sampling

  e. Purposive sampling
  f. Convenience sampling
  g. Snowballing
8. Imagine you are a DNP researcher who is interested in using survey research as the primary method of data collection for your research project. Develop a detailed scenario in which you could utilize the following survey designs for your project:
  a. Cohort study
  b. Contextual design
  c. Panel study
  d. Trend study
  e. Social network design

Resources

Allen, N., Stanley, D., Williams, H., & Ross, S. (2007). Assessing the impact of nonresponse on work group diversity effects. *Organizational Research Methods, 10*, 262–286.

Badger, F., & Werrett, J. (2005). Room for improvement? Reporting response rates and recruitment in nursing research in the past decade. *Journal of Advanced Nursing, 51*, 502–510.

Bonometti, R., & Jun, T. (2006). A dynamic technique for conducting online survey-based research. *Competitiveness Review, 16*, 97–105.

Burns, K., Kho, M., Meade, M., Adhikari, N., Sinuff, T., & Cook, D. (2008). A guide for the design and conduct of self-administered surveys of clinicians. *Canadian Medical Association Journal, 179*(3), 1–12.

Couper, M., Traugott, M., & Lamias, M. (2001). Web survey design and administration. *Public Opinion Quarterly, 65*, 230–253.

Cycota, C., & Harrison, D. (2002). Enhancing survey response rates at the executive level: Are employee- or consumer-level techniques effective? *Journal of Management, 28*, 151–176.

Cycota C., & Harrison, D. (2006). What (not) to expect when surveying executives. *Organizational Research Methods, 9*, 133–160.

Dillman, D. (2006). *Mail and Internet surveys: The tailored design method* (2nd ed.). New York, NY: John Wiley and Sons.

Dillman, D., Phelps, G., Tortora, R., Swift, K., Johrell, J., & Berck, J. (2000, May). *Response rate measurement differences in mixed mode surveys using mail, telephone, interactive voice response and the Internet.* Paper presentation at Annual Meeting of the American Association for Public Opinion Research, Montreal, Canada. Retrieved from www.sesrc .wsu.edu/dillman

Dooley, L., & Lindner, J. (2003). The handling of nonresponse error. *Human Resource Development Quarterly, 14,* 99–110.

Groves, R. (2006). Nonresponse rates and nonresponse bias in household surveys. *Public Opinion Quarterly, 70,* 646–675.

Ibeh, K., Brock, J., & Zhou, J. (2004). Drop and pick survey among industrial populations: Conceptualisations and empirical evidence. *Industrial Marketing Management, 33,* 155–165.

Morrel-Samuels, P. (2003). Web surveys' hidden hazards. *Hazard Business Review, 81,* 7, 16–18.

Porter, S. (2004). Raising response rates: What works? *New Directions for Institutional Research, 121,* 5–21.

Porter, S., & Whitcomb, M. (2006). The impact of contact type on web survey response rates. *Public Opinion Quarterly, 67*(4), 579–588.

Rogelberg, S., Conway, J., Sederburg, M., Spitzmuller, C., Aziz, S., & Knight, W. (2003). Profiling active and passive nonrespondents to an organizational survey. *Journal of Applied Psychology, 88,* 1104–1114.

Rogelberg, S., & Stanton, J. (2007). Understanding and dealing with organizational survey nonresponse. *Organizational Research Methods, 10,* 195–209.

Werner, S., Praxedes, M., & Kim, H. (2007). The reporting of nonresponse analyses in survey research. *Organizational Research Methods, 10,* 287–295.

Yoon, S., & Horne, C. (2004). Accruing the sample in survey research. *Southern Online Journal of Nursing Research, 2*(5), 1–17.

References

Baruch, Y., & Holtam, B. (2008). Survey response rate levels and trends in organizational research. *Human Relations, 61,* 1139–1160.

Black, A. E., & Deci, E. L. (2000). The effects of instructors' autonomy support and students' autonomous motivation on learning organic chemistry: A self-determination theory perspective. *Science Education, 84,* 740–756.

Brians, C., Manheim, J., Rich, R., & Willnat, L. (2010). *Empirical political analysis: Research methods in political science.* New York, NY: Addison Wesley Longman.

Kaye, B., & Johnson, T. (1999). Research methodology: Taming the cyber frontier: Techniques for improving online surveys. *Social Science Computer Review, 17,* 323–337.

Kelley, K., Clark, B., Brown, V., & Sitzia, J. (2003). Good practice in the conduct and reporting of survey research. *International Journal for Quality in Health Care, 15*(3), 261–266.

Lindsay, J. (2005). Getting the numbers: The unacknowledged work in recruiting for survey research. *Field Methods, 17,* 119–128.

LoBiondo-Wood, G., & Haber, J. (2006). Nursing Research: Methods and Critical Appraisal. St. Louis Missouri: Elsevier.

Polit, D., & Beck, C. (2006). Essentials of Nursing Research. Philadelphia: J.B. Lippincott.

Polit, D. F., & Hungler, B. P. (1999). Nursing Research: Principles and Methods (6th ed).Philadelphia: J.B. Lippincott.

Ryan, R. M., & Connell, J. P. (1989). Perceived locus of causality and internalization: Examining reasons for acting in two domains. *Journal of Personality and Social Psychology, 57,* 749–761.

Singleton, R., & Straits, B. (2009). *Approaches to social research.* New York, NY: Oxford University Press.

Williams, G. C., & Deci, E. L. (1996). Internalization of biopsychosocial values by medical students: A test of self-determination theory. *Journal of Personality and Social Psychology, 70,* 767–779.

CHAPTER 11

Data Analysis

Objectives

Upon completion of this chapter, the reader should be prepared to:

1. Describe why a researcher would be interested in descriptive statistics.
2. Describe the difference between descriptive statistics and inferential statistics.
3. Discuss the use of a frequency distribution.
4. Calculate a frequency distribution.
5. Describe three measures of central tendency: mean, median, and mode.
6. Calculate the mean, median, and mode for a set of values.
7. Discuss the four levels of measurement.
8. Describe the use of memoing as a data analysis tool.
9. Describe narrative analysis and how it can be used by a researcher.
10. Describe thematic analysis and how it can be used by a researcher.
11. Discuss the basic theme as part of thematic analysis and describe how it could be useful to a researcher.

© echo3005/ShutterStock, Inc.

12. Discuss the organizing theme as part of thematic analysis and describe how it could be useful to a researcher.
13. Discuss the global theme as part of thematic analysis and describe how it could be useful to a researcher.
14. Discuss the process of developing a thematic network.

Introduction to the Process of Data Analysis

Once the doctor of nursing practice (DNP) researcher has selected a design for his or her research project, fulfilled all of the requirements of that design such as randomized sampling and instrument design, and collected the data, the next step involves the analysis of the data to determine what the researcher has discovered. The data analysis procedure will vary depending on whether quantitative or qualitative research has been implemented (Trochim, 2006a).

Quantitative Research

When quantitative data have been collected, both descriptive and inferential statistics should be generated.

DESCRIPTIVE STATISTICS

Descriptive statistics are used to provide summaries about the sample that was used and the measures that were used to describe that sample. Just as the name implies, descriptive statistics merely describe what the data that have been collected show. If the researcher is interested in examining the characteristics of only one variable, this is known as **univariate analysis**. In comparison, **bivariate analysis** examines characteristics of more than one variable. In the interest of simplifying the discussion of statistical methods, only univariate statistics will be reviewed in this chapter. Descriptive statistics that would be used in univariate analysis include:

- *Distribution*—This is a summary of how often values appear for a variable. This could be as simple as how many students made an *A* as a letter grade on a test, how many made a *B*, and how many made a *C*. A **frequency distribution** can be developed when the values are grouped into ranges, and then the frequencies are determined.

TABLE 11-1 Example of a Frequency Table

Numerical Grade	Percentage of Students
90–100	40
80–89	30
70–79	10
60–69	10
59 and below	10

An example of a frequency distribution is shown in **Table 11-1** (Trochim, 2006a).

- *Central tendency*—This is an estimation of the center point of a distribution of values. There are three major ways to estimate central tendency:
  1. *Mean*—The average of a group of values
  2. *Median*—The score that is exactly in the middle of a group of values
  3. *Mode*—The score that occurs most frequently in a set of values

Dispersion refers to the spread of the values around the central tendency. Two measures of dispersion are commonly used: the range and the standard deviation. The range is calculated by subtracting the lowest value from the highest value. For example, if the values are dispersed as 10, 20, 30, 40, and 50, the range would be $50 - 10 = 40$. The other measure of dispersion is the standard deviation. This is calculated by finding the distance between each value and the mean. As would be imagined, the calculations obviously become more complicated at this point. The researcher is by no means advised to attempt hand calculation of any of the statistics described in this chapter. A DNP researcher in an academic setting will have the advantage of being able to consult a colleague in the mathematics department for assistance with this area of the project; the researcher in a hospital setting can certainly involve the information technology department in the project to receive its input (Trochim, 2006a).

When the question of which descriptive statistical technique is most appropriate for a study arises, the researcher must consider the level of measurement used in the study. Four levels of measurement can be used in a research project:

1. *Nominal*—This level is used to classify objects or events into categories. The numbers that are assigned to the categories are only labels and do not indicate more or less of a quantity. The nominal level uses the mode as the appropriate measure of central tendency and the range and frequency distribution as the appropriate measures of variability.

2. *Ordinal*—This level ranks objects or events so that an object in a higher category can be considered to have more of a specific attribute than an object in a lower category. The ordinal level uses the mode and median as appropriate measures of central tendency and the range and frequency distribution as appropriate measures of variability.

3. *Interval*—This level ranks objects or events on a scale with equal intervals between the numbers on the scale. The interval level uses the mode, median, and mean as the appropriate measures of central tendency and the range and standard deviation as appropriate measures of variability.

4. *Ratio*—This level ranks objects or events on a scale with equal intervals between the numbers on the scale and the presence of an absolute zero. This means the numbers represent the actual amount of the condition that an object possesses. Many of the physical characteristics that nurses typically measure in patients can be classified as occurring at the ratio level (LoBiondo-Wood & Haber, 2009).

 TOOLBOX

Imagine you are attempting to determine if one method of instruction during a senior level nursing course is more effective than another method. You have access to student grades that were achieved using both methods of instruction. Discuss the various descriptive statistics that could be obtained from such a study's results.

INFERENTIAL STATISTICS

Inferential statistics are particularly important because they allow the researcher to draw conclusions that reach far beyond a cursory examination of the data. This type of statistics is typically used either to estimate the probability that statistics found in the sample are an accurate reflection of a parameter in the population or to test hypotheses that have been developed about a population. In order for the researcher to make inferences about a population from a sample, the sample must be representative of the larger population. Another requirement for the development of inferences is the interval level of measurement. This is necessary because of the mathematics operations involved in inferential statistics (LoBiondo-Wood & Haber, 2009).

A test known as the **t-test for differences between groups** should be performed when the researcher is interested in comparing the performance of two groups on one measure to determine if a difference exists. This could consist of comparing how long obese male and female patients remained committed to adhering to a weight loss program, for example (Trochim, 2006b).

If the researcher is working with more than two groups or requires measurements to be taken more than once, the **analysis of variance (ANOVA)** can be used. In the same way as the t-test, the ANOVA tests whether group means are different, but it also considers the variation that will be present among all of the groups. This statistic takes into account that measures taken at multiple points in time will affect the range of the scores that are generated (LoBiondo-Wood & Haber, 2009).

As previously mentioned, in order for the researcher to be able to make inferences about a population, the data must be at the interval level of measurement or higher. What can a researcher do when the data are not at the interval level? The researcher can use the chi-square statistic to determine if the groups are different. As an inferential statistic, the chi-square will show if the frequency in each category is different from what would be expected to occur by chance. However, chi-square is not usable if samples are very small. Other statistical tests can be used if data are at the ordinal level, including the Kolmogorov-Smirnov test and the Mann-Whitney U test for independent groups (LoBiondo-Wood & Haber, 2009).

Researchers may be interested in examining the relationship that exists between two or more variables, and thus will use statistics such as the Pearson correlation coefficient that will determine the presence of a correlation between the variables. A correlation is literally the degree of association that exists between the variables. In this case, the researcher should use the Pearson correlation coefficient to determine if the value obtained could have been achieved by chance (LoBiondo-Wood & Haber, 2009).

 TOOLBOX

Imagine you are attempting to determine if one method of instruction during a senior-level nursing course is more effective than another method. You have access to student grades that were achieved using both methods of instruction. Discuss the various types of inferential statistics that could be obtained from such a study.

Qualitative Research

The analytic procedures used for qualitative research will vary considerably from those used with quantitative analysis, primarily because qualitative data incorporates a considerable amount of verbiage. Part of analyzing the data will include determining respondents' motivation for agreeing to participate in a focus group or provide an interview. Parry, Peel, Douglas, and Lawton (2004) found that many research subjects agreed to participate because they felt that it would benefit other people, whereas other subjects reported that interviews in particular actually were therapeutic. Parry and colleagues found that research subjects found it especially beneficial when health professionals showed an interest in hearing the patient's perspective on issues.

Data analysis for a qualitative research project tends to be **interim analysis**, meaning it will be ongoing throughout the project until either the researcher exhausts the time and resources allotted to the project or a complete understanding of the topic being researched is achieved. Qualitative data analysis can be more lengthy than quantitative analysis, because researchers using qualitative data usually engage in **memoing**, meaning they will record notes throughout each field day giving their impression of what is occurring. The memos then are transcribed into a computerized format that can be reviewed more coherently (University of South Alabama, n.d.).

Birks, Chapman, and Francis (2008) explored memoing as a precursor to data analysis and found that the technique can actually serve four important functions. It can be used to:

1. *Map research activities*—This allows the researcher to actually create a record of the decision-making process guiding the research, including the circumstances that generated a change in the direction of the research.
2. *Establish the meaning of the data*—This allows the researcher to determine what is actually occurring in the data by identifying similarities and differences, exploring relationships, and generating hypotheses.
3. *Propel the research project forward*—Because memos document the thought process behind decision making, they eliminate the need to waste valuable research time in second-guessing the logic involved in important decisions. Memos prevent the researcher from overanalyzing decisions and therefore failing to move the research project forward as needed.
4. *Maintain open communication among the research team*—Because of the memo's somewhat nonstructured approach, it can be a way to permit input and comments from all members of the research team without seeming to be judgmental or threatening (Birks et al., 2008).

Memoing can be very similar to some researchers' use of a **fieldwork journal**. Considered to be separate from field notes, the fieldwork journal allows the researcher, much as with memoing, to create a precursor to data analysis by recording relevant emotional reactions and self-reflection. The fieldwork journal can assist the researcher with the technique of participant observation, because it will record the capacity in which the researcher was present at the observation and the role he or she assumed (Arber, 2006).

Once all data are collected and transcribed, they must be carefully reviewed and then broken into analytical units. This process is known as **segmenting**. Once segmenting is completed, the researcher then must **code** the data. This means the segments of data are marked with category names. The researcher collects all of the assigned category names in a **codebook**. If multiple coders are used, the researcher must be able to show that a high degree of inter- and intracoder reliability exists. **Intracoder reliability** means that each individual coder codes all of the data consistently; **intercoder reliability** means that among the group of coders, the coding process is occurring consistently. If the researcher is able to use a set of codes that already exists, these are known as **a priori codes**; if the researcher opts to develop his or her own codes, these are referred as **inductive codes** (University of South Alabama, n.d.).

TOOLBOX

Suppose you are conducting research on the coping methods of oncology nurses who become cancer patients themselves and undergo chemotherapy. Part of the study involves you actually sitting with a nurse as he or she undergoes chemotherapy as a patient. How could memoing be effectively utilized in such a case?

NARRATIVE ANALYSIS

Narrative analysis is a qualitative data analysis technique that analyzes a chronological story; it is most effectively used for exploratory purposes. The researcher will primarily be concerned with the sequence of the elements that are included, why some elements are evaluated differently from others, how the past and present are interconnected, and how these shape the events of the future. If the narrative is collected through interviews, the interviewer and the respondent work together to create a narrative framework. The researcher will note **patterns** that actually are recurring speech groupings. Sets of these patterns are considered to be **themes**. Some researchers consider evidence of themes to be sequences of core phrases that recur in multiple interviews. It may be helpful to organize narrative material according to research subjects' chronological accounting of events to encourage the emergence of themes (Garson, n.d.).

TOOLBOX

Assume you are conducting research on the coping methods of oncology nurses who become cancer patients themselves and undergo chemotherapy. Part of the study involves interviewing several nurses who are also cancer patients in order to hear the sequence of events of their illness. How could narrative analysis be used effectively in such a case?

THEMATIC NETWORKS ANALYSIS

Thematic analysis is designed to discover the themes that exist in a narrative. **Thematic networks analysis** involves extracting basic, organizing, and global themes from text and then representing those themes as web-type maps with the relationships among them illustrated. The three classes of themes can be described as follows:

1. *Basic theme*—This is the lowest order theme that can be derived from text. It is a simple idea that is characteristic of the data.
2. *Organizing theme*—This organizes the basic theme into clusters of similar ideas.
3. *Global theme*—This is a group of organizing themes that together present a position about an issue (Attride-Stirling, 2001).

A thematic network is formulated by starting first with the basic themes and then working inward toward the global theme(s). A collection of basic themes will be classified according to the idea that is characteristic of the data. That characteristic idea will then become the organizing theme when it is used to organize the basic theme into groups of similar ideas. As more than one organizational theme develops, the global theme will emerge to represent a position that has developed about an issue. The organizing themes will be brought together to exhibit a single conclusion that will become the global theme (Attride-Stirling, 2001).

The process of creating a thematic networks analysis consists of several steps:

1. *Reduce of the data*—This is accomplished through coding and application of the explicitly defined codes to the text so it is cut into segments.
2. *Identify the themes*—The researcher should reread the text segments within the context of the classified codes so that underlying patterns are revealed. The themes are refined so as to become manageable.
3. *Arrange themes*—The various themes are arranged into similar groupings.
4. *Describe the networks*—Each network is read in sequential order to facilitate understanding of the material.

5. *Summarize*—The researcher presents a summary of the main themes and patterns characterizing the network.
6. *Compile*—This involves compiling the deductions that have been made in the summaries of all the networks along with the relevant theory that will provide more information for the themes, patterns, and structures that emerged in the text.

The process of data analysis can be a cumbersome one, depending on the type of data that have been collected and the number of resources in terms of personnel and expertise that the DNP researcher can call upon to assist. Therefore, for the novice researcher who is working with a minimum of assistance, it is recommended that either qualitative research be implemented in his or her facility of employment and on a small scale, such as pertaining to one department or unit, or quantitative research be performed using a single variable.

TOOLBOX

Suppose you are conducting research on the coping methods of oncology nurses who become cancer patients themselves and undergo chemotherapy. Part of the study involves interviewing several nurses who are also cancer patients in order to hear the sequence of events of their illness. If thematic networks analysis were utilized in this case, what types of information do you anticipate would be obtained?

Once the researcher has completed data analysis on the project, whether quantitative or qualitative in nature, the next step in the process involves writing the research report in a way compatible with the mission of peer-reviewed journals. The subsequent chapter will discuss how this process can most effectively occur.

Learning Enhancement Tools

1. Suppose you are a DNP researcher who is analyzing data gathered from a group of patients. Of the group of 25 patients:
   - 12 were discharged after being hospitalized for 3 days.
   - 7 were discharged after being hospitalized for 4 days.

- 3 were discharged after being hospitalized for 5 days.
- 2 were discharged after being hospitalized for 2 days.
- 1 was discharged after being hospitalized for 6 days.

Use this information to create a frequency distribution.

2. Imagine you are a DNP researcher who is analyzing data gathered from a group of patients. Of the group of 25 patients:
   - 12 were discharged after being hospitalized for 3 days.
   - 7 were discharged after being hospitalized for 4 days.
   - 3 were discharged after being hospitalized for 5 days.
   - 2 were discharged after being hospitalized for 2 days.
   - 1 was discharged after being hospitalized for 6 days.

   Use this information to calculate the mean, median, and mode to estimate central tendency.

3. Suppose you have obtained the following values as part of the research project you are implementing: 5, 7.5, 12.4, 15.1, 4.3, 8.3, 12.9, 30.7, 22.7, and 25.8. Use this information to calculate the range.

4. Assume you are a DNP researcher who is implementing a research project that involves assigning the various actions that occur during a code situation to specific categories for analysis. Which measure(s) of central tendency and variability will be most appropriate for this project?

5. Suppose you are a DNP researcher who is implementing a research project that involves ranking a group of patients according to their acuity levels. Which measure(s) of central tendency and variability will be most appropriate for this project?

6. Imagine you are a DNP researcher who is implementing a research project that involves analysis of the oral temperature readings of a group of patients. Which measure(s) of central tendency and variability will be most appropriate for this project?

7. Assume you are a DNP researcher who is implementing a research project that involves analysis of the blood pressure readings of a group of patients. Which measure(s) of central tendency and variability will be most appropriate for this project?

8. Suppose you are a DNP researcher who is implementing a research project to study the effectiveness of a student wellness center on a college campus. You observe the students interacting at the wellness center 3 days a week, and on alternate days, you interview students regarding their impressions of the center and the services

available to them. How could you incorporate memoing into your research project as part of your plan for data analysis?

9. Suppose you are a DNP researcher who is implementing a research project to study the effectiveness of a student wellness center on a college campus. You observe the students interacting at the wellness center 3 days a week, and on alternate days, you interview only the female students regarding their impressions of how they feel the exercise programs at the wellness center have affected their body images and self-esteem. How could you incorporate narrative analysis into your research project as part of your plan for data analysis?

10. Select a passage of text from a classic work of literature and document the basic, organizing, and global themes that you can identify.

11. Imagine you are a DNP researcher who is conducting a research project on the narratives that cancer patients have written about progressing through the grieving process after their initial diagnosis. Discuss how you could incorporate thematic analysis into your plan for data analysis.

12. Assume you are a DNP researcher who is conducting a research project on the narratives that cancer patients have written about progressing through the grieving process after their initial diagnosis. Discuss how you could develop a thematic network based on this material.

Resources

Braun, V., & Clarke, V. (2006). Using thematic analysis in psychology. *Qualitative Research in Psychology, 3,* 77–101.

Burck, C. (2005). Comparing qualitative research methodologies for systemic research: The use of grounded theory, discourse analysis and narrative analysis. *Journal of Family Therapy, 27*(3), 237–262.

Charmaz, K. (2004). Premises, principles, and practices in qualitative research: Revisiting the foundations. *Qualitative Health Research, 14*(7), 976–993.

Eaves, Y. (2001). A synthesis technique for grounded theory data analysis. *Journal of Advanced Nursing, 35*(5), 654–663.

Grinyer, A. (2004). The narrative correspondence method: What a follow-up study can tell us about the longer term effect on participants in emotionally demanding research. *Qualitative Health Research, 14,* 1326–1341.

Guest, G., & McLellan, E. (2003). Distinguishing the trees from the forest: Applying cluster analysis to thematic qualitative data. *Field Methods, 15,* 186–200.

Richards, H., & Emslie, C. (2000). The "doctor" or the "girl from the University"? Considering the influence of professional roles on qualitative interviewing. *Family Practice, 17*(1), 71–75.

Shamai, M. (2003). Therapeutic effects of qualitative research: Reconstructing the experience of treatment as a by-product of qualitative evaluation. *Social Service Review, 77*(3), 455–467.

References

Arber, A. (2006). Reflexivity: A challenge for the researcher as practitioner? *Journal of Research in Nursing, 11*(2), 147–157.

Attride-Stirling, J. (2001). Thematic networks: An analytic tool for qualitative research. *Qualitative Research, 1,* 385–403.

Birks, M., Chapman, Y., & Francis, K. (2008). Memoing in qualitative research: Probing data and processes. *Journal of Research in Nursing, 13,* 68.

Garson, D. (n.d.). *Narrative analysis.* Retrieved February 2, 2010, from http://faculty.chass.ncsu.edu/garson/PA765/narrativ.htm

LoBiondo-Wood, G., & Haber, J. (2009). *Nursing research: Methods and critical appraisal for evidence-based nursing.* St. Louis, MO: Mosby.

Parry, O., Peel, E., Douglas, M., & Lawton, J. (2004). Patients in waiting: A qualitative study of type 2 diabetes patients' perceptions of diagnosis. *Family Practice, 21,* 131–136.

Trochim, W. (2006a). *Descriptive statistics.* Retrieved from www.socialresearchmethods.net/kb/statdesc.htm

Trochim, W. (2006b). *Inferential statistics.* Retrieved from www.socialresearchmethods.net/kb/statinf.php

University of South Alabama. (n.d.). *Qualitative data analysis.* Retrieved February 3, 2010, from www.southalabama.edu/coe/bset/johnson/lectures/lec17.pdf

CHAPTER 12

Writing the Research Report for Potential Publication

Objectives

Upon completion of this chapter, the reader should be prepared to:

1. Recognize the importance of writing research reports with the intention of ultimate publication in a scholarly journal.
2. Discuss the features of a journal that would be suitable for publication of scholarly research in the DNP researcher's field.
3. Discuss the sections of a manuscript that must be included in order to make it suitable for submission for publication.
4. Analyze a completed manuscript according to the sections that it contains.

Initiating the Writing Process

Once the DNP researcher has completed all of the previously discussed steps in implementing the capstone project, the remaining hurdle is writing the research report, and in particular, writing it with the intention of publication. Submitting research for publication is important because it provides a peer review of the researcher's work; submission of the report also allows networking to occur with individuals who have similar research interests. Publication can certainly be a career boost for the researcher, particularly in academia, and can assist the researcher who is hospital based in obtaining health-related grants as well as much-needed budgetary resources for additional staff and graduate research assistants (Siedlecki, Montague, & Schultz, 2008).

WORKING WITH YOUR COMMITTEE

Your project committee will work closely with you as you write the proposal that will guide your project. Typically a DNP capstone project committee will consist of a chairperson as well as at least two other committee members, one of whom will serve as the expert on the content being researched while the other will serve as the expert on the method by which the research is implemented, such as qualitative or quantitative. Sometimes an additional faculty member may serve as a reviewer to ensure that the university's standards regarding quality of research generated are being upheld.

How do you initially choose your committee members? The choice of the committee chairperson is usually the greatest source of concern for DNP students. When considering asking a faculty member to serve as your committee chairperson, consider factors such as:

- *Is the person knowledgeable about your research topic?* If the person has little knowledge of your topic even though he or she might be otherwise an excellent chairperson, the entire venture will be a difficult and lengthy project because the chairperson will frequently need to seek guidance from other faculty who are more knowledgeable about the topic.
- *Do you interact well with the person?* Consider how the potential chairperson handles conflict or confrontation. If you have frequently seen the person lose his or her temper when a discussion becomes intense, it might be difficult for you to have the type of mentoring relationship needed to successfully move through the proposal writing and implementation process.
- *Does the person have a good working relationship with other faculty members?* If the potential chairperson has a volatile relationship with other staff members, then it may be difficult to find faculty who are willing to serve in the additional committee positions.

- *Does the person usually meet deadlines in a satisfactory manner?* Notice how soon the potential chairperson returned graded items to you or submitted your final grade for a course. This will give you a clue as to how quickly deadlines are met. The DNP capstone project completion process is essentially a series of deadlines, such as getting new revisions of the proposal to committee members and then feedback to the student, filing the forms for oral defense of the project and progression to the institutional review board, and reminding other committee members that they are overdue with a review of the proposal. The committee chairperson who does not meet deadlines in a timely manner will be a constant source of anxiety to the student.
- *How many other committees is the person serving on?* If a potential committee chairperson is serving on too many additional committees, yours may inadvertently become a lesser priority simply because there are so many other committees in the capstone project pipeline ahead of you. The chairperson who has spread himself/herself too thin serving on too many committees will be of little assistance to the student.

Continue to act as a researcher in forming your committee. Go to your DNP program's website and read everything that you can find about how the program envisions the roles of each of the committee members; then try to think of faculty members who embody those requirements. A great deal of anxiety can be relieved by knowing that you have made an informed choice rather than a blind selection when choosing your committee members.

 TOOLBOX

Do you have your committee formed for your capstone project? If not, begin considering who you would like to ask to serve as chairperson and as committee members.

WRITING YOUR RESEARCH PROPOSAL

Your research proposal is a vitally important document because it states what you intend to research and how you intend to implement your project. If the proposal is written concisely and succinctly, it can be a virtual guarantee of a smooth, expedited journey through IRB. If, however, the proposal is written so as to be confusing or conflictual, it can equally guarantee that the project remains bogged in the IRB process for weeks before finally being rejected by that entity.

If you recognize that you have difficulties writing clearly in a formal paper or adhering to APA format, locate someone to informally serve as an editor for you. This individual can be invaluable in recognizing, for example, that you are using too many lengthy quotes or that you are improperly citing your references.

Steps to Developing the Research Proposal

1. Determine:
   - Whether you can you state the purpose of your research.
   - How you intend to investigate the topic.
2. Write the introduction:
   - What is important about your topic?
   - Why should it be of vital importance to your readers?
   - Is it both timely and significant enough to cause the reader to continue to read the proposal?
3. Write the literature review:
   - Has relevant literature been included with as comprehensive a group of articles on the topic as possible?
   - Are there articles included that are both general to the field being discussed and specific to the topic being researched?
4. Write the methodology section:
   - Have you developed your hypothesis or research questions?
   - Can you describe your population and the procedure utilized for sampling?
   - Can you describe the methods used for data collection and any instruments utilized?
   - Can you describe how data analysis will occur?
   - Are there ethical considerations that could potentially occur, and have they been addressed?
   - Have generalizability, limitations, reliability, and validity been discussed adequately?

5. Analyze data:
   - How will patterns in the data be identified?
   - Are the analysis methods used appropriate for the data being collected?

Recognize that the requirements for the proposal will vary depending on the topic. Therefore, review the requirements for your program's proposal development closely to ensure that each section is formulated correctly and all deadlines are met. Build in enough time in your development timeline to allow for multiple revisions. Finally, recognize that each intervention that you intend to implement will raise an additional red flag for the institutional review board, thus ensuring that the proposal requires additional time for scrutiny. Remember that needs assessments and quality improvement plans can form the basis for highly significant projects that can gather groundbreaking data.

Choosing a Journal for Manuscript Submission

The researcher must consider several factors when evaluating the merits of journals that may be chosen for manuscript submission. One is the recognition factor of the journal. A journal that is well known and easily recognized by the researcher's peer group will allow his or her research to be seen prominently in the healthcare community. It may be listed in multiple search engines on the Internet and thus be easily accessed by other researchers who may, in turn, cite the research in additional publications (Siedlecki et al., 2008).

Another factor for consideration is the scope of the journal. It is important to know whether the journal has a clinical focus that is disease based, an educational focus that prefers articles pertaining to academia, or an experimental focus that favors research with a strong theoretical basis. The most succinctly written article will be rejected by a publication if it does not fit within the scope of the journal. A researcher who has a clear idea of the specific publication he or she wants to submit a manuscript to should research the journal carefully to determine what types of articles usually achieve acceptance, the length of the articles, their focus, and the writing style that is used (Siedlecki et al., 2008). The researcher also should review the journal's instructions to authors section very carefully.

This is the page that delineates every requirement needed for manuscript submission and, hopefully, acceptance. Some journals will not accept a manuscript that is not submitted via an electronic submission process; others still require hard copies sent via U.S. mail. A researcher who favors knowing where the journal reviewers are in the process of analyzing his or her research should select a journal that uses the electronic submission process. The electronic submission process allows the author to find out exactly where the article is in the submission process at a particular time, whether with reviewers or with the main editor. In this day of confidentiality, journals may hesitate to communicate much information by phone when there is no certainty that the publication representative is actually speaking with the actual author.

The journal instructions will usually state the acceptable font type and size to use, how tables and figures should be formatted, and how photographs can be incorporated into the article. Determine whether the journal states when the author will receive a decision regarding the manuscript. The review process for some journals can take years, requiring one revision after another, before the editors finally decide to accept or reject the article (Siedlecki et al., 2008).

As the researcher decides on the journal to use for manuscript submission, he or she should avoid the temptation to submit the article simultaneously to multiple journals in the hope that one of the group will accept the article for publication. This is considered highly unethical, and most journals have stipulations that the author must agree that the manuscript has not been submitted to another journal. The researcher should, however, prepare a list of journals that could be approached regarding publication, because it is common for an article to be rejected upon the initial submission to a journal (Rudner & Schafer, 1999).

It is important to know what manuscript reviewers will be looking for prior to your submitting a manuscript to a journal. Each journal will have specific requirements for authors that will be available on its website as well as in print form. Although some of these requirements will be individualized to each journal, there are certain areas that each reviewer will consider to be mandatory for a manuscript to be publication ready. These mandatory requirements are discussed next.

Guide to Reviewing a Manuscript for Potential Publication

1. ___ Abstract
   Does it summarize the manuscript?
   Is it understandable without reading the entire manuscript?
2. ___ Introduction
   Does it define the purpose of the study?
   Is a rationale for performing the study included?
   Are terms defined?
3. ___ Methods
   Could the study be replicated using the methods described?
4. ___ Results
   Are the results unexpected?
   Are the results clearly explained?
5. ___ Discussion
   Is the discussion too lengthy?
   Were the research questions answered, or was the hypothesis supported?
   Were limitations discussed?
6. ___ Figures and graphs
   Are the figures and graphs appropriately labeled?
   Do they depict important points of the results?
   Are the figures and graphs understandable without having to refer to the text of the study?
7. ___ Tables
   Do the tables adequately describe the results?
   Are the tables appropriately labeled?
   Are they understandable without having to refer to the text of the study?
8. ___ References
   Are there important references that are classic for the topic that were not included?
9. ___ Overview of the manuscript
   Did the study address an important area of research?
   Are there biases identified in the manuscript? (Provenzale & Stanley, 2005)

TOOLBOX

Try to identify at least three print and three online journals that potentially would be interested in your manuscript.

Formatting the Manuscript

The manuscript being formatted for submission to a peer-reviewed journal should consist of several distinct sections that will be discussed in detail. The sections consist of:

- *Title page*—The title should be specific enough to describe the contents of the paper, but not so technical as to overly narrow the scope of your audience. Authors may consist of a primary author, who performed the majority of the research discussed in the article, as well as multiple additional authors who also made a significant contribution (Columbia University, n.d.).
- *Abstract page*—This is a preview of what will be discussed in the article. It allows the readers to determine whether the article meets the needs of their practice and should then be reviewed in its entirety. Most journals require that the abstract consist of one paragraph that contains no more than 250 words. The abstract should contain the purpose of the research, the research method used, the results achieved, and the conclusions reached by the researcher (Columbia University, n.d.).
- *Introduction*—This should identify the general area of the research. The rationale for the analysis of the problem should be presented, as should the ultimate purpose of the research. The researcher should describe what he or she is trying to achieve by implementing this research (Columbia University, n.d.).
- *Literature review*—This should show how the research is building on prior knowledge in the field by summarizing what is already known about the research problem (Rudner & Schafer, 1999).
- *Method*—This section should include a description of the sample, the materials used in the research, and the procedures utilized.

Describe the research subjects, how they were selected, and how they represent the population used. Identify the research design used and the independent and dependent variables. Describe tests that were implemented as well as questionnaires or other instruments that were developed. In the case of a survey or questionnaire, describe how it was scored, validated, and interpreted. Discuss the conceptual framework if appropriate for the study. Describe the steps included in implementing the study, such as distribution of materials, observation of behaviors, and testing that was implemented. This should be clear enough that another researcher could replicate the study based on the description. Briefly discuss the statistical analysis that was performed (Rudner & Schafer, 1999).

- *Results*—This should include the techniques used in the research as well as the data analysis completed, including both descriptive and inferential statistics. Discuss any complications that were encountered, such as missing data or incomplete survey responses. If tables and graphs are included, they should be self-explanatory (Rudner & Schafer, 1999).

- *Discussion*—At this point, the researcher serves as the expert to interpret the data for the reader, describing the implications of the findings and offering recommendations. Do not overgeneralize the results; rather, allow conclusions to be the natural result of the data presented. Describe the limitations that were noted during the course of the study. Suggest problems that should be researched in order to answer new research questions that have arisen as a result of the original study. Include a discussion of the limitations that are unique to this study, implications for the nursing profession and patient care outcomes both nationally and globally, and an overall conclusion derived from the study.

- *References*—References typically are cited according to the American Psychological Association format; however, this may vary depending on the journal. The researcher must ensure that the method of formatting the references and citations in the manuscript are congruent with the requirements of the journal.

This chapter's appendix contains a manuscript that contains all of these sections.

References

Columbia University. (n.d.). *Writing a scientific research article.* Retrieved April 9, 2014 from http://www.columbia.edu/cu/biology/ug/research/paper.html#format

Provenzale, J., & Stanley, R. (2005). A systematic guide to reviewing a manuscript. *American Journal of Radiology, 185,* 848–854.

Rudner, L. M., & Schafer, W. D. (1999). How to write a scholarly research report. *Practical Assessment, Research & Evaluation, 6*(13). Retrieved April 9, 2014 from http://pareonline.net/getvn.asp?v=6&n=13

Siedlecki, S., Montague, M., & Schultz, J. (2008). Writing for publication: Avoiding common ethical pitfalls. *Journal of Wound Ostomy Continence Nursing, 35*(2), 147–150.

Critique of Clinically Based Research
Enhancing the Ruralization of Alabama's LPN Workforce

Allison J. Terry, PhD, MSN, RN
Associate Professor of Nursing
Auburn University at Montgomery
Montgomery, Alabama

Abstract

Few studies have focused on nurses in rural counties, and rarely have they centered on the licensed practical nurse. This paper uses the factors that LPNs have reported as enhancing or detracting from their job satisfaction as well as the numbers of LPNs reported to be employed in rural or urban Alabama counties to develop a model that could motivate these workers to remain in rural work environments where they could potentially achieve their maximum potential in the nursing workforce.

Keywords: job satisfaction, nurse, workforce

Introduction

Although licensed practical nurses (LPNs) have been in the workforce for years, very few studies have focused on the work environments of these nurses. As the nursing shortage continues, some healthcare facilities are focused on using more LPNs than ever before (1). These nurses are often given increasing amounts of autonomy and accountability in more rural work environments. This paper uses the factors that LPNs have reported as enhancing or detracting from their job satisfaction as well as the numbers of LPNs reported to be employed in rural or urban Alabama counties to develop a model that could motivate these workers to remain in rural work environments where they could potentially achieve their maximum potential in the nursing workforce.

Conceptual Framework

The conceptual framework used for the study was Terry and Lazarus's 2008 (2) work on the state of the licensed practical nurse in Alabama. These authors reported that a statewide survey of LPNs revealed that these nurses indicated the existence of specific factors that either enhanced or detracted from their overall job satisfaction. In descending order, the top five factors that LPNs reported making a positive impact on their current work situations were:

- Reasonable degree of autonomy/good interdependent working relations
- Security in present position
- Good administrative support
- Sufficient support staff for nonnursing duties and
- Reasonable work hours

In comparison, the top five factors that LPNs reported negatively influencing their current work situations were, in descending order:

- Extensive travel commute to work
- Lack of choice in work shift
- Lack of autonomy
- Family responsibilities and
- Inadequate benefits

Terry and Lazarus (2) stated that 52.35% of Alabama's LPNs are employed in urban counties, while 47.65% are employed in work environments located in rural counties. This finding set the stage for the introduction of the second major section of the study's conceptual framework. The Alabama Rural Health Association's (ARHA) definition of *rural* was used to provide a clear-cut distinction between rural and urban counties in the state. The ARHA uses the following criteria to define a rural county:

a. The percentage of workers in the county employed by the public school system(s); the more workers employed in school system(s), the more rural a county is considered to be since in many rural counties, the school system is the single largest employer.
b. The dollar value of agricultural production per square mile of land; the greater the value of agricultural production per square acre, the more rural the county.
c. The population per square mile of land; the fewer number of persons per square mile, the more rural the county.
d. A score derived from using the population of the largest city in the county, the populations of other cities in the county, and the population of cities that are in more than one county; counties where the largest incorporated place has a population of under 2,500 are assigned the highest index score of 25, making them the most rural (3).

Literature Review

Ulrich, O'Donnell, Taylor, Farrar, Danis, and Grady (4) surveyed both nurses and social workers regarding job satisfaction and found that being respected, being a valued member of the team, scheduling, and identification with the mission of the institution had the strongest influence on respondents' decision to remain in their current positions. This echoes Terry and Lazarus's 2008 findings regarding factors contributing or detracting from job satisfaction of LPNs.

Further information specific to nurses employed in rural counties was provided by Molinari and Monserud (5), who found that nurses who remained employed in rural areas tended to prefer a rural lifestyle, the incorporation of rural values in the practices of the organization, the role of the nurse generalist along with job variability, and patient variety. The authors expanded on the idea of patient variety by noting that rural nurses typically care for patients whose health issues differ from those in urban populations, since it has been found that rural patients tend to experience more chronic diseases as well as more occupational-related health problems. Rural patient populations have been found be more elderly and obese than urban populations, to have less health insurance, and to require medication that is more expensive. Molinari and Monserud also reported that new graduates who are employed in rural hospitals must exhibit advanced critical thinking skills as well as assessment skills that must cross multiple disciplines.

Methodology

A model was developed using both LPNs' self-reported factors that either enhanced or detracted from their job satisfaction and the factors that defined a rural Alabama county. A score was generated according to the degree of ruralization of a county, with the counties having the highest scores having the greatest need to fulfill LPNs' job satisfaction areas in order to persuade these workers to remain in practice in rural counties.

Utilization of the model consisted of initially determining the degree of ruralization of the county, using the criteria established by the Alabama Rural Health Association. Ruralization scores could range from 100 to 400, with a score of 100 generated because the county has:

- 25% of its workers employed by the public school system
- Virtually no agricultural production
- A population of 10,000 people or greater per square mile of land as well as
- A population of 10,000 people or greater in its largest incorporated place.

In comparison, a score of 400 would be generated because the county has:

- 100% of its workers employed by the public school system
- Value of its agricultural production per square acre of land above market value

■ A population under 2,500 people per square mile of land as well as
■ A population under 2,500 people in its largest incorporated place.

Once the degree of ruralization of the county was determined, the second phase of the model consisted of developing a countywide plan for incorporation of strategies to enhance LPN job satisfaction, with the expansiveness of the plan dependent upon the ruralization score. For example, the county scoring 400 points for maximum ruralization would need to incorporate multiple strategies in all five areas that LPNs have reported can enhance their job satisfaction.

Limitations

Limitations of the research were identified. A primary limitation of the project was the use of a population specific to Alabama, thus greatly decreasing generalization to other states. A secondary limitation is that the model being proposed is yet untested in a healthcare environment. In addition, it is acknowledged that a more complete picture of the overall nursing workforce and the economic impact of being employed in a rural county could be more thoroughly generated through analysis of both the LPN and RN workforce combined.

Implications

The development and potential use of the model being proposed has implications for nurse administrators, nurse educators, and the nursing profession as a whole. LPNs must initially be recruited by rural hospitals before they can begin to analyze their degree of job satisfaction in their nursing positions. Nurse administrators must recognize that although higher salaries and sign-on bonuses may not be offered by smaller rural hospitals, nurses can be offered incentives such as a slower paced lifestyle, smaller, close-knit schools with teachers who have more personal knowledge of the students, opportunities for middle management career advancement, and great variety in choice of patient assignments (4). Eldridge and Judkins (6) found that rural hospitals tend to have a lower ratio of registered nurses to LPNs and fewer nurses with bachelor's degrees, thus offering additional leadership opportunities for licensed practical nurses.

Keeping an experienced, competent LPN employed in his or her current position could potentially save thousands of dollars annually for a nursing employer who would otherwise need to recruit, orient, and retain a new employee. Recruiting nurses for positions in a medium-sized hospital has been shown to cost as much as $3 million annually; this amount could increase exponentially in a smaller rural hospital with already limited financial resources and a dwindling, frustrated staff (7). Nurse administrators must recognize that as health care continues to be in flux, their challenge will be to avoid unrealistic expectations of new nurses because of the multiple needs of patients in rural hospitals.

It was previously mentioned that new graduate nurses in rural hospitals must possess advanced critical thinking skills (5). For nursing faculty who are educating future licensed practical nurses, fostering the development of critical thinking in this group of practitioners can set the stage for not only their development as an accomplished generalist nurse who can function in a variety of hospital settings, but also for that nurse to further his or her career through additional education. Although the development of critical thinking tends to be mentioned most frequently in connection with registered nurse education, it should be fostered just as diligently in the LPN. This will produce a member of the nursing team who is proficient in his or her role and able to contribute valuable information to the registered nurse's assessment.

Finally, the enhancement of job satisfaction for LPNs localized in rural counties has implications for the overall nursing profession. The nurse who chooses to practice in a rural environment often does so because he or she is familiar with it; perhaps she grew up there and know the people and their daily hardships. The comfort derived from the provision of expert care by a practitioner who is well known to the patient over the course of several years can be immeasurable. Nurses also can receive great fulfillment from the knowledge that they are able to provide expertise to the community where they were born and reared. This may be a very apt solution to the increasing depersonalization of health care in general and the nursing profession specifically.

Conclusion

This paper used the factors that LPNs have reported as enhancing or detracting from their job satisfaction as well as the numbers of LPNs reported to be employed in rural or urban Alabama counties to develop a model that could be used to motivate these workers to remain in rural work environments. As healthcare costs continue to rise, nurse turnover, whether that of registered nurses or licensed practical nurses, must be curtailed, particularly in financially strapped rural hospitals. Application of the proposed model could potentially decrease that somewhat and ultimately save money through recruitment costs, time spent in lengthy education and training, and the time required to try to develop yet another new nurse into a dedicated employee with a commitment to the patients, the facility, and the profession.

References

1. Department of Health and Human Services. (2006). Supply, demand, and use of licensed practical nurses. Retrieved September 11, 2007 from http://www.hrsa.gov
2. Terry, A., & Lazarus, J. (2008). *Licensed practical nurses in alabama.* Retrieved from http://www.abn.alabama.gov/Content.aspx?id=304
3. Alabama Rural Health Association. (2008). What is rural? Retrieved April 30, 2008 from http://www.arhaonline.org/what_is_rural.htm
4. Ulrich, C., O'Donnell, P., Taylor, C., Farrar, A., Danis, M., & Grady, C. (2007). Ethical climate, ethics stress, and the job satisfaction of nurses and social workers in the United States. *Social Science and Medicine, 65*(8), 1708–1719.
5. Molinari, D., & Monserud, M. (2008). Rural nurse job satisfaction. *Rural and Remote Health, 8,* 1055.
6. Eldridge, C., & Judkins, S. (2002). Rural nurse administrators: Essential for practice. *Online Journal of Rural Nursing and Health Care, 3*(2). Retrieved from http://rnojournal.binghamton.edu/index.php/RNO /search/advancedResults
7. Rudner, L. M., & Schafer, W. D. (1999). How to write a scholarly research report. *Practical Assessment, Research & Evaluation, 6*(13). Retrieved from http://PAREonline.net/getvn.asp?v=6&n=13

Model for the Enhancement of Job Satisfaction of LPNs in Rural Alabama Counties

I. **Determine the degree of ruralization of the county**
   a. What percentage of workers in the county are employed by the public school system?
      Answer: 25% = Score of 25
                      50% = Score of 50
                      75% = Score of 75
                      100% = Score of 100
   b. What is the value of agricultural production per square acre of land?
      Answer: Virtually no agricultural production occurs in the county = Score of 25
                      Value is below market value = Score of 50
                      Value is equal to market value = Score of 75
                      Value is above market value = Score of 100
   c. What is the population per square mile of land?
      Answer: 10,000 people or greater = Score of 25
                      5,000 people = Score of 50
                      At least 2,500 people = Score of 75
                      Under 2,500 people = Score of 100
   d. What is the population of the county's largest incorporated place?
      Answer: 10,000 people or greater = Score of 25
                      5,000 people = Score of 50
                      At least 2,500 people = Score of 75
                      Under 2,500 people = Score of 100
      Score of 400 total = extremely ruralized county
      Score of 100 total = least ruralized county
II. **Develop county-wide plan in all counties scoring 400 points for incorporation of strategies to enhance LPN job satisfaction (for example):**
   a. Strategies to encourage reasonable degree of autonomy/good interdependent working relations:
      - Determine number of LPN charge nurse positions available in long-term care facilities
      - Determine use of LPNs in home healthcare agencies
      - Determine use of LPNs in public schools

    b. Strategies to encourage security in present position:
- Organize "town meeting" type groups periodically so that LPNs can voice concerns regarding job security
- Verify that LPNs have a clear-cut job description and concrete criteria for performance review
- Provide opportunities for additional training so that LPNs can enhance their skill level and broaden their range of job experiences

    c. Strategies to encourage good administrative support:
- Supervisors should meet with LPNs on a regular basis, apart from other nursing personnel, to allow them to discuss their concerns.
- Encourage LPNs to participate in their state and national nursing organizations.
- Develop a career ladder specific to LPNs for promotion.

    d. Strategies to encourage development of sufficient support staff for nonnursing duties:
- If funding is not sufficient to hire additional support personnel, enhance team-building with specific exercises geared toward this.
- Develop a volunteer program if none exists.
- Develop a program to utilize health career students.
- Investigate the possibility of providing support staff positions for LPN nursing students.

    e. Strategies to encourage development of reasonable work hours:
- Have multiple schedule options available.
- Develop a schedule option that is only for nurses who are in school.
- Have part-time, flex-time, job sharing, and as-needed positions available.

- Counties found to score 400 points should complete strategies to enhance LPN job satisfaction in all five areas.
- Counties found to score 300 points should complete strategies to enhance LPN job satisfaction in four of the five areas.
- Counties found to score 200 points should complete strategies to enhance LPN job satisfaction in three of the five areas.
- Counties found to score 100 points should complete strategies to enhance LPN job satisfaction in two of the five areas.

Examples of Studies/ Projects

Chapter 13: *Reducing 30-Day Hospital Readmission of the Heart Failure Patient*

Chapter 14: *A Community–Academic Collaboration to Impact Childhood Obesity*

Chapter 15: *The Impact of Evidence-Based Design*

Chapter 16: *The Lived Experience of Chronic Pain in Nurse Educators*

Reducing 30-Day Hospital Readmission of the Heart Failure Patient

An Evidence-Based Quality Improvement Project

Julie C. Freeman

© echo3005/ShutterStock, Inc.

OBJECTIVES

Upon completion of this chapter, the reader should be prepared to:

1. Prepare a gap analysis for a capstone project.
2. Prepare a SWOT analysis (strengths, weaknesses, opportunities, threats) for a capstone project.

The Institute of Medicine (IOM) report, *Crossing the Quality Chasm: A New Health System for the 21st Century* (2001), called for redesign in the methods utilized to provide care to Americans. The first recommendation states that healthcare systems must restructure to develop systems that reduce the impact of challenging healthcare issues on the patient, family, and systems. The second recommendation states that the healthcare systems must strive to assure that the care provided across America meets the following six aims: that health care should be safe, effective, patient centered, timely, efficient, and equitable. The third recommendation states that there must be a method in place to observe and record healthcare processes to determine the attainment of the six aims (Institute of Medicine, 2001). Even after the implementation of the six aims and the establishment of the Centers for Medicare and Medicaid Services (CMS) core measures, the United States of America ranks highest among eight industrialized nations with an 18% readmission rate for heart failure patients within 30 days of discharge (Westert, Lagoe, Keskimaki, Leyland, & Murphy, 2002). Therefore it is imperative for systems to develop interventions to better prepare patients for discharge from the acute care setting. The patient population selected for the quality improvement project is the patient with heart failure (HF). The quality improvement intervention selected to address the readmission of HF patients within 30 days is a standardized discharge notebook.

As the CMS does not reimburse the costs associated with readmission of HF patients within 30 days beginning in 2012, healthcare facilities must evaluate the discharge processes currently in place for the provision of efficient, cost-effective, patient-centered, and effective care (Foster & Harkness, 2010). As patient stays grow shorter and emphasis is placed on better self-management, the discharge process will take on greater significance as a viable option to improve self-management. The cost for providing care for HF patients is approaching $37 billion annually (Heidenreich, 2009). A major component of the cost is associated with readmission within 30 days of discharge (Ross et al., 2009). The individual cost associated with the initial admission is approximately $6,000 depending on the region of the nation. Readmission of HF patients within 30 days results in an additional cost of $2,500 to $4,000 in the Southeast region (Joynt & Jha, 2011; Ross et al., 2009). Mortality rates for HF patients readmitted within 30 days are higher than for patients readmitted at 60 days or 90 days (Ross et al., 2009).

As the United States faces increasing costs associated with readmission within 30 days of discharge, many organizations are evaluating interventions to determine the most effective opportunities for system change. The Institute for Healthcare Improvement (IHI), the American Heart Association (AHA), the CMS, and other healthcare agencies have recommended guidelines, developed programs, or initiated campaigns to directly address better self-management of patients with HF. An area of particular review and concern is the discharge or transition in care processes in place for the HF population.

Approximately 5 million individuals are living with HF, and almost 300,000 individuals with HF expired in 2008 (Roger et al., 2011). Poorly managed HF has resulted in a diminished quality of life, difficulty performing activities of daily living, frequent hospital admissions, and early mortality for Americans (Neilsen et al., 2008; Roger, 2011). The case for the pursuit of better discharge processes is related to the lack of primary care providers (PCPs) within the community. Montgomery County, Alabama, area and the surrounding counties are considered underserved by PCPs (Health Resources and Services Administration, 2011). Therefore, this patient population often does not have a PCP to return to upon discharge. In addition, many individuals in the Montgomery area have not completed high school and suffer from low literacy levels impacting the ability to understand the care required, recognize signs and symptoms requiring intervention, and how to go about seeking the care required. The National Center for Education Statistics (2003) estimated the low literacy level for Montgomery County to be 14%. As a result of the lack of PCPs, the emergency department (ED) is often utilized by the HF patient, and many admissions and readmissions occur through the ED. Improving the patient's ability to self-manage care through a well-constructed, literacy-appropriate discharge notebook has been acknowledged as a positive intervention regarding self-management (AHA, 2009; Boutwell, Griffin, Hwu, & Shannon, 2009; CMS, 2006, IHI, 2010; Neilsen et al., 2008). In addition, reducing readmission through improving the discharge process with a discharge notebook can result in savings of $2,000 to $6,000 per patient to both the facility and the healthcare system (Joynt & Jha, 2011).

The overall purpose of the project is to decrease readmission rates for HF patients through the development and implementation of a standardized discharge notebook. Components of the discharge notebook include education material regarding HF, activities of daily living education, exercise education, proper technique for daily weights, low sodium diet, education on signs and symptoms to report, and the follow-up plan after discharge. Patients will receive a follow-up phone call within 72 hours utilizing a telephone survey developed and based on the AHA's (2013) Get With the Guidelines Heart Failure Campaign and the IHI's (2010) *Transforming Care at the Bedside How-to Guide: Creating an Ideal Transition Home for Patients With Heart Failure* recommendations to determine level of understanding regarding self-management after receiving the discharge notebook. In addition, each patient receiving a discharge notebook will be tracked for readmission within 30 days.

Institute of Medicine Six Aims

As a component of implementing a quality improvement project, it is necessary to reflect on the Institute of Medicine six aims. The six aims provide a worthy goal for the project.

1. *Safe*—Avoiding injuries to patients and improving outcomes by providing standardized written and verbal discharge instructions via a discharge notebook to HF patients.
2. *Effective*—Provision of an evidence-based discharge education plan for all HF patients in an effort to reduce readmission within 30 days.
3. *Patient-centered*—Provision of an evidence-based discharge notebook that is culturally sensitive, is literacy appropriate and inclusive of the patient and the family in the self-management process and will help to reduce readmission within 30 days.
4. *Timely*—The quality improvement project will begin upon admission for patients with HF and will follow the patient through to the discharge to reduce readmission within 30 days.
5. *Efficient*—Developing a project that will improve self-management and reduce readmission within 30 days.
6. *Equitable*—Provision of care to all patients without consideration of gender, race, social standing, economic status, or geographic area in an effort to reduce readmission within 30 days for all HF patients.

Needs Assessment

The collaborating facility is not meeting the national benchmarks regarding readmission of HF patients within 30 days of discharge. As of this writing, the national average for readmission within 30 days is 23.8%, and the facility readmission within 30 days was 24.8 % for the time period 2007–2010 (CMS, 2010). The facility was also inconsistent in meeting the core measure for HF discharge instructions ranging from 89% to 100% from June 2010 through August 2011 (AHRQ, 2010). In June 2010, discharge instructions were provided to HF patients 89% of the time; they were provided 94.5% of the time in September 2010; 92.9% of the time in October 2010; 94% of the time in April 2011; 90% of the time in June 2011; and 91.7% of the time in July 2011. While the readmission rate is not extremely off the mark, the facility cares for many uninsured and underinsured patients, and the upcoming loss of reimbursement from the CMS for readmitted patients will add a further burden to the system. In addition, as discharge education has been identified as a key component in the reduction of readmissions, the inconsistent degree of discharge education must be addressed.

The facility is a 155-bed hospital offering medical, surgical, emergency, obstetric, and pediatric services. The facility is one of three affiliated hospitals within the region. All three facilities are a part of the same healthcare system. The facility admitted approximately 7,500 patients with a wide range of health problems in 2010. The facility is committed to serving the community, and its mission statement includes a goal of meeting the diverse needs of the community served, striving to provide programs and services that promote health and well-being across the community, collaborate with other entities to promote health and well-being, and be the first choice among the community for provision of healthcare services at a high level of quality at a reasonable cost. The facility would like to improve its discharge processes in an effort to better align with its mission statement. A strengths, weaknesses, opportunities, and threats (SWOT) analysis was completed and is seen in **Appendix 13A.** A gap analysis revealed the current resources and discharge processes available, as well as the changes necessary to move the facility toward the goal of reduced HF readmissions in 30 days. The GAP analysis is seen in **Appendix 13B**.

Approximately 90% of HF patients are admitted through the ED (Nurse manager, personal communication, August 17, 2011). The DNP student attended a meeting regarding the introduction of an express admission unit (EAU) for the ED in an effort to move admitted patients from the main ED and improve throughput. During the meeting, the nurse manager of the ED stated the ED must do a better job of capturing the data unique to patients experiencing heart failure upon their admission and indicated a goal for initiating the education necessary to improve the discharge process (Nurse manager, personal communication, August 17, 2011). The current protocol at the facility for HF patients is The Joint Commission Heart Failure Core Measure Set (Joint Commission, 2009). The current protocol and the amended protocol are seen in **Appendix 13C**. The quality improvement project will improve the process of discharge for the patient with HF. The Institute for Healthcare Improvement (2010) states a well-executed discharge begins upon admission.

The stakeholders include the chief nursing officer, the nurse manager from the ED and the nurse manager from the cardiac step-down unit that admits HF patients, the coordinator for the express admission unit (EAU), the community case management director and staff nurses, the quality improvement and risk assessment (QI) coordinator, the patients and families, and the student. The project team includes all of the above except patients and family members.

RESOURCES REQUIRED FOR CHANGE

The resources required include staff to perform the follow-up phone calls after discharge and track the patients for readmission rates and the materials needed to create the notebook. The community case management staff nurses currently call all patients within 1 week of discharge to check on the patient's weight. Now the staff nurses will call within 72 hours to complete the telephone survey and input the responses. In addition, these nurses will monitor the patient group receiving the discharge notebooks for readmissions within 30 days. The ED nurse manager and the chief nursing officer state the discharge notebook costs will be funded separately without a negative impact on the current budget (Nurse manager, personal communication, September 18, 2011).

Quality Improvement

The plan, do, study, act (PDSA) quality improvement model was chosen to develop a concept of quality and the development of the proposed discharge notebook intervention. The PDSA model has two phases that provide an opportunity for the researcher to determine the need for a quality change (IHI, 2010). The first phase includes development of the quality improvement project question, review of information indicating whether it is necessary to create the change, and if a change is needed, which change option will effect the best result (IHI, 2010). The second phase involves the development of the plan for the quality improvement project, implements the quality improvement project, reviews the results of the project, and determines if the change is needed and the best format for implementation of the quality improvement project (IHI, 2010). The PDSA model is optimal because of the well-defined format that requires the researcher to reflect and think about the motivation behind the perceived need for a quality improvement project. The determination of others interested in implementing the quality improvement project can assist the researcher in determining the reality and potential effectiveness of the project. The PDSA model also allows for data gathering from a small study that can then be extrapolated for potential impact in a larger system. The PDSA is seen in **Appendix 13D.**

The development and implementation of the discharge notebook as the quality improvement project plan meets the components of the doctor of nursing practice model through:

- Incorporation of evidence-based national guidelines from the AHA, IHI, and CMS for the discharge education for the patient with HF, which, in turn, will address the IOM six aims for provision of patient care.
- The purposeful development of a system change through evaluation of the system dynamics and identification of change champions, which will provide greater opportunity for sustainability.
- The discharge notebook, which will be a document that will meet established health literacy levels as well as be culturally and ethnically appropriate.
- Utilization of the national guidelines and the change champions to improve the discharge education with a discharge notebook, which will improve the facility's meeting of the national benchmark.
- Outcome measures that have been established and data that will be collected to determine attainment of the expected outcomes.
- A result in a reduction in readmission within 30 days for patients with HF.

The doctor of nursing practice (DNP) project planning model is seen in **Appendix 13E.**

SYSTEM TO CHANGE

The quality improvement project requires a change at the microsystem level. The patients served by the microsystem are patients with HF.

Over 80% of HF patients are admitted through emergency departments (EDs) across the United States (Weintraub et al., 2010). The professionals involved in the quality improvement project include the nursing staff, administration, and case management team. The change will impact the nursing personnel in the ED and the patient care unit that provides care for the HF patients. The institutional review committee (IRC) for the facility has approved the IRC application.

An example of a value proposition would be the standardized discharge process based on evidence and established recommendations/guidelines that provide value (better patient outcomes/improved health/quality of life) through provision of high-quality patient education with a measurable outcome (reduced readmissions within 30 days) and a reduction in costs associated with readmissions within 30 days (savings of $2,500 to $5,000 per readmission) (Ross et al., 2009).

Evidence-Based Model

The Academic Center for Evidence-Based Practice (ACE) star model is selected to guide the development of the project. The model provides a clear outline through the first stage, the discovery or identification of the problem. The second stage includes the evidence summary or review of the evidence available on the problem identified. The translation stage provides guidance for recognizing and identifying the evidence-based guidelines for clinical practice related to the problem. The integration stage establishes the components necessary to work within and without the system to best implement the change identified. The evaluation stage requires measurement of the outcomes identified to determine the impact of the change, which then allows for modification as needed for the intervention (Academic Center for Evidence-Based Practice, 2010).

Review of the Evidence

A literature search was conducted to provide research articles relating to heart failure patients, transition in care, self-management, and readmission within 30 days. The University of South Alabama Medical Library, PubMed, Google Scholar, and the Cochrane Library were utilized for the literature search. The search returned 67 articles. Twenty articles met the criteria for review. Inclusion criteria were articles related to transitions in care for any patient with a complex chronic illness, articles discussing strategies to reduce readmission within 30 days for HF patients, and articles discussing research regarding interventions related to patient education for HF patients upon discharge. Exclusion criteria included articles discussing interventions for complex chronic illnesses other than HF and those articles that were focused on the medical treatment for HF. The search terms utilized were *discharge process, heart failure, self-management,* and *heart failure readmission.* The level of evidence utilized for the review of the literature is seen in **Appendix 13F.** The evidence matrix is provided in **Appendix 13G.**

LEVELS OF EVIDENCE/CRITICAL APPRAISAL

The review of the literature revealed strong evidentiary support for the improved transition in care processes including the development and implementation of a well-planned, structured discharge process for patients with HF. The Agency for Healthcare Research and Quality (2010), Balaban, Weissman, Samuel, and Woolhandler (2008); Barach and Johnson (2006); Dunlay et al. (2010); IOM (2001); Johnson, Sanford, and Tyndall (2008); and Joynt and Jha (2011) state that greater attention must be given to the transition of care from the acute care setting to home for patients with complex chronic illnesses.

Boutwell, Griffin, Hwu, and Shannon (2009); Clancy (2009); Dunlay et al. (2010); Friedman, Cosby, Boyko, Hatton-Bauer, and Turnbull (2011); Gardetto and Carroll (2007); Hill (2009); Jack et al. (2009); Johnson et al., (2008); Joynt and Jha (2011); Neilsen et al. (2008); Phillips et al. (2004); Sauvard, Thompson, and Clark (2011); VanSuch, Naessens, Stroebel, Huddleston, and Williams (2006); Vreeland, Rea, and Montgomery (2011); and Weintraub et al. (2010) identify ineffective transition processes, inaccurate discharge processes, inconsistent discharge instructions, and inconsistent follow-up as some of the major reasons for readmission within 30 days for HF patients. The inconsistent processes included patient education that was dependent on the individual nurse or physician's level of knowledge and interest in providing a comprehensive review of the patient's discharge instructions. The lack of a structured, consistent education format often left the patient without a clear understanding of which symptoms should be reported, whom to contact, or where to go to seek care. A lack of familiarity with the medications prescribed and a lack of interest in seeking the necessary medication knowledge required to provide the patient with a thorough understanding of administration was also identified as an issue during the discharge education. The patients often left the acute care setting unsure of whether to continue all previous medications or take a combination of newly prescribed and previously prescribed medications.

Overall, the researchers recommend a well-planned and coordinated multidisciplinary discharge process, a standardized education plan to begin upon admission and continue through discharge including the teach-back method, the inclusion of both the patient and the family members or care providers, the provision of both verbal and written discharge instructions, and the provision of a discharge notebook for the patient and care providers to refer to after discharge.

POTENTIAL RISKS/ALTERNATIVE STRATEGIES

Potential risks to the patient are minimal as the quality improvement project is primarily based on improving the education of the patient upon admission continuing through the discharge process.

Phases of the Project

Phase 1 included the research and development of the material to be incorporated into the discharge notebook. In addition, a telephone survey has been developed to evaluate the patients' understanding of the heart failure discharge education provided. The patient education materials have been selected from guidelines/protocols established by the AHA, IHI, and CMS. The patient education materials and protocol will be submitted to administration, the quality improvement coordinator, nurse manager for the pilot unit, the ED nurse manager, and the change champions. The estimated timeline for phase 1 is October through January. Upon receiving feedback on the selected components for the discharge notebook and the protocol, phase 2 will begin.

Phase 2 includes the production of the discharge notebook and protocol upon institutional review board (IRB) approval and the staff education regarding the protocol and the use of the discharge notebook. The timeline is expected to be December through January. The education will be provided through handouts; PowerPoint presentations; and regular communication with the primary change champions, nurse manager of the cardiac step-down unit, nurse manager of the ED and community case management coordinator, the general nursing staff for the EAU; cardiac step-down unit; and the community case management team. The education for the staff in the EAU, community case management staff, and on the cardiac step-down unit will take place in January on four dates at 7:30 a.m. and 2:00 p.m. The communication with the primary change champions will occur through weekly e-mail and in-person discussion once a week for the first 4 weeks. After 4 weeks, the communication with primary change champions will take place via weekly e-mail and telephone or face-to-face meetings at a minimum of every other week. The general nursing staff communication will take place on-site once a week for 4 weeks and then at a minimum of every other week. The communication schedule with the general nursing staff will be adjusted as needed dependent on compliance with the discharge notebook protocol.

The implementation of the quality improvement project, phase 3, is targeted to begin in January and complete in May. Upon completion of the staff education, the facility will begin to utilize the discharge notebook and protocol for the admitted HF patients. The nursing staff initiating the protocol will be the RNs admitting the HF patients through the EAU. The EAU RNs will utilize the current HF admission protocol, which includes documentation of the patients being admitted with HF. The current hospital protocol for the admission of HF patients includes an automatic consult generated through the electronic healthcare record for the community case management team. The EAU staff will provide the patients with the discharge notebook and begin the initial review of the notebook with the patients. The discharge notebook is seen in **Appendix 13H**. The staff nurses on the cardiac step-down unit will continue to review the patient education within the discharge notebook with the patient and additional family or friend care provider. The community case management staff nurses will note the date of discharge and will follow up within 72 hours of discharge and conduct the telephone survey. The telephone survey is seen in **Appendix 13I**. The community case management staff nurses will monitor the discharged HF patients for hospital readmission within 30 days.

Phase 4 will include gathering the data identified, analyzing the data, and developing the manuscript and formal presentation as well as submission of the materials for faculty and administrative review of the results of the project. The telephone survey will be scored for retention of the discharge education.

Plan for Evaluation

An evaluation plan is included as part of this material as a means of evaluating patient outcomes.

DEFINED OUTCOMES

The expected outcome of the quality improvement intervention is a reduction in the readmission within 30 days for patients discharged after a diagnosis of HF.

DATA MANAGEMENT

The facility collects data regarding the care provided to all patients admitted with CMS-designated core measures including HF. Readmission within 30 days of discharge is being recorded and will, therefore, be readily available for the patient population during the time frame of the intervention. The outcome measures to be evaluated include both quantitative and qualitative data. The quantitative data that will be collected and analyzed to determine the success of the discharge notebook intervention will include tracking the readmission within 30 days rate for patients receiving the discharge notebook. In addition, the data collected from the intervention from January to May will be compared against the readmission rates in the months of January to May. The data collected will allow for comparison to determine if there was any difference in the readmission rates with and without the quality improvement project.

Qualitative data will be sought through a follow-up telephone survey within 72 hours seeking patient/family evaluation of the efficacy of the discharge notebook. The community case management nurses will be responsible for calling the patient. These nurses will have a copy of the discharge notebook and the patient discharge summary with pertinent information regarding the discharge including, for example, the follow-up PCP appointments. These staff members will complete the telephone survey and input the data upon completion of the survey. The telephone survey was developed following the guidelines and recommendations of the AHA Target Heart Failure Program (2010) and the IHI *Transforming Care at the Bedside How-to Guide: Creating an Ideal Transition Home for Patients With Heart Failure* (2010). The telephone survey will seek responses that evaluate the level of understanding the patient/caregiver has of the steps to an accurate daily weight, patient/caregiver ability to name at least three warning signs requiring the patient/caregiver to notify the PCP, patient/caregiver ability to name three food items low in sodium as established by the AHA and IHI guidelines, patient/caregiver ability to provide the name of the person to call if the patient is experiencing problems, and patient/caregiver ability to provide the date, time, and location for the first follow-up appointment. A balance scorecard was developed and is seen in **Appendix 13J.** The evaluation grid is seen in **Appendix 13K.**

Identification of Performance Measures

In selecting a process measure, the student selected evaluation for the discharge notebook for whether readmission occurred within 30 days. The facility measures and documents the CMS core measures for HF including discharge instructions. Each HF patient is tracked throughout the three-facility system in order to capture any readmissions within 30 days. The documentation within the medical record and the follow-up telephone survey will provide confirmation of receipt of the discharge notebook. Positive impact from the intervention will be determined to have occurred if the patient is not readmitted within 30 days. Reviewing the performance measures of the selected outcomes is important to the stakeholders, the facility seeking to improve performance, and the CMS and third-party payers. The selected measures are scientifically sound as demonstrated by the evidentiary support that indicates a reduction in cost occurs when readmission rates within 30 days are lowered. The selected measures are feasible as the data is currently collected and available for analysis during and after the quality improvement project.

Retrieval of Data

As core measure data is currently collected regarding the readmission of the HF patient, the quantitative data will be retrieved through a retrospective measure (Geary & Clanton, 2011). The time frame for the implementation will occur January through May based on the academic schedule for the spring semester requirements. The telephone survey will provide guidance for the collection of the qualitative data as there will be several staff members collecting the data (Geary & Clanton, 2011). Qualitative data analysis will require telephone surveys that are implemented with a standard set of questions within 72 hours. It will be necessary to provide all staff members with education regarding the telephone survey to increase the probability of gathering the data in a consistent manner.

Data Analysis

The line graph will be an effective analytical tool. Geary and Clanton (2011) state line graphs can measure changes produced during the intervention. The line graph will allow the student to indicate the HF patients readmitted. In addition, a bar chart will be an effective means of presenting the number of patients readmitted within 30 days before the intervention and the number of HF patients readmitted after the intervention (Geary & Clanton, 2011).

SUSTAINABILITY

There is strong support for the quality improvement project and belief that the project can be expanded to include many other complex chronic diagnoses. The stakeholders recognize that improving the patient's and family members' ability to better manage care after discharge will save money and provide the patient a better quality of life. As patient stays grow shorter and greater emphasis is placed on self-management, the patients and family members must understand the discharge process. The discharge notebook has been utilized in other regions of the country with great success (Boutwell et al., 2009; Jack et al., 2009; Neilsen et al., 2008).

There are multiple change champions willing to begin the process of providing the patient with the discharge notebook. The team appears to be flexible and willing to evaluate the project and make changes needed after evaluation to ensure the best outcomes for patients. The impact for the facility will be reduced readmission rates within 30 days for HF patients.

References

Academic Center for Evidence-Based Practice. (2010). University of Texas Health Science Center School of Nursing. *ACE star model*. Retrieved from http://www.acestar.uthscsa.edu/index.asp

Agency for Healthcare Research and Quality (AHRQ). (2010). Heart failure (HF): Hospital 30-day, all-cause, risk-standardized readmission rate (RSRR) following HF hospitalization. *National Quality Measures Clearinghouse.* Retrieved from http://www.qualitymeasures.ahrq.gov/content.aspx?id=27444

American Heart Association. (2013). Get with the guidelines-HF overview. Retrieved from https://www.heart.org/HEARTORG/Healthcare Research/GetWithTheGuidelinesHFStrokeResus/GetWithThe GuidelinesHeartFailureHomePage/Get-With-The-Guidelines-HF-Overview_UCM_307806_Article.jsp

Balaban, R. R., Weissman, J. S., Samuel, P. A., & Woolhandler, S. (2008). Redefining and redesigning hospital discharge to enhance patient care: A randomized control study. *Journal of General Internal Medicine, 23*(8), 1228–1233. doi:10.1007/s11606-008-0618-9

Barach, P., & Johnson, J. K. (2006). Understanding the complexity of redesigning care around the clinical microsystem. *Quality Safe Health Care, 15*, i10–i16. doi:10.1136/qshc.2005.015859

Boutwell, A., Griffin, F., Hwu, S., & Shannon, D. (2009). *Effective interventions to reduce rehospitalizations: A compendium of 15 promising interventions.* Institute for Healthcare Improvement. Retrieved from http://www.ihi.org

Centers for Medicare and Medicaid Services (CMS). (2006). *Report to Congress improving the Medicare quality improvement organization program—Response to the Institute of Medicine study.* Retrieved from http://www.cms.gov/QualityImprovementOrgs/downloads/QIO_Improvement_RTC_fnl.pdf

Clancy, C. M. (2009). Reengineering hospital discharge: A protocol to improve patient safety, reduce costs, and boost patient satisfaction. *American Journal of Medical Quality, 24*, 343–346. doi:10.1177/1062860609338131

Dunlay, S. M., Gheorghiade, M., Reid, K. J., Allen, L. A., Chan, P. S., Hauptman, P. J., . . . Spertus, J. A. (2010). Critical elements of clinical follow-up after hospital discharge for heart failure: Insights from the EVEREST trial. *European Journal of Heart Failure, 12*, 367–374. doi:10.1093/eurjhf/hfq019

Foster, D., & Harkness, G. (2010). Healthcare reform: Pending changes to reimbursement for 30-day readmissions. Retrieved from http://thomsonreuters.com/content/healthcare/pdf/pending_changes_reimbursements

Friedman, A. J., Cosby, R., Boyko, S., Hatton-Bauer, J., & Turnbull, G. (2011). Effective teaching strategies and methods of delivery for patient education: A systematic review and practice guideline recommendations. *Journal of Cancer Education, 26*, 12–21. doi:10.1007/s13187-010-0183-x

Gardetto, N. J., & Carroll, K. C. (2007). Management strategies to meet the core heart failure measures for acute decompensated heart failure: A nursing perspective. *Critical Care Nursing Quarterly, 30*(4), 307–320.

Geary, M., & Clanton, C. (2011). Developing metrics that support projects and programs. In J. L. Harris, L. Roussel, S. E. Walters, & C. Dearman (Eds.), *Project planning and management: A guide for CNLs, DNPs and nurse executives* (pp. 119–144). Sudbury, MA: Jones & Bartlett Learning.

Health Resources and Services Administration (HRSA). (2011). *Healthcare provider shortage areas.* Retrieved from http://hpsafind.hrsa.gov/HPSASearch.aspx

Heidenreich, P. (2009). *Readmission for heart failure.* Health Services Research and Development Service. Retrieved from http://www.hsrd.research.va.gov/publications/forum/may09/may09-5.cfm

Hill, C. A. (2009). Acute heart failure too sick for discharge teaching? *Critical Care Nursing Quarterly, 32*(2), 106–111. Retrieved from http://journals.lww.com/ccnq/pages/default.aspx

Institute for Healthcare Improvement (IHI). (2010). Transforming care at the bedside how-to guide: Creating an ideal transition home for patients with heart failure. Retrieved from http://www.ihi.org/knowledge/Pages/Tools/TCABHowToGuideTransitionHomeforHF.aspx

Institute of Medicine. (2001). *Crossing the quality chasm: A new health system for the 21st century.* Washington, DC: National Academies Press.

Jack, B. W., Chetty, V. K., Anthony, D., Greenwald, J. L., Sanchez, G. M., Forsythe, S. R., . . . Culpepper, L. (2009). A reengineered hospital discharge program to decrease rehospitalization: A randomized trial. *Annals of Internal Medicine, 150*(3), 178–187. Retrieved from http://annals.org/

Johnson, A., Sanford, J., & Tyndall, J. (2008). Written and verbal information versus verbal information only for patients being discharged from acute hospital settings to home (Review). *The Cochrane Collaboration, 4*, 1–18. Retrieved from http://www.thecochranelibrary.com/view/0/index.html

Joint Commission, The. (2009). *Heart failure core measure set.* Retrieved from http://www.jointcommission.org/assets/1/6/Heart%20Failure.pdf

Joynt, K. E., & Jha, J. K. (2011). Who has higher readmission rates for heart failure, and why? Implications for efforts to improve care using financial incentives. *Circulation: Cardiovascular Quality and Outcomes, 4*, 53–59. doi:10.1161/CIRCOUTCOMES.110.950964

National Center for Education Statistics. (2003). State and county estimates of low literacy. Retrieved from http://nces.ed.gov/naal/estimates/StateEstimates.aspx

Neilsen, G. A., Barteley, A., Coleman, E., Resar, R., Rutherford, P., Souw, D., & Taylor, J. (2008). Transforming care at the bedside how-to guide: Creating an ideal transition home for patients with heart failure. Retrieved from http://www.ihi.org

Phillips, C. O., Wright, S. M., Kern, D. E., Singa, R. M., Shepard, S., & Rubin, H. R. (2004). Comprehensive discharge planning with post-discharge support for older patients with congestive heart failure: A meta-analysis. *Journal of the American Medical Association, 291*(11), 1358–1367. Retrieved from http://jama.ama-assn.org/

Roger, V. L., Go, A. S., Lloyd-Jones, G. M., Adams, R. J., Berry, J. D., Brown, T. M., . . . Wylie-Rosett, J. (2011). Heart disease and stroke statistics: Our guide to current statistics and the supplement to our heart and stroke facts. *Circulation: Journal of the American Heart Association, 123*, e18–e209. doi:10.1161/CIR.0b013e3182009701

Ross, J. S., Chen, J., Lin, Z., Bueno, H., Curtis, J. P., Keenan, P. S., . . . Krumholz, H. M. (2009). Recent national trends in readmission rates after heart failure hospitalization. *Circulation Heart Failure, 3*(1), 97–103. doi: 10.1161/CIRCHEARTFAILURE.109.885210

Sauvard, L. A., Thompson, D. R., & Clark, A. M. (2011). A meta-review of evidence on heart failure disease management programs: The challenges of describing and synthesizing evidence on complex interventions. *Trials Journal, 12*, 194–203. Retrieved from http://www.trialsjournal.com/content/12/1/194

VanSuch, M., Naessens, J. M., Streobel, R. J., Huddleston, J. M., & Williams, J. R. (2006). Effect of discharge instructions on readmission of hospitalized patients with heart failure: Do all of the Joint Commission on Accreditation of Healthcare Organizations heart failure core measures reflect better care? *Quality Safe Health Care, 15,* 414–417. doi:10.1136/qshc.2005.017640

Vreeland, D. G., Rea, R. W., & Montgomery, L. L. (2011). A review of the literature on heart failure and discharge education. *Critical Care Nursing Quarterly, 34*(3), 235–245. doi:10.1097/CNQ06013e31821ffe5d

Weintraub, N. L., Collins, S. P., Pang, P. S., Levy, P. D., Anderson, A. S., Arslanian-Engoren, C., . . . Gheorghiade, M. (2010). Acute heart failure syndromes: Emergency department presentation; Treatment and disposition: Current approaches and future aims; A scientific statement from the American Heart Association. *Circulation: A Journal of the American Heart Association, 122,* 1975–1996. doi:10.1161/CIR.0b013e3181f9a223

Westert, G. P., Lagoe, R. J., Keskimaki, I., Leyland, A., & Murphy, M. (2002). An international study of hospital readmissions and related utilization in Europe and the USA. *Health Policy, 61,* 269–278. doi:10.1016SO168-8510(01)00236-6

SWOT Analysis

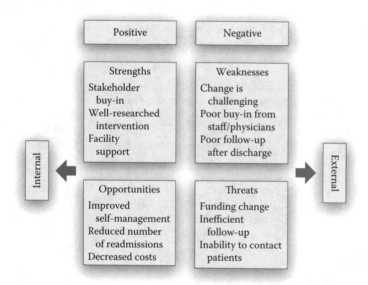

Gap Analysis

Current Experience	Planned Intervention	Desired Outcome	Gap Identified
Patients with heart failure (HF) receive unstructured, inconsistent discharge instructions from registered nurses throughout the facility. The discharge education is not based on any of the recommended guidelines provided by the American Heart Association, Agency for Healthcare Research and Quality, Centers for Medicare and Medicaid Services, Institute for Healthcare Improvement, or The Joint Commission.	Patient discharge education will be provided based on established guidelines and recommendations by a variety of registered nurses who have received education via a formal structured guideline for HF discharge education based on best evidence and guidelines.	The patient will experience an increased ability to self-manage care after discharge, leading to a reduction in the readmission within 30 days rate for the HF patients at the facility.	Discharge education is provided in an inconsistent manner by the nursing staff and without assurance that the education provided is evidence based and recommended by the American Heart Association, Agency for Healthcare Research and Quality, Centers for Medicare and Medicaid Services, Institute for Healthcare Improvement, and The Joint Commission.

Protocol for Quality Improvement Project

Reducing 30-Day Hospital Readmission of the Heart Failure Patient

Current protocol for management of the congestive heart failure patient is the Congestive Heart Failure Core Measure Set, which includes the following:

1. Discharge instructions

Modification of the current protocol will address the process of providing discharge instructions. The patient/caregiver will receive a standardized consistent discharge education process through the discharge notebook. The project will take place January through June.

A telephone questionnaire will be administered within 72 hours to measure the retention of the education provided during the discharge education process (Society of Hospital Medicine, 2008).

Reference

Society of Hospital Medicine. (2008). Retrieved from http://www.hospitalmedicine.org/ResourceRoomRedesign/RR_HeartFailure/html_HF/05Track/02_Care.cfm

Plan, Do, Study, Act Model

Aim: Improve discharge education process and reduce readmission rates for heart failure patients.

Describe your first (or next) test of change:	Person Responsible	When to Be Done	Where to Be Done
Redesign the discharge process for patients with heart failure (HF)	Julie Freeman	August–October	Name of facility

Plan

List the tasks needed to set up this test of change	Person Responsible	When to Be Done	Where to Be Done
1. Evaluation of current discharge processes	Julie Freeman	August–November	Name of facility
2. Perform a literature search to determine best practice, guidelines, and evidence for the discharge of HF patients			
3. Determine from literature review the best evidence for discharge processes for HF patients			
4. Develop the discharge process identified as best practice			

Predict what will happen when the test is carried out.	Measures to determine if prediction succeeds
1. Patient knowledge of at-home management will be improved. 2. The facility will see a reduction in the rate of readmission within 30 days for HF patients.	1. Postdischarge telephone survey 2. Review data to determine number of patients readmitted within 30 days

Do

Describe what actually happened when you ran the test.

1. Utilizing the discharge notebook provided standard, consistent HF education for the patient/caregiver.
2. Follow-up telephone interview indicated the patient and/or caregiver had better understanding of the appropriate manner of weighing, warning signs and symptoms, who to contact in case of warning signs and symptoms, diet, activity, and follow-up appointments.

Study

Describe the measured results and how they compared to the predictions.

Act

Describe what modifications to the plan will be made for the next cycle from what you learned.

Project Planning Model

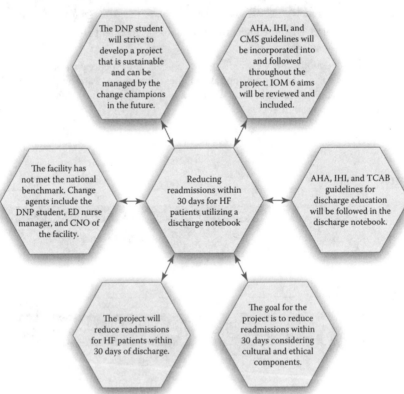

The DNP student will strive to develop a project that is sustainable and can be managed by the change champions in the future.

AHA, IHI, and CMS guidelines will be incorporated into and followed throughout the project. IOM 6 aims will be reviewed and included.

The facility has not met the national benchmark. Change agents include the DNP student, ED nurse manager, and CNO of the facility.

Reducing readmissions within 30 days for HF patients utilizing a discharge notebook

AHA, IHI, and TCAB guidelines for discharge education will be followed in the discharge notebook.

The project will reduce readmissions for HF patients within 30 days of discharge.

The goal for the project is to reduce readmissions within 30 days considering cultural and ethical components.

Notes: CNO = chief nursing officer. TCAB = *Transforming Care at the Bedside.*

Review of the Literature

Author/Year/Title	Level/Grade	Design	Sample/Data Collection	Findings	Limitations	Recommendations
Balaban, R. B., Weissman, J. S., Samuel, P. A., & Woolhandler, S. (2008). Redefining and redesigning hospital discharge to enhance patient care: A randomized controlled study.	Level 1 Grade B	Randomized control study	Diverse patients admitted with a diagnosis of HF between June 2006 and January 2007 (122 total eligible)	Utilizing a simple discharge form only 25.5% of patients experienced one or more undesirable outcomes when compared to 55.1% of concurrent patients and 55% of historical controls. Only 14.9% of patients receiving the intervention failed to follow up with care provider within 21 days compared to 40.8% of concurrent patients.	Single small study	Simple inexpensive printed discharge materials improve patient transition, understanding, and compliance with discharge instructions and reduce the incidence of complication including readmission.
Bernheim, S. H., Grady, J. N., Lin, Z., Wang, Y., Wang, Y., Savage, S. V., . . . Krumholz, H. M. (2010). National patterns of risk-standardized for acute myocardial infarction and heart failure: Update based on publicly reported outcomes measures based on the 2010 release.	Level 1++ Grade A	Meta-analysis	Hierarchical logistic regression model was utilized with Centers for Medicare and Medicaid Services data from approximately 4,500 facilities over 3 years reviewing the hospital referral regions for those hospitals with better than expected and those with worse than expected rates for mortality and readmission	There was a difference between the number of readmissions between facilities in the 95th percentile and the 5th percentile with the higher risk-standardized readmission rates in the eastern, southeastern, and midwestern states.	The report only includes FFS Medicare patients and therefore the data cannot necessarily be extrapolated to other populations due to their lack of inclusion.	There continues to be an opportunity for hospitals to improve the discharge processes for patients to reduce the risk-standardized mortality and risk-standardized readmission rates for patients with heart failure.

Blanck, A. W., & Marshall, C. (2011). Patient education materials from the layperson's perspective: The importance of readability.	Level 3 Grade D	Nonrandomized control trial	Convenience sample from nonclinical employees, volunteer services, senior center partner, and patients in the ambulatory surgical center	Printed education materials developed by healthcare professionals based on evidence but reviewed for ease of understanding by laypersons is beneficial.	As a convenience sample was utilized, there were no patients with very low literacy levels on the panel. Some respondents provided no feedback, therefore the committee could not ascertain the depth of review by the panel member.	Healthcare facilities should utilize laypersons or nonclinical individuals in reviewing formal evidence-based patient education materials to assure that the materials exhibit an appropriate literacy level, are free of jargon, and are able to be understood by a range of nonhealthcare persons.
Clancy, C. M. (2009). Reengineering hospital discharge: A protocol to improve patient safety, reduce costs, and boost patient satisfaction.	Level 4 Grade D	Commentary	N/A	Reorganizing the discharge process to include both written and verbal discharge instructions improves patient outcomes, safety, efficacy, and satisfaction.	N/A	Hospitals should consider redesigning the discharge processes for patients with heart failure to include a structured written discharge instruction.

(continues)

Author/Year/Title	Level/Grade	Design	Sample/Data Collection	Findings	Limitations	Recommendations
Coleman, E. A. (2011). What will it take to ensure high quality transitional care?	Level 4 Grade D	Expert opinion/ commentary	N/A	Multiple areas of improvement in the discharge process including written discharge instructions can offer better transition in the discharge process and self-management for the patient/family.	N/A	Complex chronic illnesses require greater consideration when transitioning the patient from the acute care setting to self-management
Foote, M. (1997). Heart failure: Helping your patient help herself.	Level 4 Grade D	Expert opinion/ commentary	N/A	Several actions can improve the patient's ability to better manage his or her heart failure.	N/A	Assessing the patient's functional status, improving knowledge, and encouraging compliance should be included in a discharge notebook for the patient with heart failure.

Citation	Level/Grade	Design	Sample	Results	Limitations	Implications
Friedman, A. J., Cosby, R., Boyko, S., Hatton-Bauer, J., & Turnbull, G. (2011). Effective teaching strategies and methods of delivery for patient education: A systematic review and practice guideline.	Level 1++ Grade A	Systematic reviews and meta-analyses were evaluated utilizing the AMSTAR tool	Review of research studies that evaluated teaching strategies for patients with complex illnesses (cancer)	The use of structured, well-defined multiple teaching strategies was more effective in retention of knowledge regarding self-management.	The limitations include the variability among the various studies regarding the specific outcomes chosen for measurement and the wide variety of disease processes addressed in the differing studies.	Structured, culturally appropriate and patient-specific education is more effective than off-the-cuff patient education.
Gardetto, N. J., & Carroll, K. C. (2007). Management strategies to meet the core heart failure measures for acute decompensated heart failure: A nursing perspective.	Level 3 Grade D	Commentary/ expert opinion	N/A	Well-organized and structured processes to assure compliance with core measures reduce mortality and readmission and reduce costs and improve quality of life.	N/A	Structured education processes begun at admission can improve the discharge process. The structured education should address discharge instructions and begin upon admission.

(continues)

Author/Year/Title	Level/ Grade	Design	Sample/Data Collection	Findings	Limitations	Recommendations
Hill, C. A. (2009). Acute heart failure too sick for discharge teaching?	Level 4 Grade D	Commentary/ expert opinion	N/A	Short hospital stays and high education needs require an organized and standardized process to best meet the needs of the HF patient.	N/A	Develop dedicated strategies to provide the high level of education needs for the HF patient to better prepare them for discharge home and self-management.
Jack, B. W., Chetty, V. K., Anthony, D., Greenwald, J. L., Sanchez, G. M., Johnson, A. E., . . . Culpepper, L. (2009). A reengineered hospital discharge program to decrease rehospitalization: A randomized trial.	Level 1++ Grade A	Randomized trial	Block randomization of 6 and 8. Randomly arranged index cards were placed in opaque envelopes, labeled consecutively with study numbers, and participants were assigned a study group by revealing the index card (749 English speaking)	Participants with HF in the intervention experienced a reduction in length of stay and reduced readmission rates compared to the HF patients receiving the usual discharge process.	Single-center study in which not all potentially eligible patients could be enrolled, and outcome assessment sometimes relied on participant report.	Discharge processes should be reevaluated for HF patients and other patients with complex chronic illnesses to include individual management during admission and in preparation for discharge including planning and making follow-up appointments as needed, medication reconciliation, HF education, and an individualized discharge notebook that can be utilized with PCP.

Citation	Level/Grade	Design	Findings	Limitations	Recommendations
Johnson, A., Sanford, J., & Tyndall, J. (2008). Written and verbal information versus verbal information only for patients being discharged from acute hospital settings to home (Review).	Level 1+ Grade A	Meta-analysis	Literature review of randomized control trials or clinical trials that provided comparison between written and verbal discharge instructions for the patient discharged from the acute care setting	Standardized verbal and written discharge instructions provided greater patient/family member satisfaction and understanding of discharge plan of care.	Included the lack of trials that met the inclusion criteria.	More studies are needed to determine efficacy of standardized verbal and written discharge instructions.
Kripalani, S., Jackson, A. T., Schnipper, J. L., & Coleman, E. A. (2007). Promoting effective transitions of care at hospital discharge: A review of issues for hospitalists.	Level 4 Grade D	Expert opinion/ recommendation	N/A	Transitions in care are identified as very vulnerable times for the patient, in particular the discharge process from the acute care setting to home produces at least one medication error per patient.	N/A	Transitions in care should be well organized and structured to improve the patient's ability to self-manage care and reduce potential harm after discharge.

References

Balaban, R. R., Weissman, J. S., Samuel, P. A., & Woolhandler, S. (2008). Redefining and redesigning hospital discharge to enhance patient care: A randomized control study. *Journal of General Internal Medicine, 23*(8), 1228–1233. doi:10.1007/s11606-008-0618-9

Bernheim, S. H., Grady, J. N., Lin, Z., Wang, Y., Wang, Y., Savage, S. V., . . . Krumholz, H. M. (2010). National patterns of risk-standardized for acute myocardial infarction and heart failure: Update based on publicly reported outcomes measures based on the 2010 release. *JAMA, 309*(6), 587–593.

Blanck, A. W., & Marshall, C. (2011). Patient education materials from the layperson's perspective: The importance of readability. *Journal for Nurses in Staff Development, 27*(2), E8–E10.

Clancy, C. M. (2009). Reengineering hospital discharge: A protocol to improve patient safety, reduce costs, and boost patient satisfaction. *American Journal of Medical Quality, 24*, 343–346. doi:10.1177/1062860609338131

Coleman, E. A. (2011). What will it take to ensure high quality transitional care? *Annual Review of Gerontology & Geriatrics; 31*, preceding p1.

Foote, M. (1997). Heart failure: Helping your patient help herself. *Nursing, 27*(4), 32aaa–32ddd.

Friedman, A. J., Cosby, R., Boyko, S., Hatton-Bauer, J., & Turnbull, G. (2011). Effective teaching strategies and methods of delivery for patient education: A systematic review and practice guideline recommendations. *Journal of Cancer Education, 26*, 12–21. doi:10.1007/s13187-010-0183-x

Gardetto, N. J., & Carroll, K. C. (2007). Management strategies to meet the core heart failure measures for acute decompensated heart failure: A nursing perspective. *Critical Care Nursing Quarterly, 30*(4), 307–320.

Hill, C. A. (2009). Acute heart failure too sick for discharge teaching? *Critical Care Nursing Quarterly, 32*(2), 106–111. Retrieved from http://journals.lww.com/ccnq/pages/default.aspx

Jack, B. W., Chetty, V. K., Anthony, D., Greenwald, J. L., Sanchez, G. M., Forsythe, S. R., . . . Culpepper, L. (2009). A reengineered hospital discharge program to decrease rehospitalization: A randomized trial. *Annals of Internal Medicine, 150*(3), 178–187. Retrieved from http://annals.org/

Johnson, A., Sanford, J., & Tyndall, J. (2008). Written and verbal information versus verbal information only for patients being discharged from acute hospital settings to home (Review). *The Cochrane Collaboration, 4,* 1–18. Retrieved from http://www.thecochranelibrary.com/view/0/index.html

Kripalani, S., Jackson, A. T., Schnipper, J. L., & Coleman, E. A. (2007). Promoting effective transitions of care at hospital discharge: A review of issues for hospitalists. *Journal of Hospital Medicine, 2*(5), 314–323.

Grading System Used by New Zealand Guideline Group in Cardiac Rehabilitation Guideline[1]

Levels of Evidence

1++   High-quality meta-analyses, systematic reviews of randomized control trials (RCTs), or RCTs with a very low risk of bias

1+   Well-conducted meta-analyses, systematic reviews of RCTs, or RCTs with a low risk of bias

1 -   Well-conducted meta-analyses, systematic reviews of RCTs, or RCTs with a high risk of bias

2++   High-quality systematic reviews of case-control or cohort studies with a very low risk of confounding or bias and a high probability that the relationship is causal

2+   Well-constructed case-control studies with a low risk of confounding or bias and a moderate probability that the relationship is causal

2-   Case-control or cohort studies with a high risk of confounding or bias and a significant risk that the relationship is not causal

---

[1] New Zealand Guidelines Group. (2002). Cardiac rehabilitation guideline. Wellington: New Zealand Guidelines Group http://www.health.govt.nz/publication/cardiac-rehabilitation-guideline

3   Nonanalytical studies (case reports, case series)
4   Expert opinion

Grades of Recommendations

A   At least one meta-analysis, systematic review, or RCT rated as 1++ and directly applicable to the target population, OR a body of evidence consisting principally of studies rated as 1+, directly applicable to the target population, and demonstrating overall consistency of results

B   A body of evidence including studies rated as 2++, directly applicable to the target population, and demonstrating overall consistency of results, OR extrapolated evidence from studies rated as 1++ or 1+

C   A body of evidence including studies rated as 2+, directly applicable to the target population, and demonstrating overall consistency of results, OR extrapolated evidence from studies rated as 2++

D   Evidence levels 3 or 4, OR extrapolated evidence from studies rated as 2+, or expert opinion

APPENDIX **13H**

Heart Failure Education Packet

Julie C. Freeman, MSN, RN
University of South Alabama
College of Nursing

Table of Contents

Section One: What Is Heart Failure?
Section Two: Warning Signs and Symptoms and Whom to Contact
Section Three: Weighing Every Day
Section Four: Your Medication
Section Five: Diet
Section Six: Activity
Section Seven: Questions for My Healthcare Provider

Section One: What Is Heart Failure?

The diagnosis of heart failure does not mean that your heart has stopped functioning or that your heart is about to stop functioning. Heart failure does mean that you will need to make changes to your lifestyle because heart failure is a very serious health problem that requires medical care.

Heart failure is a condition in which the heart muscle is unable to pump enough blood throughout the body to meet the needs required.

Sometimes the heart is unable to fill with enough blood to pump throughout the body. In some patients, the heart muscle is unable to produce enough force to move the blood throughout the rest of the body. Some patients have a problem with the heart muscle's strength to pump the blood and the heart's ability to fill with blood.

Heart failure occurs over a period of time because the heart muscle loses the ability to pump as strongly. Heart failure may affect the right side of the heart only, or heart failure can affect both sides of the heart. Most patients with heart failure have involvement of both the right and left side of the heart.

The right side of the heart experiences heart failure when the heart cannot pump enough blood to the lungs to pick up oxygen. The left side heart of the heart experiences failure when the heart cannot pump enough of the oxygen-rich blood to the rest of the body.

If you have right-side heart failure, you may have fluid collect in your feet, ankles, legs, liver, abdomen, and the veins in your neck. Both right-side and left-side heart failure can cause shortness of breath and fatigue (tiredness).

Coronary artery disease, high blood pressure, and diabetes are diseases that contribute to a patient developing heart failure.

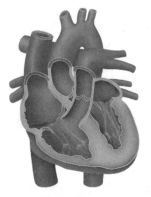
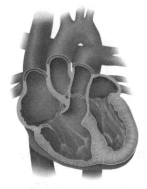

Healthy Heart   Congested Heart

Section Two: Warning Signs and Symptoms and Whom to Contact

Remember FACES

Fatigue
- Feeling very tired
- Having less energy
- Needing more rest periods than usual

Activities
- Unable to perform usual activities around home
- Unable to perform usual errands outside of home

Chest congestion/cough
- Frequent dry, hacking cough

Edema
- Weight gain of 3 pounds in 1 day
- Weight gain of 5 pounds in 1 week
- More swelling in your stomach, legs, ankles, and feet

Shortness of breath
- Difficulty breathing while performing usual activities
- Waking up from sleep with shortness of breath
- Unable to lie flat to sleep
- Use three or more pillows to sleep

Who do I call if I have any of the warning signs?

Healthcare provider: _____

Phone number: _____

Emergency department: _____

Immediate assistance: 911

Section Three: Weighing Every Day

Gaining weight is often one of the first warning signs that your heart is having more difficulty pumping blood throughout your body. When you have heart failure you must:

- Weigh yourself every day
- Weigh at the same time of day

- Many patients find it best to weigh when they wake up in the morning
- Weigh in the same type of clothes
  - Weighing in the morning in the same type and weight of clothes such as a nightgown or pajamas
- Weigh on the same scales
  - This is important because it will be the most accurate weight

Weighing yourself in this manner allows you to keep a closer eye on whether you are maintaining your weight at the weight your healthcare provider believes is best for you.

Record your weights in a log like the one that follows. Record any swelling in your feet, ankles, or abdomen. Write down how you felt that day in the comments section, such as felt good, short of breath or winded, tired, or sleepy.

Date	Weight	Swelling in Feet, Ankles, or Abdomen (Please Circle)	Comments
		New Same More	
		New Same More	
		New Same More	
		New Same More	
		New Same More	
		New Same More	
		New Same More	

Section Four: Your Medication

List your current medications according to the date they are prescribed below. Also note the name of the prescribing physician and any changes that are made in the dosage.

Date Medication Prescribed	Prescribing Physician	Date Dosage Changed

Section Five: Diet

You should eat foods that are low in salt (sodium). Some types of foods that are low in salt include fresh fruit and vegetables. Some examples of fresh or frozen fruit you can eat include oranges, bananas, grapes, and apples. Some examples of fresh or frozen vegetables you can eat include green beans, broccoli, cauliflower, corn, and collard and turnip greens unless you have been told these vegetables will interfere with the medications you take. You may eat canned fruits and vegetables if you check the sodium content on the label or choose canned products labeled as low sodium.

Food that has a lot of salt will cause you to gain fluid weight. This extra fluid makes your heart work harder. Limit foods that have a lot of salt such as salty snacks. Examples of salty snacks include potato chips, popcorn, and pretzels. You should not eat cured meats, such as bacon, ham, sausages, or smoked meats. You should not eat vegetables such as olives, pickles, or pickled okra. This includes any foods prepared in a brine solution.

Sometimes salt is hidden in foods such as canned fruits or vegetables, diet sodas, and prepackaged or fast foods. Learn to look at the nutrition label on packaged and canned foods so that you have an idea of the amount of salt the food contains. Keep the salt shaker away from the table and do not add extra salt when cooking. You may try some of the nonsalt substitutes if you like.

It is best if you eat lean meat such as fish or chicken. Eat three to four servings of fresh or frozen vegetables and fruit each day.

NUTRITION LABEL

Look on the nutrition labels to find the amount of salt (sodium) in the food you plan to buy.

Serving Size
This tells you what amount equals one serving of the product. Every other nutrient value listed on the label is based on this amount.

Calories
Calories are a unit of energy. Calories in food come from carbohydrates, protein, and fat. Because calories give us energy, we need them to be able to think and be active.

% Daily Value
This tells you the percentage of the recommended daily value for a nutrient that you get in one serving. A food that has more than 20% of the Daily Value of a certain nutrient is a good source of that nutrient.

Cholesterol
Cholesterol is a substance found only in animal products. Eating too much cholesterol is not healthy for your heart.

Total Carbohydrate
Carbohydrates give your muscles and brain energy. Certain types of carbohydrates are sometimes listed on the label.

Fiber: Helps with digestion and keeps you full between meals.

Sugars: Give you instant energy, but eating too much added sugar can be unhealthy.

Nutrition Facts

Serving Size
Servings per Container

Amount per serving
Calories   Calories from Fat

                         % Daily value*
Total Fat
    Saturated Fat
    Trans Fat
    Polyunsaturated Fat
    Monounsaturated Fat
Cholesterol
Sodium
Total Carbohydrate
    Dietary Fiber
    Sugars
Protein
Vitamin A   Vitamin C
Calcium   Iron

*Percent Daily Values are based on a 2,000 calorie diet. Your daily values may be higher or lower depending on your caloric needs:

		Calories	2,000	2,500
Total Fat	Less than	65g	80g
Sat. Fat	Less than	20g	25g
Cholesterol	Less than	300mg	300mg
Sodium	Less than	2,400mg	2,400mg
Total Carbohydrates		300g	375g
Dietary Fiber		25g	30g

Calories per gram:
Fat 9 • Carbohydrate 4 • Protein 4

Footnote
This reminds us that all of the Daily Values come from the recommendations for a 2,000-calorie meal plan. Your needs may be higher or lower based on your height, genetics, and activity level. Keep in mind this is just an average, these daily value percentages (%) are not for everyone.

Servings Per Container
This tells you how many servings you can get from one package. Some containers have a single serving, but most have more than one serving per package.

Calories from Fat
This is the number of calories that come from fat. It is not the percent of fat in the food.

Total Fat
Fat is essential in our bodies. There are 4 kinds of fat. Monounsaturated and polyunsaturated fat are the kinds of fat that are heart healthy. These kinds of fat may not be included on the food label. Saturated fat and *trans* fat are unhealthy for your heart, and should be limited.

Sodium
Sodium tells you how much salt is in the food. People with high blood pressure are sometimes told to follow a low sodium diet.

Protein
This nutrient is used to build muscle and fight infections.

Vitamins/Minerals
This tells you the percent Daily Value for vitamin A, vitamin C, calcium, and iron you are getting from this product. Other vitamins and minerals may be included in this section.

Source: ©Center for Young Women's Health, Boston Children's Hospital. All rights reserved. Used with permission. http://www.youngwomenshealth.org

Section Six: Activity

It is important to keep moving! Our physical therapists will pay you a visit to evaluate your level of activity and to work with you. Your activity level should be guided by how you feel each day. But it is important to remember that staying active will help you stay strong and keep your joints flexible, and it can help reduce feelings of sadness. So, try to perform some activities of daily living each day.

It is best to begin with small levels of activity and add more as you are able to tolerate it. For example, one day you may not feel like dressing, but you can bathe or shower. If you do not feel well enough to bathe or shower then wash your face and brush your hair and teeth.

You need to understand that you may feel different each day of the week, but taking your medication as prescribed, staying as active as possible, and eating a proper diet can all help you feel stronger. Feeling stronger will help you to be more active every day.

Section Seven: Questions for My Healthcare Provider

Circle any of the areas listed below and write notes to remember what to discuss with your healthcare provider.

I have questions about:

My medication. _____

My test results. _____

My level of pain. _____

Feeling stressed. _____

Other questions or concerns. _____

Resources

American Heart Association. (2009). *Target heart failure: Taking the failure out of heart failure.* Retrieved from http://www.heart.org/idc /groups/heart-public/@wcm/@private/@hcm/@gwtg/documents /downloadable/ucm_310295.pdf

Bouffard, L. D. (2011). Nursing management: Heart failure. In S. L. Lewis, S. R. Dirksen, M. M. Heitkemper, & L. Bucher (Eds)., *Medical-surgical nursing: Assessment and management of clinical problems* (8th ed., pp. 797–817). St. Louis: MO. Elsevier Mosby.

Institute for Healthcare Improvement. (2008). *How-to guide: Improved care for patients with congestive heart failure.* Retrieved from http:// www.ihi.org/knowledge/Pages/Tools/HowtoGuideImprovedCarefor- PatientswithCongestiveHeartFailure.aspx

Institute for Healthcare Improvement. (2010). *Transforming care at the bedside: How-to guide: Creating an ideal transition home for patients with heart failure.* Retrieved from http://www.ihi.org/knowledge /Pages/Tools/TCABHowToGuideTransitionHomeforHF.aspx

Jack, B. W., Chetty, V. K., Anthony, D., Greenwald, J. L., Sanchez, G. M., Forsythe, S. R., . . . Culpepper, L. (2009). A reengineered hospital discharge program to decrease rehospitalization: A randomized trial. *Annals of Internal Medicine, 150*(3), 178–187. Retrieved from http://annals.org/

National Institutes of Health. (2011). *What is heart failure?* National Heart, Lung, and Blood Institute. Retrieved from http://www.nhlbi .nih.gov/health/health-topics/topics/hf/

Neilsen, G. A., Barteley, A., Coleman, E., Resar, R., Rutherford, P., Souw, D., & Taylor, J. (2008). *Transforming care at the bedside how-to guide: Creating an ideal transition home for patients with heart failure.* Retrieved from http://www.ihi.org

Telephone Survey

Date, time, and person conducting the telephone survey: _____
_____

Please tell me how you weigh yourself:

- Weigh yourself every day
- Weigh at the same time of day
  - Many patients find it best to weigh when they wake up in the morning.
- Weigh in the same type of clothes
  - Weighing in the morning in the same type and weight of clothes such as a nightgown or pajamas
- Weigh on the same scales
  - This is important because it will be the most accurate weight

Are you keeping a written record of your daily weights? Yes _____ No _____

If not, why? _____

Please name three warning signs that you should report to your primary care provider. Remember FACES.

Fatigue
- Feeling very tired
- Having less energy
- Needing more rest periods than usual
Activities
- Unable to perform usual activities around home
- Unable to perform usual errands outside of home

Chest congestion/cough
- Frequent dry, hacking cough

Edema
- Weight gain of 3 pounds in 1 day
- Weight gain of 5 pounds in 1 week
- More swelling in your stomach, legs, ankles, and feet

Shortness of breath
- Difficulty breathing while performing usual activities
- Waking up from sleep with shortness of breath
- Unable to lie flat to sleep
- Use three or more pillows to sleep

Please tell me who you will contact if you have warning signs and symptoms:

Healthcare provider: _____
Phone number: _____

Please name three food items that you should avoid:

1. _____
2. _____
3. _____

Please tell me why you need to eat a diet low in salt/sodium:

Food that has a lot of salt will make me gain fluid weight.
The extra fluid makes my heart work harder.
Other: _____.

What are the date, time, and location for your follow-up appointment? Does this match the discharge summary?

Date: _____
Time: _____
Location: _____
With: _____

Balance Scorecard

Customers/Partners

| Reengineer discharge processes to reduce readmission | → | Improve selfmanagement of heart failure |

Improved financial resources due to the potential savings of $2,500 to $4,000 per patient not readmitted within 30 days

Financial

| HF core measures reduce readmission rate of HF patients | → | Reduce nonreimbursable charges |

Intervention/Internal Processes

| Improve discharge processes | ↔ | Better patient understanding | ↔ | Improve compliance with IOM aims to provide efficient, effective, patient-centered care and meet core measures |

Organization Capacity

| Cohesive discharge process followed by staff | ↔ | Interdisciplinary collaboration | ↔ | Improve staff knowledge/buy-in regarding compliance with core measures through staff education |

APPENDIX **13K**

Evaluation Grid

Goal for Quality Improvement Project	IOM Aims	Benchmark (CMS)	Method of Measurement		Data Collection and Timeline	Evaluation Method	Data Display
			Numerator	Denominator			
No readmission for heart failure (HF) within 30 days of discharge	Safe Effective Timely Efficient Equitable Patient-centered	100% no readmission for HF within 30 days	Number of patients readmitted within 30 days with HF	Number of patients admitted within the 30-day period	Retrospective review of medical records after completion of quality improvement (QI) project	Quantitative Benchmark met for February/March: No 30-day readmissions Summative Retrospective review of number of patients d/c with dx of HF and 30-day review for readmission in February/March	Bar graph
Standardization of discharge education	Safe Effective Timely Efficient Equitable Patient-centered	100% of patients to be provided with scripted HF discharge education	Number of patients receiving the scripted discharge education during the QI project	Number of patients admitted with HF during the QI project	Follow-up telephone survey within 72 hours to determine the discharge education was provided and retrospective review of medical records after completion of QI project	Summative Quantitative Documentation that 44 notebooks were given out in February/March but only two patients received the telephone survey; one phone number was a fax machine; seven patients did not answer the phone Qualitative	Pie chart

Retention of discharge education	Safe Effective Timely Efficient Equitable Patient-centered	100% better self-management of HF through discharge education	Number of patients able to identify specific criteria asked through the telephone survey and number of patients unable to identify specific criteria asked through the telephone survey	Number of patients admitted with HF during the QI project	Follow-up telephone survey within 72 hours to evaluate retention of discharge education (See telephone survey)	Summative Barriers were present preventing follow-up for each patient Of the 44 notebooks provided in February/ March, 2 patients received the telephone survey; 1 phone number was a fax machine; 7 patients did not answer the phone Qualitative One survey indicated the notebook was only partially covered by staff	Bar graph

Notes: d/c = discharge; dx = diagnosis.

CHAPTER 14

A Community–Academic Collaboration to Impact Childhood Obesity

Lois "Ginny" Langham

OBJECTIVES

After review of this material, a reader should be able to:

1. Discuss the incidence of childhood obesity in rural areas of Alabama.
2. Identify an appropriate BMI for a child.
3. Define the terms "overweight" and "underweight" for a child.

Abstract

Healthcare professionals are challenged with reversing the current childhood obesity epidemic as well as preventing its occurrence among future generations. This paper describes a community–academic partnership that implemented clinical guidelines in a medically underserved elementary school in Alabama. Quantitative and qualitative evaluation methods, pretests, posttests, health screenings, and surveys were used to establish a screening and prevention program and to create a collaboration between a rural county school system and a local school of nursing university.

Outcomes indicate this evidence-based, multipronged approach may accelerate the progress toward the prevention of childhood obesity.

Alabama's youth have an alarming obesity rate of 17% with a national comparison rate of 13.6% in 2011 within the United States (Centers for Disease Control and Prevention [CDC], 2012d; n.d.). Trending data of the past 30 years have revealed a tripling of childhood obesity rates and its prominence as the most common nutritional problem among the pediatric population (Alabama Department of Public Health [ADPH], 2005; CDC, 2012c). Alabama is currently ranked among the top four states in the prevalence of adult obesity at 32% (CDC, 2012a). The World Health Organization ([WHO], 2012) has estimated that over 300 million adults worldwide are presently obese and that the United States ranks first globally as having the highest incidence of obesity. According to recent literature, childhood obesity is often a precursor to adult obesity; obese children are at higher risk of developing comorbidities such as heart disease, stroke, diabetes and arthritis; and that school-based interventions are effective (American Academy of Pediatrics [AAP], 2005; CDC, 2011d, 2012c; Institute of Medicine [IOM], 2012a; Nihiser et al., 2009; Peterson & Fox, 2007; WHO, 2012). Consequently, numerous organizations and agencies have identified the need to address this significant public health issue. The steady rise of obesity rates has challenged healthcare professionals with reversing the current obesity epidemic, as well as preventing its occurrence among future generations.

A quality improvement project was designed to establish a community partnership among public school leaders, school nurses, and a university nursing program to provide childhood obesity screenings and a health educational intervention for third graders in a rural, medically underserved Alabama elementary school. The goals of this collaborative endeavor were to address childhood obesity by establishing a screening and prevention program and to create an ongoing community–academic partnership between a rural county school system and a local school of nursing. The foundation of this project was designed to incorporate clinical protocols and guidelines into the public school system through the utilization of baccalaureate nursing students to augment the heavy workloads of public school nurses in identifying obese children and those at risk for obesity. Additionally, the promotion of healthy living habits was emphasized in an age-appropriate health education-teaching program.

The purpose of this paper is to describe and explore the development and implementation of this quality improvement project.

Background

In 2001, the Institute of Medicine (IOM) published a critical account of substandard health care entitled, *Crossing the Quality Chasm: A New Health System for the 21st Century*. Despite technological progress and significant advances within health sciences, the provision of patient care was considered to be of poor quality (Stevens, McDuffie & Clutter, 2009). As a result, a fundamental transformation of the U.S. healthcare system began to occur in an attempt to improve quality of care. The IOM (2001) identified six areas of emphasis: safety, effectiveness, patient-centeredness, timeliness, efficiency, and equity. When one or more of the IOM aims are integrated within an improvement program, the efficacy and value are strengthened. The quality improvement initiative described herein is based upon a framework of effectiveness, timeliness, and equity.

The *effectiveness* goal is aimed at the identification of treatments that result in improved patient outcomes (IOM, 2001). This goal is supported in the quality improvement project through the integration of clinical guidelines regarding annual childhood obesity screenings as recommended by the AAP (2005), the CDC (2011a), and the United States Preventive Services Task Force ([USPSTF], 2010). Annual obesity screenings in children can help track weight status while also providing longitudinal data. Additionally, the development of community–academic partnerships has shown promising potential in promoting health behaviors and healthy choices among children (Agency for Healthcare Research and Quality, 2010; American School Health Association, 2011; CDC, 2005, 2008, 2009; IOM, 2004, 2006, 2012b; Jayaratne, Kelaher, & Dunt, 2010; Lesser & Oscor-Sanchez, 2007; Teutsch & Briss, 2005). Furthermore, any combination of these factors increases the likelihood of positive outcomes (Gonzalez-Suarez, Worley, Grimmer-Somers, & Dones, 2009; Lavelle, Mackay, & Pell, 2012; Peterson & Fox, 2007). Indeed, a comprehensive approach would appear warranted given the magnitude of the issue. Through an analysis of evidence, the most effective methods can be translated into practice and thereby address many of the *Healthy People*

2020 leading healthcare initiatives (United States Department of Health and Human Services [USDHHS], 2012).

The *timeliness* aim is targeted toward providing appropriate patient care without harmful delays (IOM, 2001). Healthcare treatments are centered upon evidence provided through scientific research. There is often a delay, however, in the implementation of the most current evidence to the patient bedside. Lavelle and colleagues (2012) asserted that if children learn healthy habits early in life, there is a greater likelihood that maintenance of these behaviors will continue into adulthood. Conversely, Lavelle et al. (2012) also concluded that if children learn unhealthy eating habits, there is a greater likelihood of obesity and other health problems to be present in adulthood. Efforts have been made to concentrate on interventions targeting the population of children due to the steadily rising childhood obesity rates and because obesity increases the risk of numerous other comorbidities. Moreover, WHO (2000, 2012) has identified a public health approach to obesity prevention as one of the most effective strategies. The timeliness aim is supported through recognition that early intervention can yield more positive outcomes regarding childhood obesity.

The *equity* aim is targeted at providing high quality care to everyone regardless of gender, socioeconomic status, ethnicity, or geographic location (IOM, 2001). All 67 counties of Alabama have been designated as medically underserved areas and/or being composed of medically underserved populations (USDHHS, n.d.). Documented factors that negatively impact the health of local rural residents include a lack of healthcare providers, limited personal transportation, inadequate public transportation, and lack of health insurance (ADPH, 2007, n.d.b). The equity aim is supported in the quality improvement project by the provision of health screenings and education to rural, medically underserved elementary school children.

An examination of Alabama public schools revealed that 67 county school systems and 65 city school systems comprised 1,499 total public schools for the 2011–12 school year with an enrollment of nearly 745,000 students (Alabama State Department of Education, 2012). During that period, the Alabama Department of Education employed 1,381 full-time nurses to provide health services for all public school children. This included 815 registered nurses (RNs) and 566 licensed practical nurses

(LPNs). The resulting state ratio is one school nurse for every 539 students. Initially, this would seem a satisfactory ratio given the federal recommendation of one school nurse for every 750 students (CDC, 2011d). However, the ratios widely vary when extrapolated among the numerous county and city school systems.

School nurses are challenged with daily responsibilities that include medication administration, the management of chronic disease, the creation and ongoing maintenance of individual student health records, providing emergency care for illness or injury of students and school personnel, the prevention and control of communicable diseases and other health conditions, health education, and providing counseling opportunities (National Association of School Nurses, 2011). With the additional federal requirements for scoliosis screenings, the maintenance of immunization records, and the increasingly complex medical issues of students, the school nurse has little time to incorporate teaching and individual counseling sessions into the daily schedule.

A selected Alabama county public school system currently operates 15 schools with an enrollment of over 11,000 students within 5 rural communities. Twelve school nurses are employed with a resulting ratio of 1 nurse for every 916 students, well under the CDC's recommendation of 1:750 (CDC, 2011d). With unrelenting annual reductions in funding, public agencies continue to struggle in finding ways to make every education dollar stretch further in order to provide current services. The resulting impact has created a devastating perfect storm among state programs. Mandatory decreases in state funding have caused many school systems to lay off school nurses and impose hiring freezes. Increased numbers of children with special healthcare needs are being mainstreamed into the public school classroom. Additionally, the recent general downturn of the economy has forced many parents to withdraw children from private school and enroll them in public schools. Consequently, fewer school nurses are faced with caring for greater numbers of children who have a wider variety of health issues than ever before.

A baccalaureate school of nursing in close proximity to the county school system recently experienced a change in curriculum that resulted in an increased need for pediatric and population-based clinical experiences. Additionally, the university identified the need to actively search for community outreach opportunities. Meetings with potential stakeholders from the county school system and the school of nursing were successful in garnering support for the quality improvement project. Key personnel involved in these meetings included the county assistant superintendent, the school nurse coordinator, the principal and teachers of a selected elementary school, as well as the associate dean, faculty, and nursing students of the university. Numerous follow-up meetings ensued to review existing school health data, to dialogue about the obesity status among the rural county public school children, and to present evidence-based strategies in addressing childhood obesity. A needs assessment revealed that no aggregate student data was tracked by the school system. Additionally, a desire was noted within the school system to address childhood obesity, yet a sense of powerlessness prevailed. Despite possessing adequate information, knowledge, and recognition of obesity's long-term significance, no attempts to address the clinical health issue within the school system had been made. A contextual issue existed in this rural population regarding a lack of community resources and a lack of community collaboration. The patterns of need that emerged revealed gaps of provided healthcare services to children, especially regarding obesity screening.

The measurement of an individual's body mass index (BMI) is the most common method utilized to assess weight status (CDC, 2012b). In the pediatric population, however, BMI fluctuates with age and is gender specific. The variances between adult and pediatric BMIs necessitate the determination of BMI-for-age percentiles among children and adolescents (CDC, 2011a). This process involves plotting data on either a girl's or boy's CDC BMI-for-age growth chart (CDC, 2000). Percentiles are used to compare a child's BMI among children of the same sex and age. The weight status categories reflected on the CDC growth charts for children and teens are underweight, healthy weight, overweight, and obese (CDC, 2011a). For children aged 2–19 years of age, *underweight* is defined as a BMI less than the 5th percentile; *healthy weight* is defined as a BMI at or above the 5th percentile and lower than the 85th percentile; *overweight* is defined as a BMI at or above the 85th percentile and less than the 95th percentile; and *obese* is defined as a BMI equal to or greater than the 95th percentile for children of the same age and sex (Barlow et al., 2007; CDC, 2011a).

The AAP (2005), the CDC (2011a), and the USPSTF (2010) recommend annual obesity screenings for children over 2 years of age. An assumption may exist that children will receive such screenings at yearly checkups with their primary care physician; yet, in rural areas, many children lack such a provider and frequently receive services from the county public health department. Despite recommendations from pediatric experts for annual obesity screenings, adherence may be problematic for rural populations.

An opportunity exists for evidenced-based healthcare interventions to be implemented within school settings, as children are present for up to 6 hours a day, two daily meals are served, and physical education classes are conducted (Benjamins & Whitman, 2010; CDC, 2011d; Gonzalez-Suarez et al., 2009; Kanekar & Sharma, 2008; Lavelle et al., 2012; Luttikhuis et al., 2009; Peterson & Fox, 2007; Sharma, 2006). Early interventions are significant and have proven to greatly reduce the incidence of complex health issues associated with a sedentary lifestyle, poor nutrition, and obesity (AAP, 2005). Literature has shown that the promotion, encouragement, and implementation of physical activities along with the use of nutritional education can make an impact on obesity levels (Benjamins & Whitman, 2010; CDC, 2011d; Gonzalez-Suarez et al., 2009; Lavelle et al., 2012; Luttikhuis et al., 2009; Peterson & Fox, 2007; Sharma, 2006). Recommendations for interventions include strategies that increase knowledge of dietary significance, increase fruit and vegetable intake, limit fat intake, decrease consumption of fast food, increase awareness of portion sizes, and increase daily water intake. The United States Department of Agriculture ([USDA], 2012b) updated school meal nutrition standards to include more whole-grain products, less processed foods, and more varieties of fruits and vegetables. Continued adherence to providing healthy food options through the cafeteria in schools will help address the childhood obesity epidemic.

Project Overview

Noninvasive health screenings were provided to third graders in a rural, underserved elementary school. The screenings consisted of height, weight, BMI-for-age, BMI percentile, and blood pressure measurements. A short pretest was administered regarding current knowledge and awareness of nutrition, physical activity, and healthy behaviors. A health teaching program, lasting approximately 30 minutes, was presented by baccalaureate nursing students along with an interactive game. After

10 weeks, a posttest was administered to assess knowledge retention, and the health screenings were repeated. The aim was to positively impact child health, utilizing an IOM framework of quality improvement strategies. Additionally, a collaboration survey was administered to stakeholders of the public school system and the school of nursing at the completion of the project.

Method

The project was completed using a descriptive study design involving a retrospective review as well as the collection and analysis of information obtained through health screenings and a pretest/posttest. Participants were third graders of a selected elementary school. Following the distribution of parental information/permission forms to 6 third grade classes, 45% ($n = 57$) of the forms were signed and returned. Participants included 32 males and 25 females ranging from 8 to 9 years of age. Inclusion criteria encompassed any child enrolled in the third grade at the selected elementary school, English literacy and a signed parental consent form. Exclusion criteria included any child with known identified special needs such as a high-acuity health issue. Public school administrators and the elementary school principal granted permission for the project to be implemented at the selected location. Parents and participants were provided with written correspondence, which included the purposes of the project, a detailed description of the process, that participation was voluntary, and that confidentiality would be maintained.

The health teaching program, which focused on childhood obesity prevention, was developed in conjunction with expert guidelines and recommendations (AAP, 2005; CDC, 2011a; USDA, 2012b; USDA & USDHHS, 2010; USPSTF, 2010). Topics of the program included an explanation and description of calories, the importance of water to our bodies, examples of healthy/unhealthy food choices, risk factors of heart disease, and an explanation of aerobic exercise with an active component that required students to engage in a series of structured physical exercises. The program concluded with tips on being a healthy kid: choose to eat healthier foods, increase physical activity, eat a nutritious breakfast, and reduce time watching television and playing computer/video games.

Additionally, an interactive game entitled, "Let's Go Shopping" was created and implemented. A long table was covered with a red and white checked tablecloth and filled with a variety of simulated food items such as meats, fruits, vegetables, pizza, potato chips, and desserts. Several third graders were given a plastic grocery bag and instructed to "go shopping" and select three healthy food items. Following their selections, the bags were inspected and, as a group, dialogue occurred about what they picked and why. This provided an opportunity to discuss healthy vs. unhealthy options in a nonthreatening environment.

When calculating BMI and BMI for age for large groups of children, the CDC has developed an effective and helpful instrument. The Children's BMI Tool for Schools is an Excel spreadsheet and database for date of birth, sex, height, weight, and date of measurement (CDC, 2011b). This tool was utilized during the project. All collected data was coded and password protected to ensure confidentiality. Local agencies were contacted to assist in providing health-related items to the students as a means of positive reinforcement. Participants received treat bags containing donated items such as pencils, toothbrushes, temporary tattoos, and stickers.

Data Collection

Data collection began in a semisecluded area outside of the school's gymnasium. The screenings were performed one homeroom at a time with an average cohort of 8–10 students per class with a total of 57 participants. The third graders were escorted to the screening area with a signed parental consent form in hand as the "ticket" to enter the scheduled event. After a greeting and brief explanation of the agenda, the pretest was administered. Upon completion, the students rotated to one of two stations for height, weight, and blood pressure measurement. While awaiting their turn to be screened, participants interacted with nursing students who utilized visual teaching aids of food portion replicas and body fat/muscle replicas to briefly dialogue about healthy behaviors. Each assessment station was positioned behind privacy screens. Participants received a verbal explanation of the screening process. If a student was wearing shoes that could provide a false measurement of height (for example, high heels), he/she was asked to remove them prior to screening procedures. Stadiometers and digital weight scales were utilized by nursing students for height and weight measurement. Blood pressure readings were obtained with manual sphygmomanometers. Questionable readings were verified by the project leader. Abnormal findings of BMI-for-age percentiles or blood pressures were reported to the school nurse and the county school nurse coordinator for follow-up. The project leader entered individual data into the database. When all students within the group had been screened, the health teaching program was administered by the nursing students, and the "Let's Go Shopping" game was played. When these activities were concluded, the participants returned to class, and another set of participating students were escorted to the screening area. Individual measurements were documented on a parental notification letter that included explanations of the measurements following noted recommendation guidelines (CDC, 2011a, 2011b; Hockenberry & Wilson, 2009).

After 10 weeks, baccalaureate nursing students returned to the elementary school and administered a posttest to the participating third graders in order to assess knowledge retention. Additionally, the health screenings were repeated (height, weight, BMI for age, BMI percentile and blood pressure), utilizing the previously described procedure. Again, the project leader entered individual data into the Children's BMI Tool for Schools. Abnormal findings of BMI-for-age percentiles or blood pressures were reported to the school nurse coordinator for follow-up. The referral criteria for BMI-for-age percentiles were based on the CDC's guidelines of weight status categories (CDC, 2011a; 2011b). Hockenberry and Wilson (2009) provided the pediatric blood pressure referral criterion utilized in the project.

The pretest/posttest was composed of 12 multiple choice questions regarding healthy behaviors, foods, and physical activities as shown in **Appendix 14A**. Additionally, 4 items captured demographic information. Questions on the pretest/posttest were adapted from materials published by the USDA (2012b) and the partnership of the USDA with the USDHHS (2010). The test items are specifically aimed at empowering youth regarding nutrition and physical activity.

Appendix 14B depicts the survey utilized to measure the effectiveness of collaboration and stakeholder satisfaction. The survey is composed of 13 statements that utilize a Likert scale of 1–7, with 1 representing strongly disagree and 7 representing strongly agree. These measurements are an adaptation of the Levels of Collaboration scale developed by Frey,

Lohmeier, Lee, and Tollefson (2006). The tool allowed participating stake-holders to rate their partners on levels of collaboration and corresponding attributes in order to gauge overall satisfaction of the project and willing-ness to continue the community–academic partnership.

Data Analysis

The IBM SPSS Statistics Version 20 software was utilized to analyze results from the pretest and posttest. The Children's BMI Tool for Schools devel-oped by the CDC (2011b) was utilized to compare the 2 sets of anthropo-metric measurements of height, weight, BMI for age, BMI percentile, and blood pressure. All 57 participants were present on each day of the screen-ings. At the conclusion of the project, each of the key stakeholders willingly participated in the collaboration survey and the results were assessed ($n = 5$).

Results

A paired t-test was used to compare the number of correct responses on the pretest and posttest composed of 12 multiple choice questions. There was a significant difference in the correct responses on the pretest (M = 30.17, SD = 14.17) and the correct responses on the posttest (M = 42.08, SD = 11.94); $t(11) = 4.07$, $p = 0.002$. The mean percent of change for cor-rect responses was 39.45% among the 57 participants. These results sug-gest that the obesity prevention program had a positive impact on the knowledge level and retention of third graders regarding healthy behav-iors and nutrition.

An analysis of the BMI-for-age measurements also revealed an overall improvement. The prevalence of children in the overweight category was reduced from 19% to 18%; with the incidence of those in the obese cat-egory decreased from 7% to 5%. A further difference was noted, however, upon an examination by gender of prevalence of overweight and obesity. The baseline measurements disclosed 19% of males and 20% of females in the overweight category; with 6% of males and 8% of females within the obese category. After 10 weeks, the repeated screenings resulted in 13% of males and 24% of females in the overweight category; and 6% of males and 4% of females in the obese category as shown in **Table 14-1**.

TABLE 14-1 Summary of Children's BMI for Age Preimplementation and Postimplementation

	Boys Preimplementation	Boys Postimplementation	Girls Preimplementation	Girls Postimplementation	Total Preimplementation	Total Postimplementation
Number of children assessed	32	32	25	25	57	57
Underweight (< 5th percentile)	9%	9%	4%	4%	7%	7%
Healthy weight (5th–85th percentile)	72%	78%	76%	72%	74%	75%
Overweight or obese (≥ 85th percentile)*	19%	13%	20%	24%	19%	18%
Obese (≥ 95th percentile)	6%	6%	8%	4%	7%	5%

*Terminology based on: Barlow, S. E and the Expert Committee. (2007). Expert committee recommendations regarding the prevention, assessment, and treatment of child and adolescent overweight and obesity: Summary report. *Pediatrics*, *120*(suppl 4), s164–s192.

Modified from Centers for Disease Control and Prevention. (2011b). *Children's BMI tool for schools: Assessing your weight.* Retrieved from http://www.cdc.gov/healthyweight/assessing /bmi/childrens_BMI/tool_for_schools.html

The third grade students reported learning valuable information and appeared to enjoy interacting with the nursing students. Many questions were asked about college, and the nursing students took the opportunity to emphasize the importance of earning good grades and completing high school. Because several of the participating nursing students were male, comments were overheard from the third graders such as, "I didn't know boys could be nurses." Potential long-term results could impact not only health outcomes but education and career outcomes as well. The third grade teachers reported that nonparticipating students enviously expressed sentiments such as, "I wish my mom had signed my permission form!" The teachers, principal, and school nurse coordinator verbalized appreciation for the establishment of an effective collaboration and the forthcoming assistance in addressing an important health issue that had been, heretofore, out of reach. The baccalaureate nursing students overwhelmingly expressed positive comments and recommended that the activity be continued for other nursing students. According to the collaboration survey, 100% of the respondents ($n = 5$) reported the alliance produced positive influences on their organization, expressed a strong desire to continue the partnership, and indicated strong overall satisfaction regarding the project. Such approaches support the emergence of community collaborations and partnerships as a potentially successful strategy in implementing healthcare interventions and improving health outcomes (American Public Health Association, 2010; American School Health Association, 2011; Carney, Maltby, Mackin, & Maksym, 2011; CDC, 2005, 2008, 2009; IOM, 2004, 2006, 2012c, 2012d; Peterson & Fox, 2007; Resnick et al., 2009; Teutsch & Briss, 2005).

Value Propositions

The direct monetary cost to implement the quality improvement project was minimal. Nondisposable items such as weight scales, stadiometers, blood pressure cuffs, stethoscopes, and privacy screens can be purchased for approximately $850.00. However, the county school system and the university school of nursing already possessed these items and were willing to donate their use for this project. Both partners also donated disposable supplies including gloves and copy paper as well as making needed copies of permission forms and parental notification letters.

Potential monetary benefits from the project include a major reduction in healthcare costs. Healthcare costs for obese individuals are at least $1,429.00 more per year than for nonobese individuals (CDC, 2010). It has been estimated that an annual amount of $263 billion in healthcare costs is associated with obesity and diabetes (CDC, 2010, 2011c). The foremost cause of death in Alabama is heart disease, and it results in more than 12,000 deaths annually (ADPH, 2007, 2010). The prevalence of modifiable risk factors for cardiovascular disease is significant in Alabama with 27.2 % of adults being affected by hypertension, 12.2% by diabetes, and 32% by obesity (ADPH, 2007, 2010; CDC, 2012a). If fewer children entered adulthood with obesity, hypertension and/or diabetes, a significant savings in annual healthcare costs could be achieved.

Nonmonetary potential benefits include the positive promotion of healthy behaviors, increased awareness of nutrition and exercise, and the assurance of current and accurate health education. Another benefit would be improved health choices and behaviors of children resulting in a fewer number entering adulthood with health concerns. Furthermore, Alabama has identified a need to improve rural health outcomes, partly due to a high prevalence of mortality related to diabetes and heart disease (ADPH, 2007, n.d.a). The implementation of interventions that promote healthy behaviors and lifestyles can be seen as a nonmonetary benefit for such rural and underserved populations.

The successful implementation of the quality improvement project resulted in positive outcomes for all stakeholders involved. For the public school system, advantages included the assistance for overburdened school nurses, the identification of obese children and those at risk, and the potential for improved child health outcomes. Participation by the school of nursing yielded benefits that include pediatric and population-based clinical experiences for baccalaureate nursing students, increased skill competence and confidence of nursing students, outreach and research opportunities for nursing faculty, and an increased school of nursing presence within the community. Advantages for the community included increased knowledge and awareness of healthy behaviors among children, increased parental awareness of child health issues, potential decrease and/or prevention of childhood obesity, and improved overall health of community. The project plan is a mutually beneficial endeavor that meets resource needs of school nurses, meets health needs of a vulnerable population, and meets learning needs of nursing students.

Limitations

One limitation of the project included the small number of participants. The target population of third graders at a selected elementary school was made up of 126 students among 6 classes. Of those, 57 permission forms were returned. It is the researcher's observation that utilization of the term *childhood obesity* within the permission form may have hindered some parents from allowing their children to participate. Therefore, the accuracy of the obesity prevalence rates obtained is questionable. Replication of the project using the term *health screening* or *screening for health behaviors* as part of the permission form may result in increased numbers of children included in the project. More precise data could be collected and tracked if the project is sustained and inclusive of all students in the elementary school.

Another limitation not identified until late into the project implementation was the wording of some questions on the 12-item pretest/posttest. During the posttest, several children asked for clarification of terms. It is interesting to note that no such questions were posed during the administration of the pretest. Perhaps the third graders felt intimidated or afraid to ask during the first encounter, but by the second meeting a more relaxed atmosphere was perceived. The nursing students surmised that some children may have merely guessed on questions that were not actually understood appropriately. The reading level of the pretest/posttest was found to be on a 5.9 grade level instead of a 3.0 grade level. The weakness of this measurement makes accurate validation difficult, and readers are cautioned in the utilization of the existing pretest/posttest without age-appropriate revisions.

Conclusion and Implications

Findings indicate that third graders have limited knowledge of healthy behaviors or of risk factors to heart disease. The implementation of projects as described herein, however, could increase knowledge, influence individual behaviors, and improve child health outcomes. The community will be served by improving the overall health of public school students in rural and medically underserved areas of the state through the implementation of childhood obesity screenings and an obesity prevention health teaching program emphasizing nutrition and physical activity. Results support the use of school-based collaborations to implement best practices guidelines and thereby impact childhood obesity.

As an outcome of this project, the collaboration between a rural county school system and a nearby school of nursing is ongoing. Stakeholder satisfaction with the project indicates a willingness to possibly expand the project of the selected elementary school to include kindergarten through sixth grade students. The potential exists to expand such an initiative within the entire county school system. Effective, meaningful collaboration is necessary for population-based interventions to succeed, for the potential sustainability and expansion of the project, and for the collection of longitudinal data on the health status of a vulnerable population.

The rates of childhood obesity continue to escalate along with the worsening of the financial burden and the related comorbidities. Addressing the obesity epidemic will require a long-term and multifaceted approach. This paper presented the implementation of an obesity screening and prevention intervention among third graders in one elementary school through a community–academic partnership utilizing the manpower of baccalaureate nursing students. The framework of this quality improvement project was based on effective, timely, and equitable health care to rural, underserved public school children, thus strengthening the overall impact and success of a population-based initiative.

This community health endeavor benefited underserved public school children, provided assistance to school nurses, assisted undergraduate nursing students in experiential opportunities, and promoted strategies of population-based health care. Such an evidenced-based, multipronged approach may accelerate the progress toward the prevention of childhood obesity.

References

Agency for Healthcare Research and Quality. (2010). *The community health promotion handbook: Action guides to improve community health.* Retrieved from http://innovations.ahrq.gov/content .aspx?id=2954

Alabama Department of Public Health (ADPH). (2005). *Alabama obesity task force: Strategic plan for the prevention and control of overweight and obesity in Alabama.* Retrieved from http://adph.org/NUTRITION /assets/ObesityPlan.pdf

Alabama Department of Public Health (ADPH). (2007). *Selected indicators of health status in Alabama.* Retrieved from http://www.adph .org/ruralhealth/assets/ARACCombinedSelectedIndicators.pdf

Alabama Department of Public Health (ADPH). (2010). *The risk of heart disease and stroke in Alabama burden document: Finding the path to cardiovascular health.* Retrieved from http://www.adph.org/cvh /assets/2010_HeartDiseaseStroke_Alabama_Burden.pdf

Alabama Department of Public Health (ADPH). (n.d.a). *Healthy Alabama 2010.* Retrieved from http://www.adph.org/administration/ha2010.pdf

Alabama Department of Public Health (ADPH). (n.d.b). *The Alabama community health resource guide.* Office of Primary Care and Rural Health. Retrieved from http://www.adph.org/ruralhealth/assets/ALCommHealthResGuide.pdf

Alabama State Department of Education. (2012). *Alabama 2011–12 quick facts.* Retrieved from http://www.alsde.edu/general/QuickFacts_11-12.pdf

American Academy of Pediatrics (AAP). (2005). Screening and interventions for overweight in children and adolescents: Recommendation statement. *Pediatrics, 116,* 205–210. doi:10.1542/peds.2005-0302

American Public Health Association. (2010). Toolkit for intervention of overweight children and adolescents. Retrieved from http://www.apha.org/programs/resources/obesity/proresobesitykit.htm

American School Health Association. (2011). Core beliefs. Retrieved from https://netforum.avectra.com/temp/ClientImages/ASHA1/6eb77696-7e60-4128-ae9e-844290967c2d.pdf

Barlow, S. E., & the Expert Committee. (2007). Expert committee recommendations regarding the prevention, assessment, and treatment of child and adolescent overweight and obesity: Summary report. *Pediatrics, 120,* S164–S192. Retrieved from http://pediatrics.aappublications.org/content/120/Supplement_4/S164.full.html

Benjamins, M. R., & Whitman, S. (2010). A culturally appropriate school wellness initiative: Results of a 2-year pilot intervention in 2 Jewish schools. *Journal of School Health, 80,* 378–386. Retrieved from http://www.suhichicago.org

Carney, J. K., Maltby, H. J., Mackin, K. A., & Maksym, M. E. (2011). Community–academic partnerships: How can communities benefit? *American Journal of Preventive Medicine, 41,* S206–S213.

Centers for Disease Control and Prevention (CDC). (2000). CDC growth charts. Retrieved from http://www.cdc.gov/growthcharts/

Centers for Disease Control and Prevention (CDC). (2005). *Public health strategies for preventing and controlling overweight and obesity in school and worksite settings: A report on recommendations of the task force on community preventive services.* Retrieved from http://www.cdc.gov/mmwr/preview/mmwrhtml/rr5410a1.htm

Centers for Disease Control and Prevention (CDC). (2008). *Make a difference at your school.* Retrieved from http://www.cdc.gov/healthy youth/keystrategies/pdf/make-a-difference.pdf

Centers for Disease Control and Prevention (CDC). (2009). *Recommended community strategies and measurements to prevent obesity in the United States.* Retrieved from http://www.cdc.gov/mmwr/preview /mmwrhtml/rr5807a1.htm

Centers for Disease Control and Prevention (CDC). (2010, August). Adult obesity. *Vital signs.* Retrieved from http://www.cdc.gov/VitalSigns /pdf/2010-08-vitalsigns.pdf

Centers for Disease Control and Prevention (CDC). (2011a). *About BMI for children and teens.* Retrieved from http://www.cdc.gov/healthy-weight/assessing/bmi/childrens_bmi/about_childrens_bmi.html

Centers for Disease Control and Prevention (CDC). (2011b). *Children's BMI tool for schools: Assessing your weight.* Retrieved from http:// www.cdc.gov/healthyweight/assessing/bmi/childrens_BMI/tool_for _schools.html

Centers for Disease Control and Prevention (CDC). (2011c). *National diabetes fact sheet, 2011.* Retrieved from http://www.cdc.gov/diabetes /pubs/pdf/ndfs_2011.pdf

Centers for Disease Control and Prevention (CDC). (2011d). *School health guidelines to promote healthy eating and physical activity.* Retrieved from http://www.cdc.gov/mmwr/preview/mmwrhtml/rr6005a1 .htm?s_cid=rr6005a1_w

Centers for Disease Control and Prevention (CDC). (2012a). *Adult obesity facts.* Retrieved from http://www.cdc.gov/obesity/data/adult.html

Centers for Disease Control and Prevention (CDC). (2012b). *Basics about childhood obesity.* Retrieved from http://www.cdc.gov/obesity /childhood/basics.html

Centers for Disease Control and Prevention (CDC). (2012c). *Childhood obesity facts.* Retrieved from http://www.cdc.gov/healthyyouth/obesity /facts.htm

Centers for Disease Control and Prevention. (2012d). *Obese youth over time.* Retrieved from http://www.cdc.gov/healthyyouth/obesity /obesity-youth-txt.htm

Centers for Disease Control and Prevention (CDC). (n.d.). *Alabama 2011 and United States 2011 results.* Retrieved from http://www.cdc.gov /obesity/data/adult.html.

Frey, B. B., Lohmeier, J. H., Lee, S. W., & Tollefson, N. (2006). Measuring collaboration among grant partners. *American Journal of Evaluation, 27*, 383–392. doi: 10.1177/1098214006290356

Gonzalez-Suarez, C., Worley, A., Grimmer-Somers, K., & Dones, V. (2009). School based interventions on childhood obesity: A meta-analysis. *American Journal of Preventive Medicine, 37*, 418–427. doi:10.1016/j.amepre.2009.07.012

Hockenberry, M. J., & Wilson, D. (2009). *Wong's essentials of pediatric nursing* (8th ed.).St. Louis, MO: Mosby Elsevier.

Institute of Medicine (IOM). (2001). *Crossing the quality chasm: A new health system for the 21st century.* Washington, DC: National Academy Press.

Institute of Medicine (IOM). (2004). *The health-care sector and providers can play a role in preventing childhood obesity.* Retrieved from http://www.iom.edu/~/media/Files/Report%20Files/2004/Preventing-Childhood-Obesity-Health-in-the-Balance/FactSheetHealthcare FINALBitticks.pdf

Institute of Medicine (IOM). (2006). *Progress in preventing childhood obesity: How do we measure up?* Retrieved from http://www.iom.edu /Reports/2006/Progress-in-Preventing-Childhood-Obesity—How -Do-We-Measure-Up.aspx

Institute of Medicine (IOM). (2012a). *Accelerating progress in obesity prevention: Solving the weight of the nation.* Retrieved from http://www .iom.edu/Reports/2012/Accelerating-Progress-in-Obesity-Prevention.aspx

Institute of Medicine (IOM). (2012b). *Alliances for obesity prevention: Finding common ground: Workshop summary.* Retrieved from http:// www.iom.edu/Reports/2012/Alliances-for-Obesity-Prevention-Finding-Common-Ground.aspx

Jayaratne, K., Kelaher, M., & Dunt, D. (2010). Child health partnerships: A review of program characteristics, outcomes and their relationship. *BMC Health Services Research, 10*, 172. doi:10.1186/1472-6963-10-172

Kanekar, A., & Sharma, M. (2008). Meta-analysis of school-based childhood obesity interventions in the UK and US. *International Quarterly of Community Health Education, 29*, 241–256.

Lavelle, H. V., Mackay, D. F., & Pell, J. P. (2012). Systematic review and meta-analysis of schoolbased interventions to reduce body mass index. *Journal of Public Health*, pp. 1–10. doi: 10.1093/pubmed/fdr116

Lesser, J., & Oscor-Sanchez, M. A. (2007). Community–academic research partnerships with vulnerable populations. *Annual Review of Nursing Research, 25,* 317–337.

Luttikhuis, H. O., Baur, L., Jansen, H., Shrewsbury, V. A., O'Malley, C., Stolk, R. P., & Summerbell, C. D. (2009). Interventions for treating obesity in children. *Cochrane Database of Systematic Reviews, 1.* Retrieved from http://summaries.cochrane.org/CD001872 /treating-obesity-in-children

National Association of School Nurses. (2011). *Role of the school nurse: Position statement.* Retrieved from http://www.nasn.org/portals/0 /positions/2011psrole.pdf

Nihiser, A. J., Lee, S. M., Wechsler, H., McKenna, M., Odom, E., Reinold, C., . . . Grummer-Strawn, L. (2009). BMI measurement in schools. *Pediatrics, 124,* S89–S97. Retrieved from http://pediatrics.aappublications.org/content/124/Supplement_1/S89.full.pdf+html

Peterson, K. E., & Fox, M. K. (2007). Addressing the epidemic of childhood obesity through school-based interventions: What has been done and where do we go from here? *Journal of Law, Medicine & Ethics, 35,* 113–130. Retrieved from http://www.ncbi.nlm.nih.gov/pubmed /17341220

Resnick, E. A., Bishop, M., O'Connell, A., Hugo, B., Isern, G., Timm, A., . . . Geller, A. C. (2009). The CHEER study to reduce BMI in elementary school students: A school-based, parent-directed study in Framingham, Massachusetts. *Journal of School Nursing, 25,* 361–372. doi: 10.1177/1059840509339194

Sharma, M. (2006). School-based interventions for childhood and adolescent obesity. *Obesity Reviews, 7,* 261–269. Retrieved from http:// www.ncbi.nlm.nih.gov/pubmed/16866974

Stevens, K. R., McDuffie, K., & Clutter, P. C. (2009). Research and the mandate for evidence based practice, quality and patient safety. In M. A. Mateo & K. T. Kirchhoff (Eds.), *Research for advanced practice nurses: From evidence to practice.* pp. 43–70. New York, NY: Springer Publishing Company.

Teutsch, S., & Bliss, P. (2005). Spanning the boundary between clinics and communities to address overweight and obesity in children. *Pediatrics, 116*(1) 240–241. doi:10.1542/peds.2005-038

United States Department of Agriculture (USDA). (2012a). *Empowering youth with nutrition & physical activity*. Retrieved from http://www.fns.usda.gov/tn/Resources/empoweringyouth.html

United States Department of Agriculture (USDA). (2012b). *Nutrition standards in the national school lunch and school breakfast programs*. Retrieved from http://www.gpo.gov/fdsys/pkg/FR-2012-01-26/pdf/2012-1010.pdf

United States Department of Agriculture and United States Department of Health and Human Services (USDA & USDHHS). (2010). *Dietary guidelines for Americans* (7th ed.). Washington, DC: U.S. Government Printing Office.

United States Department of Health and Human Services (USDHHS). (2012). *About healthy people*. Retrieved from http://healthypeople.gov/2020/about/default.aspx

United States Department of Health and Human Services (USDHHS). (n.d.). *Find shortage areas: MUA/P by state and county*. Retrieved from http://muafind.hrsa.gov/index.aspx

United States Preventive Services Task Force (USPSTF). (2010). *Screening for obesity in children and adolescents*. Retrieved from http://www.uspreventiveservicestaskforce.org/uspstf10/childobes/chobesrs.htm

World Health Organization (WHO). (2000). *Obesity: Preventing and managing the global epidemic; Summary*. Retrieved from http://apps.who.int/bookorders/WHP/detart1.jsp?sesslan=1&codlan=1&codcol=10&codcch=894

World Health Organization (WHO). (2012). *Global strategy on diet, physical activity and health: Obesity and overweight*. Retrieved from http://www.who.int/mediacentre/factsheets/fs311/en/

Pretest/Posttest

Today's Date: _____ **Homeroom Teacher:** _____

Sex: _____Male _____Female

Race: _____Caucasian (white) _____African American

_____Hispanic _____Asian _____Other

Instructions: Circle the best answer for each of the following items.

1. The human body needs calories for:
   A. Nothing—calories are bad for you.
   B. Your body to operate properly.
   C. A good cholesterol level.
   D. Making choices from every food group.
   E. All of the above.

2. If you eat more calories than your body needs, the leftover calories change into:
   A. Energy.
   B. Sugar.
   C. Protein.
   D. Fat.
   E. All of the above.

3. Which activity does NOT count as active exercise?
   A. Playing kickball
   B. Dancing
   C. Reading a difficult book
   D. Riding your bike
   E. All of the above

4. Aerobic exercise is a kind of activity that requires your heart to need and use more:
   A. Oxygen.
   B. Sweat.
   C. Fruits and vegetables.
   D. Strength.
   E. All of the above.

5. More than half of your body weight is made up of:
   A. Water.
   B. Calories.
   C. Internal organs.
   D. Muscle.
   E. All of the above.

6. Which are the healthiest foods and are good to eat almost any time?
   A. Pancakes and waffles
   B. French fries and pizza
   C. Bananas and apples
   D. Ice cream and cookies
   E. All of the above

7. Which are the least healthy foods and should only be eaten once in a while?
   A. Pancakes and waffles
   B. French fries and pizza
   C. Bananas and apples
   D. Low-fat milk and cookies
   E. All of the above

8. A major cause of deaths that occur every year is from:
   A. Car accidents.
   B. Physical exercise.
   C. Plane crashes.
   D. Heart disease.
   E. All of the above.

9. Which activity uses the most energy?
   A. Playing tennis
   B. Sleeping
   C. Doing homework
   D. Playing video games

10. High blood pressure, being overweight, and physical inactivity are all risk factors for:
    A. Low BMI.
    B. Lung disease.
    C. Heart disease.
    D. High self-esteem.
    E. All of the above.
11. The amount of food a person eats should match:
    A. The amount of energy he or she uses.
    B. His or her age.
    C. Stored fat.
    D. Each food label.
    E. All of the above.
12. I can be a healthy kid by:
    A. Increasing physical activity.
    B. Eating a nutritious breakfast.
    C. Eating a variety of foods.
    D. Reducing TV time.
    E. All of the above.

Collaboration Survey

A community–academic partnership is a mechanism for advancing nursing practice to improve the health of the public. This type of intentional and formalized relationship has been established between the Elmore County Board of Education and the Auburn Montgomery School of Nursing in order to test an ongoing childhood obesity screening and prevention program for school-aged children. The following survey will help indicate the level of collaboration that was achieved. Thank you for participating.

Please circle the organization you represent:
Elmore County Board of Education
Auburn Montgomery School of Nursing

Circle the number that best indicates your feelings regarding the statements that follow:

	Strongly Disagree 1	Somewhat Disagree 2	Disagree 3	N/A 4	Agree 5	Somewhat Agree 6	Strongly Agree 7
This collaboration has positively influenced your organization's services or operations.	1	2	3	4	5	6	7
Professional philosophies between the organizations make it difficult for you to work together.	1	2	3	4	5	6	7
Your organization is familiar with the programs and operations of the partner organization.	1	2	3	4	5	6	7
The organizations share information that strengthens each of you.	1	2	3	4	5	6	7
You feel what your organization brings to the collaboration is appreciated and respected by the partner organization.	1	2	3	4	5	6	7
The organizations work through differences to arrive at win-win solutions.	1	2	3	4	5	6	7

	1	2	3	4	5	6	7
The collaboration hinders your organization from meeting its own organizational mission.	1	2	3	4	5	6	7
The people who represent the partner organization in the collaboration are trustworthy.	1	2	3	4	5	6	7
Your organization can count on the partner organization to meet its obligations to the collaboration.	1	2	3	4	5	6	7
Your organization has difficulty getting in touch with the partner organization when you need to contact it.	1	2	3	4	5	6	7
Frequent communication occurs to ensure the collaboration functions well.	1	2	3	4	5	6	7
Your organization feels it is worthwhile to stay and work with the partner organization rather than leave the collaboration.	1	2	3	4	5	6	7
Overall, your organization is satisfied with the collaboration.	1	2	3	4	5	6	7

CHAPTER 15

The Impact of Evidence-Based Design

Heather Hardin

Objectives

Upon review of this information, the reader will be able to:
1. Define the use of a "no interruption zone" in medication preparation.
2. Discuss the incidence of medication errors in the modern health-care community.
3. Define the use of an evidence-based design and the importance of it in the modern health-care community.

Abstract

Evidence-based design (EBD) is a multidisciplinary process that utilizes design principles based on the best evidence to achieve the best possible outcomes. Hospital design features are an essential element in patient and employee safety. The purpose of the project is to implement elements of evidence-based design in improvement of medication safety.

Results suggest that greater emphasis on a no interruption zone is an effective method of reducing interruptions during medication preparation.

The numbers and types of interruptions were presented pre- and postinterventions. The data reveals most interruption categories had a drop in interruptions after the interventions. After the implementation, nursing staff reported an increased understanding and compliance with the no interruption zone. This project demonstrates that evidence-based design must include educating staff, as well as a cultural shift within the organization for success.

CONCLUSION

Implementation of evidence-based design includes not only arrangements that positively influence outcomes by enhanced physical layout, but also incorporation of knowledge about human behavior. Data from this project provides further evidence to support the benefits of implementation of a no interruption zone and the impact of evidence-based design in medication safety.

The Impact of Evidence-Based Design

The idea that the environment influences health began in the days of Hippocrates, continued through Florence Nightingale, and is still present today (Edvardsson, Sandman, & Rasmussen, 2005). The Joint Commission sets recommendations for the environment of care, and the International Building Code has recommendations for facility design (Ecoff & Brown, 2010). The five goals identified by The Joint Commission for effective facility design and management include: (1) reduce the environmental risks; (2) prevent accidents; (3) maintain safety; (4) maintain an environment that is patient centered; and (5) reduce environmental stress (Brown & Ecoff, 2011).

Evidence-based medicine prompted of the utilization of evidence as a basis for patient care. The intention of evidence-based medicine is to improve outcomes by conscientious use of the best evidence in making decisions about patient care (Moore & Geboy, 2011). Medicine is moving toward evidence-based practice, applying research-based evidence into clinical practice to promote the best outcomes, and now, hospitals are following this trend (Bliss-Holtz, 2007). Evidence-based design (EBD) is a natural parallel to evidence-based medicine (Moore & Geboy, 2011). EBD is the process of basing decisions about the built environment on credible research to achieve the best possible outcomes. Utilizing design principles based on the best research improves patient safety, patient outcomes, and staff outcomes. Environmental design can be divided into two groups: structural and nonstructural. Some of the dimensions of environmental design include single rooms, lighting, acoustics, ergonomic designs, floor layouts, and unit layout (Ulrich et al., 2008). These design features are important in patient infection rates, patient safety data, and employee satisfaction and retention. EBD incorporates a multidisciplinary team including architects, builders, engineers, designers, and healthcare professionals.

The United States will spend over $180 billion for new hospitals in the next five years. Healthcare construction was projected to exceed $70 billion in 2011 (Ulrich et al., 2008). The hospitals and hospital renovations that are being built will remain for decades. The ultimate goal of evidence-based design is to create a healing environment that promotes safety, quality of care, and patient satisfaction.

Approximately 44,000 people die every year in American hospitals as a result of preventable medical errors (Chaudhury, Mahmood, & Valente, 2009). Errors can be both environmental and nonenvironmental. A recent study found noise, lighting, ergonomics, and design/layout to be the key environmental contributors to medical errors. The project will explore the impact of evidence-based design on an inpatient hospital setting. Through an evidence-based practice framework, the EBD project will be developed. The project will explore the impact of evidence-based design on system failures, and more specifically, the effect of interruptions on medication errors. In his landmark article, Leape (1994) noted that medication errors occur in as many as 14 percent of patients admitted to hospitals. He also noted the design of work environments can minimize the occurrence of errors (Leape, 1994).

Background and Significance

Nurses work in a fragmented and unpredictable environment. Nursing is dynamic, and it requires a significant amount of coordination. Nurses serve a primary role in medication administration, and they play a pivotal role in medication management and patient safety. However, nurses frequently experience operation failures such as missing medications and broken equipment. This causes interruptions ultimately affecting productivity, accuracy, and morale.

A medication error is defined as the administration of the wrong medication to the wrong patient, at the wrong time, or failure to administer the drug in the manner prescribed (Armitage & Knapman, 2003). Medication errors represent at least 20 percent of all medical errors (Joanna Briggs Institute, 2009). Because medication administration involves several steps, it is a complex system, and complex systems, even with protocols in place are not, unfortunately, incapable of error (Pape, 2003). Medication errors are not the result of individual performance. They are the result of production, process, or system failures. Human error is not a cause; it is a consequence (Armitage & Knapman, 2003). Increased hospital stays, legal expenses, and further medical treatments as a result of medication errors increase costs. The contributing factors of medication errors are nurse distractions, poor communication, and failure to follow protocol (Pape, 2003). Because nursing and medication administration are complex, designing processes and environments that are robust to resist nurse distractions can reduce errors (Tucker & Spear, 2006).

A Proposed Project

This project will be aimed at assisting nurses in delivering safe, high quality care to patients, thereby improving their current state of health and satisfaction with their care. Nurses are faced with increasingly complex patients, illnesses, technology, and information synthesis. Nurses are charged with patient care, improving quality, maintaining safety, developing policy, training, cost containment, and communication. The healthcare environment is often chaotic. Attempting to reduce distractions and interruptions is necessary to decrease the complexity of nursing work and place patients in a safer environment. One strategic innovation is the introduction of a no interruption zone for medication preparation. Identifying a designated quiet area around the medication dispensing machine allows the nurses to concentrate solely on medications without interruptions, ultimately reducing potential for medication errors. The goal of the project is to reduce distractions and therefore reduce medication errors.

TARGET POPULATION AND LOCATION

The targeted population will be nurses and patients. This focus is on the utilization of evidence-based design at a local community hospital, identified as the "project hospital," on a 36-bed medical-surgical floor.

PURPOSE

The purpose of the project is to uncover the role that evidence-based design plays in the safety of patients in an inpatient setting. More specifically, the project will explore the impact of evidence-based design on medication preparation. This project hopes to answer the PICO question: During medication preparation in hospital-based patient care environments (P), does implementation of evidence-based design, a red carpet for a no interruption zone with education (I), compared to no education with the carpet (C), result in a reduction of interruptions and medication errors (O)?

Theoretical Framework

Florence Nightingale noted that nurses were to create an environment conducive to health (Edvardsson et al., 2005). Appropriate light, warmth, cleanliness, fresh air, and sound are some of the healing properties she recognized in the physical environment. Over 150 years ago, Nightingale recognized the importance of the integration of the environment with care delivery. She hypothesized that ensuring the best possible environment facilitated the reparative processes of the patient.

There are several models available to form a systematic approach to evidence-based design. Evidence-based design is influenced by many different specialties such as architects, engineers, healthcare employees, regulations, and patients. Because of this diverse influence, the utilization of evidence-based decision making in evidence-based design is appropriate (Brown & Ecoff, 2011). A systematic approach to evidence-based decision making is the evidence-based information cycle. When applying this to evidence-based design, eight steps are noted (Brown & Ecoff, 2011). The eight steps begin with a catalyst, and they include assessing, asking, acquiring, appraising, applying, analyzing, adopting, and advancing (Brown & Ecoff, 2011; see **Figure 15-1**). These will be discussed throughout this chapter.

Catalyst

The catalyst is the trigger for the need of an evidence-based process. This could be a problem or an issue within a setting. Regulations and regulatory

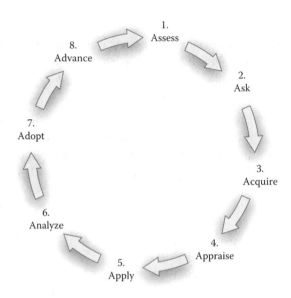

FIGURE 15-1 Evidence-based decision making model applies to evidence-based design.

agencies such as the International Building Code and The Joint Commission have detailed guidelines for the healthcare environment. Outcomes from setting which are relevant to the safety and satisfactions of patients may signal the need to address the built environment (Brown & Ecoff, 2011).

The catalyst for this proposed project is the number of sentinel events that occur as a result of medication errors. A sentinel event is defined as an error that results in patient death, paralysis, or coma (Pape, 2003). When one of the seven rights is violated, there is a potential for a medication error. According to Pape (2003), the number of medication errors that occur in this country is comparable to two plane crashes per day.

Assessing

After the catalyst, the problem is assessed. Once a problem is confirmed as clear concern and it is deemed important to address, the right question must be asked. This allows the scope of the problem to be narrowed enough that clarity of the issue is revealed. The PICO(T) question is a structure used to produce a narrow, searchable, answerable question (Brown & Ecoff, 2011). The research question guides the search for evidence.

Asking

EVIDENCE-BASED PRACTICE QUESTION

In the standard PICOT definition, P is defined as population, I is the intervention, C is the comparison, O is the outcome, and T is the time. However, when applying the PICOT format to architecture and design, nurses may make modifications to the evidence-based practice process (Ecoff & Brown, 2010). For example, when asking the PICOT question, space or occupants may be interchanged with patient or problem (Brown & Ecoff, 2011). I is interventions within the built environment. C is the alternative design or the existing element of design. O is still outcomes, but in design, it is in relation to the built environment.

PICO(T)

In an attempt to uncover the impact of evidence-based design, a PICOT question has been developed. The PICO(T) question for this project takes the design adaptations into account. As stated previously, the PICO question is: During medication preparation in hospital-based patient care environments (P), does implementation of evidence-based design, a red carpet for a no interruption zone with education (I), compared to no education with the carpet (C), result in a reduction of interruptions and medication errors (O)?

Time (T) is not addressed in this particular question. However, a more detailed question could include the impact of improved efficiency and increased patient safety during a particular shift such as night shift or day shift. With so many facets of hospital design, asking an effective, specific question becomes imperative.

Acquiring

After a narrow, searchable, and answerable question has been formulated, a framework for inquiry is developed; the next step becomes acquiring the best evidence to answer the question. Keywords and database searches lead to appropriate evidence. Databases used for this paper include CINAHL (Cumulative Index to Nursing and Allied Health Literature), Academic Search Premier, Alt HealthWatch, Art & Architecture Complete, Business Source Premier, ERIC, Health Source: Nursing/Academic Edition, Communication Abstracts, EDS Foundation Index, Education

Research Complete, Professional Development Collection, Philosopher's Index, PsycARTICLES, PsycINFO, MEDLINE, InformeDesign, SUM-search, Trip database, and Ripple database. Several articles were identified after a search in Google Scholar and the Institute of Healthcare Improvement databases. References within the articles were used to uncover other applicable articles. The keywords included *design, environment and nursing, quality, medication errors, evidence-based design, hospital environment, medication, safe zone,* and *no interruption zone.*

Appraising

Evidence-based medicine prompted the development of a hierarchy of evidence (Moore & Geboy, 2010). Each study has a level of evidence based on the methods and design of the study. Systematic reviews, meta-analyses, and randomized controlled trials have the lowest potential for bias and are therefore considered the highest level of evidence (Brown & Ecoff, 2011). Appraising the evidence has two functions. It is important to determine if there is evidence to apply and if the applicable evidence is reliable. There are three possible answers to this question: First, there is definite evidence; second, there is inconclusive evidence; or third, there is little evidence. Healthcare decision makers are exposed to a wide range of information in regard to the effects of environmental design on patients. Unfortunately, not all the information can be substantiated with a high level evidence (Stichler, 2010).

EBD involves basing decisions about the built environment on the best research to achieve the best outcomes in patient care (Moore & Geboy, 2011). A more inclusive definition of evidence should be considered in reference to the development of knowledge with the potential to inform the design process (Moore & Geboy, 2011). Furthermore, Moore and Geboy insist that while traditional empirical evidence is important in applied science, within the design community, interpretivism and intuitionism should also be included in evidence. This is similar to the evidence-based nursing definition of evidence, which defines knowledge as extrapolated information from a variety of sources that is found to be credible (Moore & Geboy, 2011).

Conversely, Stichler (2010), states that assessing the level of evidence in literature reviews is critical. She states that architects, healthcare providers, and executives may make eloquent arguments about specific designs based on case studies, but decisions, especially those with significant project and operational cost implications, should be based on strong evidence.

LEVELS OF EVIDENCE FOR THE PROPOSED PROJECT

In the search for evidence for this project, studies were excluded because they were nonempirical, or there was a lack of discussion in regards to patients, the environment, or nursing. For this project, nine studies were reviewed. There was one study that was a level 1. Two quasi-experimental studies were included, and they were level 3 studies. There were four studies that were level 4 (See **Figure 15-2**). Two literature reviews, which have a low level of evidence, were included. They were scored at a level 5. Each study was purposeful, and each showed a unique relationship to this project.

There were nine studies utilized for evidence in the development of this proposal; three specifically point to the benefits of a no interruption zone (see **Appendix 15A**). However, a clear relationship was developed between the studies.

The systematic review referred to for this proposal discusses the effects of the environment in healthcare settings on the health of patients (Dijkstra, Pieterse, & Pruyn, 2006). The review divided 30 studies into multiple environmental studies and single environmental studies. This review included studies of 17 different environmental stimuli. This study has a high level of evidence (level 1); however, it does not include data on the impact of the environment on the hospital staff. The strength of the article is in the conclusive evidence of the impact of the environment on the well-being of patients (Dijkstra et al., 2006; see Appendix 15A).

Hendrich, Chow, Skierczynski, and Zhenqiang (2008) studied how the environment affects nurses. They investigated the time of clinical nurses

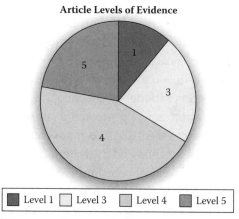

Article Levels of Evidence

Level 1   Level 3   Level 4   Level 5

FIGURE 15-2 The nine studies used in this project and their levels of evidence.

in the hospital work environment. This study identified the impact of the hospital environment on nurses and attempted to identify the causes of inefficiencies in nursing practice. The results revealed that nurses spend a considerable amount of time on medication administration, and approximately one third of that time was spent on medication preparation. The article suggests that this process should be streamlined because of apparent fragmentation. Documentation, care coordination, and medication administration were the three main categories of nursing processes that were identified in this study as targets for improving efficiency of nursing care (Hendrich et al., 2008; see Appendix 15A). Westbrook, Woods, Rob, Dunsmuir, and Day (2010) uncovered the directly proportional relationship between interruptions and medication errors.

An article by Tucker and Spear (2006) describes the work systems within the nursing environment. The article cites the five most frequent types of failures in nursing work systems. They include medications, orders, supplies, staffing, and equipment. Two conclusions are drawn in this article. First, improvement processes are necessary, and second, processes must be robust to interruption to prevent errors (see Appendix 15A).

Whereas Tucker and Spear (2006) uncover operational failures and the impact of interruptions, Armitage and Knapman (2003) specifically address medication administration errors. The article cites the system as the cause of the error as opposed to the individual. Several potential contributing factors to errors are discussed, including nurse distractions and interruptions. The study revealed that approximately one third of the study sample thought that interruptions were a factor in medication errors (see Appendix 15A).

Similarly, Biron, Lavoie-Tremblay, and Loiselle (2009) discussed the characteristics of nurse interruptions during medication administration. Whereas the article by Tucker and Spear (2006) focused on failures in the work system, this article narrowed in on failures during medication administration. This observational study concluded that the process of medication administration is not protected against interruptions. Furthermore, this study uncovered that the main cause of work interruptions were nurse colleagues followed by system failures. The study cites the necessity for system-level interventions to stop interruptions leading to errors (Biron et al., 2009, p. 335; see Appendix 15A).

An additional study addressing interruptions was an empirical study of the relationship between interruptions and medication administration errors (Westbrook et al., 2010). The study implicitly found that the more interruptions nurses experienced, the greater the number of errors committed, and the more a nurse was interrupted within one medication administration, the greater the severity of the medication error. This study solidified the necessity and importance implementing systematic changes within the hospital environment in order to decrease interruptions and ultimately decrease medication errors (see Appendix 15A).

The two other articles included in this review refer to specific interventions to the environment as an avenue to decrease medication errors. These two quasi-experimental studies examine the use of a no interruption zone on medication administration (Anthony, Wiencek, Bauer, Daly, & Anthony, 2010; Pape, 2003). These two studies revealed that changes in environmental design had the potential to reduce medication errors, improve nurse efficacy, and significantly impact patient safety (see Appendix 15A).

The utilization of a no interruption zone is modeled after the sterile cockpit rule within the aviation industry. Because of the complexities of take-offs and landings, in 1981, the Federal Aviation Administration implemented policies that prohibited nonessential communication by aircraft crews during flights below 10,000 feet (Anthony et al., 2010). Adapting effective safety measures from other industries and applying proven policies to health care reduces errors.

In a quasi-experimental study by Pape (2003), a visible symbol during medication administration was found to reduce nursing distractions and ultimately reduce medication errors. Based on these findings, The Institute for Safe Medication Practices has recommended the no interruption zone as a strategy for the reduction of medication errors (Safe practice environment chapter proposed by USP, 2008).

The United States Pharmacopeia, an institution for the reporting of medication errors, published a proposal on the physical environment that promotes medication safety. It cites five important areas for medication safety based on evidence, which include illumination, interruptions, sound, physical design, and medication safety zones (Safe practice environment chapter proposed by USP, 2008). A review article from the National Nursing Research Unit in London cited that the implementation of interventions to reduce interruptions during medication preparation and administration reduced interruptions by 89 percent and medication errors by 60 percent (Interruptions to nurses during medication administration, 2010; see Appendix 15A). Finally, the AHRQ recommended no interruption zones in its book; a 64 percent reduction in interruptions was found with the implementation of a safety zone.

CRITICAL APPRAISAL OF EVIDENCE

Overall, the weakness of these articles lies in the lower level of evidence. The four observational studies could have been impacted by the very nature of observation or the Hawthorne effect. Additionally, the ability to determine the exact number of medication errors either before or after an intervention is completely dependent on reporting; therefore, calculating a reliable rate of error is difficult. Furthermore, causation of errors is difficult because of variables and complexity.

The strength of the evidence is a result of a clear trend of supporting data indicating that the environment impacts well-being. A clear linear relationship has developed from these studies and can be extrapolated into purposeful evidence for recommendations. (See **Figure 15-3**.) Overall,

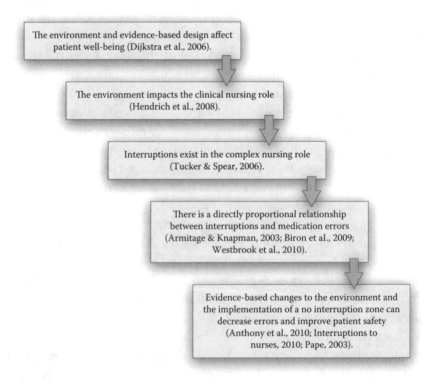

FIGURE 15-3 The literature in this project proposal has a clear relationship in order to answer the PICO(T) question.

the literature for this project proposal included one systematic review that discussed the specifics of evidence-based design and two quasi-experimental studies that addressed the no interruption zone. There were four observational studies and two literature reviews. Further discussion of these studies can be found in Appendix 15A.

At this point in the model, recommendations are formed. The recommendations are graded according to the quality, quantity, and consistency of the evidence on which they are based (Joanna Briggs Institute, 2009).

The application of evidence to practice must include a multidisciplinary team in addition to patient preferences, clinical expertise, and resources (Brown & Ecoff, 2011). Because knowledge doesn't always flow from science to practice, direct experiential learning and practice-based knowledge should also be incorporated (Melnyk & Fineout-Overholt, 2011). Several recommendations have evolved as a result of the literature review for this project proposal.

- Unnecessary conversation during medication preparation should be discouraged. (Grade B)
- Education and teamwork should be utilized to reduce distractions. (Grade B)
- Visual symbols within the environment should be utilized during medication administration. (Grade B)
- Checklists should be utilized as a reminder. (Grade C)
- Other sources of distraction should be eliminated or limited. (Grade B)
- The use of a pharmacy wait zone could be utilized. (Grade C)
- A medication nurse could be utilized. (Grade C)

These recommendations are based on the literature cited in this proposal. Because there are no systematic reviews or clinical practice guidelines specifically addressing interruptions during medication preparation and administration, no grade A was given. Grade C was given to three of the recommendations because, although these interventions were mentioned, they did not have sufficient evidence to warrant a grade B recommendation.

The relationship between interruptions and the potential for errors and the implementation of a no interruption zone are comparable to the aviation industry. Safety in aviation has been institutionalized by the

Federal Aviation Administration (FAA) and the National Transportation Safety Board. Safety in medicine has never been institutionalized (Leape, 1994). However, the Institute for Safe Medication Practices, the United States Pharmacopeia, the National Nursing Research Unit in London, and the AHRQ currently recommend the implementation of a no interruption zone for the reduction of interruptions during medication preparation.

Applying

Evidence should be balanced with stakeholder values and the designers' expertise to create a plan for a small test of change (Brown & Ecoff, 2011). After a needs assessment is complete, primary stakeholders must be willing to address the political and cultural obstacles that are inherent within any organizational change.

Needs Assessment

There has been extensive research on in-patient medication errors. There is at least one medication error per hospital patient every day in the United States (Rabinowitz, 2008). Across the country, the most common medication errors are related to wrong dose (Hodgkinson, Koch, Nay, & Nichols, 2006). The financial burden of preventable medication errors is between 17 and 29 billion dollars per year (Hodgkinson et al., 2006).

ORGANIZATIONAL DATA

The project hospital is no exception. The hospital collects monthly data on the numbers, locations, and types of medication errors. Unfortunately, in fiscal year 2010, the project hospital had over 350 reported medication errors. Reports indicated that there was no decrease in errors in 2010 from 2009. As a result of increasing errors and the level of those errors, stakeholders decided to take action. A series of four rapid-improvement events based on lean methodology identified ways to decrease medication errors. One idea that evolved from these sessions was the installation of a red carpet to identify a no interruption zone. The red carpet area was named the "red zone," and it was to signal an area where disruptions and interruptions should be eliminated.

Unfortunately, in casual observation, the red zone was not respected, and it was not perceived as a legitimate safety tool. Many nurses agreed prior to the implementation of this project that the red zone, while it may be effective in theory, was not being observed, and it did not work.

One reason for the insufficient compliance was related to a lack of appropriate information. There was one small, plain sign to indicate the purpose for the red carpet. The white sign had a small font, and it was not particularly appealing. Once, when three nurses were asked about the red zone, they did not know what it was. After the sign was pointed out to them, they admitted they had never seen the sign. When asked about the purpose of the red carpet, several nurses thought that it was for leg support during medication preparation (See **Figure 15-4**).

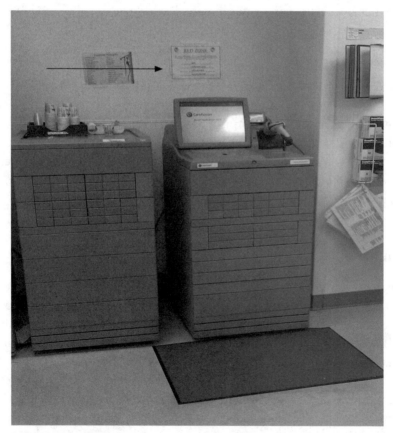

FIGURE 15-4 The current sign above the medication dispensing machine at the project hospital is small, unattractive, and ambiguous.

CARE DELIVERY PROCESSES

Work processes must be designed to reduce interruptions during medication preparation (Cohen et al., 2011) Well-designed environments provide the opportunity to prevent errors, but steps must also be taken to enhance the performance of staff members. These steps include provision of education about the environmental changes and a plan to sustain change. While education and visually striking signs can encourage behavior change, true sustainment must occur within the organizational culture. Senior management teams that facilitate change, manage stress, and promote safety are pivotal in creating environments that are conducive to safety measure implementations (Cohen et al., 2011). Cohen et al., (2011) also suggest that understanding how people react to systems and how they integrate them into their mental structures reveals new ways of enhancing workflow and environmental work spaces.

STAKEHOLDERS

Stakeholders have a perspective that may allow them to foresee challenges that individuals and designers may overlook (Brown & Ecoff, 2011). The director of pharmacy in the project hospital is passionate about the reduction of medication errors, and he is eager to implement error reduction strategies. The manager of the unit impacted, patient safety management, the education department, and the director of nursing are also stakeholders in this study.

Implementation

Medicine and the design of medical facilities are about making choices. Ideally, choices are based on the best information. While there is no guarantee for perfection, decisions are accountable to the best evidence (Gillis, 2010). Because decisions about the medical environment affect patient safety, they cannot be open ended, and they cannot be deterministic without consistent evaluation (Gillis, 2010). The nine studies utilized for evidence in the development of this proposal created a strong foundation for this project. Because medication errors were identified as an area of opportunity for the project hospital, this project proved important to stakeholders, staff, and patients.

PROCESS OF IMPLEMENTATION

The environmental change based on evidence-based design for this project is the installation of a red carpet in front of the medication dispensing machines. Because the machine is loaded by pharmacy based on clients' needs, drug availability, and formulary, there is opportunity for error. Additionally, Akansel and Kaymakci (2008) state nurses' stations are responsible for the highest level of noise compared to other areas on the unit. Unfortunately, the dispensing machines for this project are located within the nursing stations, which potentiate a need to address noise that leads to interruptions.

The red carpet is a design element that serves as a visual cue to decrease interruptions during medication preparation. The project hospital calls this area the red zone. The area has a small sign posted above the medication dispensing machine to remind staff that conversation should be eliminated during medication preparation. This design change was implemented as a result of a rapid improvement event that identified, although not statistically, a need to address medication safety. The implementation occurred without providing education to the staff; therefore, it has not been effective.

A SMALL TEST OF CHANGE VERSUS A FULL IMPLEMENTATION

The small test of change proposed for this project was the implementation of additional signs and additional education about the red zone around the medication dispensing machines to increase compliance and reduce interruptions during medication preparation. Prior to the implementation of additional signs and education, interruptions during 10 medication preparation cycles were recorded on a modified medication administration dispensing observation sheet (MADOS) developed and validated by Pape (2003). Next, an educational session was held and reinforced with additional signs around the medication dispensing machine. Finally, interruptions were counted during 10 medication cycles again. Using SPSS Statistics software, a t-test was performed to determine if there is any significant difference in the number of interruptions prior to and then after education and environmental changes (poster implementation).

The small test of change for this project was only slightly different from a full implementation of this project. A full implementation would provide more extensive data collection over a longer period of time, and it would allow for the collection of medication errors in relation to interruptions. For a full project implementation, more medication cycle interruptions would be observed on varying shifts and in varying units. In addition to interruptions, an extended project would allow for the collection of medication error data to observe a potential correlation between interruptions during medication preparation and medication errors. In the formula to determine such a correlation, the number of inpatients in each unit would be the denominator while the number of medication errors would be the numerator. This would eliminate the potential for the census to impact the collected data. Large, costly architectural changes are not reasonable for the scope of this project; however, this small test of change produces evidence to answer the original PICO(T) question. Because of the time limitations, this project is limited to a small test. This paper discusses the implementation of a small test of change; however, references to a full implementation are also included.

POPULATION

Participation in any part of this study was voluntary, and all subjects provided consent. Ten high-volume medication administration cycles were observed prior to the education, and 10 were observed after the education. A high volume medication cycle began as the nurse stepped onto the red carpet to prepare her medications for 1 patient. The cycle ended when she walked out of the medication room. Additionally, 10 surveys were administered prior to education, and 10 surveys were administered posteducation. The surveys were completely anonymous.

Education is essential for compliance with a design implementation. Without education, the staff members were unaware of the potential gains associated with compliance. To the casual observer, the current state of the no interruption zone was simply noncompliance. The zone was not acknowledged by the staff, managers, or senior leaders. The small test of change for this project included education with reinforced signs about the red zone (See **Figure 15-5**).

Ultimately, for a full evidence-based practice implementation, reeducation would be necessary at regular intervals to impress a cultural change. Evidence shows that changes in the environment to promote safety must

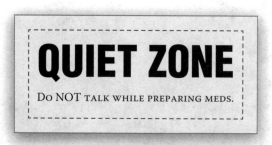

FIGURE 15-5 The implementation includes additional signs and further education to encourage compliance.

be reinforced with education and supportive organizational dynamics (Cohen, 2010). Furthermore, Cama (2009) suggests that success of the evidence-based design decisions require the alignment of operational goals and architectural solutions while overcoming challenges. Cama states that the political and cultural challenges can be the most difficult. In this case, a cultural change must occur. The success of the no interruption zone requires a behavior modification by the staff. A lack of compliance with the design change hinders positive results.

THE SMALL TEST OF CHANGE

Prior to implementation, a meeting was conducted with the managers, assistant managers, patient care coordinators on each shift, and the educator within the unit. Education provided included information concerning importance and potential gains associated with compliance of the no interruption zone. A 15-slide slideshow was displayed to address multiple learning styles. Information was provided explaining the evidence that suggests the implementation of the red zone reduces errors if the staff members are compliant. An opportunity for questions was also provided.

Next, the small test of change was implemented according to a timeline (see **Appendix 15B**). The timeline was an important addition to this project because of the time limitation for completion of the small test. The small test began with administering an assessment questionnaire to ascertain staff perception of the no interruption zone. Next, 10 medication preparation cycles were observed utilizing the modified MADOS sheet designed by Pape, 2003. Then, a large, colorful poster was installed

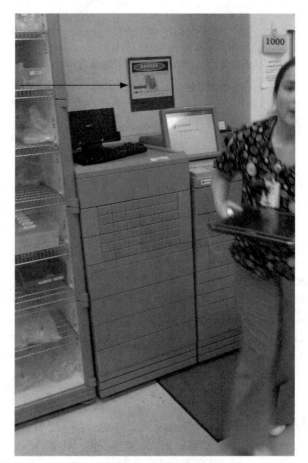

FIGURE 15-6 Observation of medication preparation and interruptions.

above all of the medication dispensing machines indicating the red zone area (See **Figure 15-6**). Flyers similar to the large poster were prepared and disseminated for additional education. The reinforced signs were large, colorful posters. Temporarily, additional posters were placed in the lounge to further engage employees. The objective of the posters was to draw attention to the red zone and to avoid the "wallpaper syndrome" that occurs as a result of monotony.

Once approval was granted through the institutional review board of the university and the project hospital, there were two implementations for this project. First, education on the red zone was provided, and second, additional signs and posters were installed to reinforce the education concerning the red zone. An assessment questionnaire was anonymously administered before and after the education to assess the response of the nurses to the education (see **Appendix 15C**). Utilizing the modified MADOS tool, interruption observations were collected prior to the implementations and then, again, after the implementations to determine if the two implementations were impactful. The questionnaire data were collected and analyzed on a locked personal computer after consent was achieved. Only the investigator had access to the data. No personal or identifying information was included on the questionnaire. A small budget was necessary for implementation (see **Appendix 15D**).

POTENTIAL BARRIERS TO IMPLEMENTATION

While every effort was made to minimize the impact of potential variables, there were several barriers to this small test of change. First, the amount of time to implement the project necessitated strict adherence to a proposed timeline for completion. Next, according to the IRB, informed consent was necessary for every observation. Finally, a lack of formal departmental meetings essentially eliminated the possibility of a formal educational session.

The time limitation was a significant obstacle to overcome (see **Appendix 15E**). The small test of change incorporated the time limitation; however, there were some unpredictable impacts during the small test of change. For example, the limited amount of time reduced the time available for the nurses to complete the assessment questionnaire and the amount of time for observation of interruptions.

The timeline answered this challenge because it became an outline to ensure completion of the project in a timely manner. While the timeline provided rigid due dates, it also allowed flexibility in the display of results. As opportunities emerged to present preliminary results, the timeline allowed for explanation of the process of the project, and it provided stakeholders with clarity of the progress of the project.

Because the project was implemented on a medical-surgical floor that did not hold staff meetings, educating the staff simultaneously was a challenge. The education session became individualized or group based. This was ultimately beneficial because staff developed ownership of the reduction of interruptions during medication preparation. These small educational sessions provided group discussions and incorporated active learning, which is pivotal to deep learning.

According to the IRB, informed consent was necessary from each participant. This presented a challenge because of staff awareness of observation. The Hawthorne effect was an identified potential weakness of the project as a result of direct observation for interruptions; therefore, the interruption tracking was performed in small increments by the educator. In the end, informed consent was actually beneficial to the overall success of the project because staff were aware of the importance of data collection as a result of the explanation of the project. The informed consent process actually allowed for additional education. Staff displayed a willingness to help facilitate the observation of the data.

UNINTENDED CONSEQUENCES

In an attempt to collect the number of unnecessary interruptions, a definition of appropriate interruptions was essential. For example, because the project hospital encouraged teaching, it was important to develop a standard that acknowledged the role of a nurse speaking with a student or preceptor about medication while on the red carpet.

Additionally, it was imperative to acknowledge and support the importance of communication while on the red mat for wasting narcotics and returning narcotics. These actions must be confirmed by two nurses and require communication. Discouraging appropriate communication that revolves around safe medication preparation and dispensing would be inappropriate and not the intention of this project. Additionally, there may appear to be an increase in medication errors after implementation of an intervention because of increased vigilance and improved reporting.

Analyzing

The analysis is the change between the baseline and the outcome data. In this phase, the effectiveness of the evidence-based initiative is analyzed using the SPSS Statistics software. Beyond the qualitative data, the qualitative analysis of the assessment questionnaire also provided valuable information about the perception of interruptions by the staff.

OUTCOMES AND EVALUATION

Two outcomes were evaluated in this small test of change (see **Appendix F**). First, the number of interruptions within 10 medication preparation cycles were counted pre- and posteducation. Second, a staff assessment and willingness to comply was measured with a 5-question assessment survey pre- and posteducation. The 3 categories of outcome evaluations are behavioral, clinical, and health outcomes. The behavioral outcome for this project was based on staff member compliance with the red zone that was measured through the survey. The clinical outcome was the total number of interruptions. Because interruptions can lead to medication errors, the overall health outcome is the number and level of medication errors. This small test of change did not measure the number of medication errors; however, for a fully implemented project additional medication cycles could be observed and data from the safety registry could provide the total number of medication errors (see **Table 15-1**).

INTERRUPTIONS

The initial plans for specific implementation included the collection of data from one medical-surgical unit at the project hospital. Initial data was collected about the compliance of the unit with the no interruption zone. Prior to any changes, 10 cycles of medication preparation were observed, and the number of interruptions were recorded using the modified Medication Administration Distraction Observation Sheet (MADOS) designed by Pape (2003). This validated tool contained definitions of distraction categories, and it was utilized to reduce bias for the observational portion of this project (Pape, 2003). The types of interruptions collected during this project were categorized into: physician, other personnel, phone calls, patients,

TABLE 15-1 A Plan for Measuring Red Zone Success

Outcome	Measurement	Source
Interruptions/types of interruptions	Raw numbers, 10 medication preparations before education and 10 after education	Direct observation
Assessment	Descriptive information	Assessment questionnaire
Number of medication errors (only for full implementation—not for small test of change)	Raw numbers, categorized	Clinical pharmacy manager or patient safety management

visitors, missing medications, wrong dose medications, emergencies, conversations, and external noise. Consent for observation was obtained, and interruptions were measured by cycles to maintain confidentiality. After an educational session and the implementation of additional signs, another 10 cycles of medication preparation were observed with the number of interruptions. Finally, a survey was conducted regarding the implementation of the red carpet, which contributed qualitative data to the results.

Ideally, for a full-scope evidence-based design project, in an equation, the number of interruptions could be the numerator while the number of minutes of medication preparation could be the denominator. This would produce a ratio or percentage of interruptions per hour of medication preparation. Because of the time constraint and data collection challenges associated with this small test of change, a raw number of interruptions was sufficient. The posteducation data were analyzed using the SPSS Statistics software with the data obtained prior to the education and poster implementation. A t-test was utilized in the statisical analysis.

MEDICATION ERRORS

Interruptions are related to a process; however, this data provided an accurate measurement of an improved process that was a result of an implementation of an evidence-based design feature. An additional outcome measure for a full-scope project would include the total number of medication errors; unfortunately, because the medication errors are collected quarterly, medication errors would not be accurately available for the scope of this project. For a full implementation, medication error information could be obtained from the patient safety database where medication errors are inputted by nurses. Accurate data on the number of medication errors committed by a nurse is difficult to obtain based on the perceived potential disciplinary action for reporting an error. Therefore, measuring the number of interruptions related to each intervention may prove more accurate.

DATA MANAGEMENT

In order to determine the impact of the red zone on the number of interruptions, data must be collected and analyzed appropriately. Healthcare professionals are inundated with decisions; the importance of correct data and analysis is imperative. The art of statistical thinking requires clear, measurable operational definitions, objectives, and data (Carey & Lloyd, 2001). The results must be interpreted correctly, and a chart or graph must be appropriate for the display of the results. While descriptive statistics were used to organize and summarize data, inferential statistics were used to evaluate the statistical significance of the data.

RESULTS

A literature search conducted prior to the small test of change revealed important information about the no interruption zone. Studies showed that interruptions were a problem during medication preparation, and interruptions could lead to medication errors. Implementing a no interruption zone could reduce the opportunity for interruptions during medication preparation (Pape, 2003). The results of this small test of change were congruent with those findings.

Most categories' interruptions decreased after the education. However, some interruptions were unaffected by the education. For example, the institutional phones carried by the nurses were still ringing during medication preparation. The nurses did not want to answer during medication preparation; it was highly distracting to them. The most significant and obvious changes in the preeducation and posteducation data occurred in the total interruptions category and other personnel category. The education created a temporary awareness on the unit about interruptions during medication preparation.

Most nurses found interruptions during medication preparation irritating. Moreover, all of the assessment surveys with one exception revealed that the nurses did not have confidence in the ability of the red carpet to reduce interruptions independently. Interruptions within these medication rooms were complex and multidimensional. A cumulative solution that included ongoing education, administrative support, design changes, and cultural infusion of the impact of interruptions was necessary.

The staff clearly recognized the importance of reducing interruptions even after only one brief educational session. There were two main issues. First, there were interruptions that were beyond the control of the nurse, which included the phone and overhead pages. Second, the size and the layout of the medication room prevented the reduction in interruptions. Because the room is a large, multipurpose room, it was physically impossible for the nurse on the red carpet to remain uninterrupted as staff members revolved through the doors of the supply room. This promoted an atmosphere of camaraderie and conversation. In order to address this change, the unit will need ongoing education and reinforcement of the importance of reducing interruptions.

DATA ANALYSIS

The data analysis in this project revealed interesting information. While the majority of interruption categories showed a decrease in the raw number of interruptions, only two categories showed a statisically significant decrease in interruptions after the interventions. This data brings an awareness to the importance of statistical inference as opposed to the reliance on raw numbers when addressing the validity of evidence in evidence-based practice (see **Figure 15-7**).

The posteducation data was analyzed in the SPSS Statistics software with the data obtained prior to the education and poster implementation. A t-test was utilized in the statisical analysis. A liberal alpha was utilized

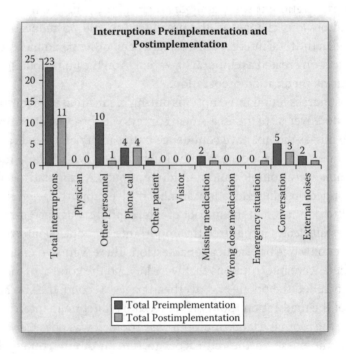

FIGURE 15-7 The change in the raw number of interruptions.

TABLE 15-2 Statistical Differences in Interruptions and Difference in Raw Numbers of Interruptions

Interruption Type	T-Test	Mean Difference	Raw Data Difference in Interruptions
Total interruptions	0.0615	1.2	12
Other personnel	0.046	0.9	5
Phone calls	0.5	0	1
Other patients	0.172	0.1	0
Missing medication	0.279	0.1	1
Emergency situation	0.172	−0.1	−1
Conversation	0.194	0.2	2
External noises	0.331	0.1	0
Visitors	0	0	0
Physicians	0	0	0
Wrong dose medication	0	0	0

because of the small sample size. With a 90 percent confidence interval, the total interruptions category and the other personnel category had a statistically signficant decrease in interruptions (see **Table 15-2**).

COMPLIANCE

Beyond the significance of the quantitative data analysis and the statistically significant reduction in interruptions, the survey questionnaire provided qualitative data. In addition to the observerance of interruptions, a preeducation assessment was administered randomly and confidentially to the nurses of the unit concerning compliance with the red zone. This assessment provided valuable information to address within the educational sessions. Next, an educational session was provided, and more effective posters were installed above the medication dispensing machine and in high-traffic areas around the unit. After the educational session, a postsession survey was administered to determine staff awareness and willingness to comply.

Staff members reported via the survey that the most imposing interruption during medication preparation was their institutional phone

(IP). Even while attempting to provide education about the no interruption zone, the nurse conducting the education was interrupted several times during different education sessions because of work-related phone calls. These institutional phones had purpose; however, phone calls were causing observable interruptions to the nurses' workflow, and the abundance of incoming calls was causing visible frustration in the nurses. This frustration was not isolated to the medication room. The impact of interrupted workflow spills over into multiple facets of nursing care.

Additionally, the assessment questionaire specifically asked if the nurse thought that the red carpet was effective in reducing distratctions. On a scale of 1–5 with 1 being not at all effective, the average answer prior to education on the surveys was 1.9. The average response after the education was 2.2. Meanwhile, there was no change in nurses' opinion that distractors cause errors.

While nurses agreed that distractions could provide an opportunity for medication errors, prior to education, they felt that the red carpet or the no interruption zone was not an effective way of reducing distractions. After an educational session, the nurses' perception of the ability of the red carpet to reduce interrruptions changed. After an explanation of the value of the no interruption zone, nurses recognized the impact that reducing interruptions could have on patient safety and the reduction of medication errors. This small test of change exhibited the importance of a cultural awareness of evidence-based practice. Nurses and staff want to implement safe and effective standards of care, but they want to know that the changes are based on valid, reliable evidence.

Adopting and Advancing

Adopting the project is the consideration of taking the small test of change or the pilot throughout the organization. Finally, advancing involves the dissemination of the findings to a broader area (Brown & Ecoff, 2011). Evidence-based design projects are important to disseminate in order to facilitate growth in the field of design and contribute to the evidence related to EBD. Currently, the pharmacy clinical manager and the director of patient safety have shown interest and provided guidance for this project. These stakeholders are pivotal in the dissemination of this information and the adaptation of these environmental changes throughout the hospital. The findings from this project were presented to the clinical unit manager. A poster was created for the visual display of evidence.

Discussion

Evidence supports that the implementation of evidence-based design, such as a red zone, reduces nursing interruptions and medication errors. This project was important to understanding the impact that design had on distractions, interruptions, and medication errors. Design evidence included not only arrangements that positively influence outcomes by enhanced physical layout, but also how humans respond to the environmental changes. Additionally, in order to foster support, changes based on the best evidence must be accompanied by education, accountability, and a sustainment plan. Ultimately, a systems approach to evidence-based design is imperative. Trained, supportive staff and adopted policies combined with environmental changes will achieve successful outcomes (Morrill, Taege, & Slater, 2010). Measuring interruptions and nursing satisfaction provides feedback to the original PICO question. Because this was not a stagnant process, changes can, and should be, implemented and reassessed as hospitals move toward error-free environments.

Florence Nightingale recognized the importance of the environment on the health and well-being of patients. Environmental psychology has emerged as a scientific discipline with a focus on the understanding of the relationship between humans and the environment (Moore & Geboy, 2010). Literature supports the link of the physical environment in the promotion of health and safety (Brown & Ecoff, 2011). Drawing from evidence-based practice models in medicine and nursing, a systematic approach can be applied to evidence-based design (Brown & Ecoff, 2011). The model of evidence-based decision making can be applied to design. This eight-step model helped achieve desired results by focusing on and evaluating outcomes. The process encouraged addressing the catalyst in a structured manner, and the use of a PICO(T) question identified an answerable and appropriate question.

For this project proposal, interruptions and medication errors were examined in the context of the influence of the environment. A clear linear relationship was identified between the complexity of the nursing role, the complexity of medication administration, the frequency of interruptions, and the directly proportional relationship of interruptions to medication errors. Changes in the design of the environment based on evidence had an impact on the distractions of nurses during medication administration. Ultimately, environmental changes caused a significant reduction in interruptions during medication preparation, resulting in a reduction of medication errors.

Presenting evidence of the impact of the no interruption zone produced predictable apprehension and resistance from the nursing staff. According to Groccia (1997), learning involves discomfort and disequilibrium. Groccia further acknowledges that conflicts occur when new information or new perspectives are uncovered. This makes a cultural shift within the organization all the more important in evidence-based medicine.

While the red carpet was already in place, a prospective view of evidence-based design was achieved by implementing education and an ongoing sustainment plan. The number and types of unnecessary interruptions provided statistical information on the potential impact on patient safety as a result of the implementation of environmental changes. Data from this proposed red zone project provided evidence to support the benefits of implementation of a red zone or a no interruption zone protocol in other facilities. Data collection and analysis from the implementation of the no interruption zones indicated a potential impact of hospital design on patient safety.

Findings

This project explored the impact that evidence had on the design of the medication room, and more specifically, the impact of a zone devoted specifically to medication preparation would have on the reduction of medication errors. The raw data from the small test of change concluded that interruptions can be reduced with education and environmental changes such as a no interruption zone. Categorically, interruptions during medication preparation were reduced in this small test of change after education was provided. There was a statistically significant difference in the overall number of interruptions. Additionally, the category known as "other personnel" also saw a statistically significant drop in interruptions. This reinforces the need for education throughout the staff and cultural changes throughout the institution. While the nurses were the only staff members to receive the education, other personnel were clearly impacted by the additional signage and discussions surrounding the no interruption zones.

Utilizing evidence to make the best decisions serves two purposes. Uncovering evidence for any change ensures the validity of the improvement, but also the dissemination of the evidence serves as a tool to promote organizational support. Through evidence, leaders, clinicians, and institutional staff can see the impact that changes have on their institution. This creates a cultural shift to incorporate evidence-based practice into the institution.

IMPLICATIONS

Important implications have been identified within this project. First, evidence-based design impacts the quality and safety of organizations. This small test of change identified a statistically significant difference in interruptions during medication preparation with the implementation and education of a no interruption zone.

Beyond the design changes that are implemented, the leadership of the hospital must create a vision that incorporates evidence-based practice into their mission and cultural values. Education that extends beyond displaying evidence can assist with transformative changes within an organization. Education should consist of assessment and evaluation, teaching, and active learning. In this sense, educating staff about the evidence that supports institutional change serves as a marketing tool in order to get buy-in from the clinician, staff, and patients. Education that extends beyond specific organizational changes and promotes the incorporation of evidence-based practice creates a cultural awareness of the ongoing drive for excellence.

FURTHER RESEARCH

Further research in consideration of evidence-based design should include the impact of lean and the organizational culture. Because performance improvement cannot occur in a vacuum, senior leaders and champions must be involved for sustained success of evidence-based design. The built environment is one aspect of quality patient care. Changing operational processes and physical environment within an organization involves a change in the culture of the organization also. Empowering people makes quality and improvements more successful and sustainable (Morrill et al., 2010). Senior leaders, clinicians, and patients should be included in the aspects of evidence-based design and the journey to quality care.

Increasing evidence in evidence-based design is necessary. Moreover, specific design changes need further exploration. Evidence supports the necessity of a no interruption zone; however, there is a need for further research in consideration of the medication room. A comparison of locked medication rooms that only allow for one to two nurses at a time could be compared to large open medication rooms that expose the medication nurse to noise, interruptions, and open access. In this particular project, the expanse of the medication room with open access significantly impacted the ability of the nurse to concentrate. Furthermore, the large medication room significantly reduced the amount of control of medications. The constant barrage of multiple and interdisciplinary healthcare providers created a chaotic environment that was simply not conducive to reducing and eliminating distractions. Furthermore, The Joint Commission standards insist on medication rooms that have controlled access.

Additionally, further research is necessary to evaluate specific methods for the incorporation of evidence-based practice changes into the organization. Evidence to support changes that promote quality and safety of patient care is essential, but without proper support and implementation of the changes, the evidence is virtually useless. Organizations that create a vision and culture of continuous quality and safety improvement are essential for the ongoing implementation of evidence-based design and the pursuit of excellence in care.

Conclusion

In the end, this project extended far beyond evidence-based design and evidence-based practice. The process of gathering evidence to support a small test of change, implementing the small test of change, interpreting the data collecting, and disseminating the information revealed important considerations. The importance of education and organizational awareness of evidence-based practice was exposed. Human behavior contributes to the science of nursing as much as evidence, the environment, or scientific study. Nurse educators have the ability to reach beyond the rhetoric of lectures and enhance the quality of the patient experience by tapping into the unique individual qualities of future healthcare providers. With so much information about the advances in healthcare and the move for reform, ultimately, the care of humans remains constant across organizational, cultural, and national boundaries. While much of what we, as healthcare professionals, do is a science, but as Nightingale said, nursing remains an art of caring. Nurse educators tap into a unique blend of caring for patients, students, and the science of nursing.

References

Akansel, N., & Kaymakci, S. (2008). Effects of intensive care unit noise on patients: A study on coronary artery bypass graft surgery patients. *Journal of Clinical Nursing, 17*(12), 1581–1590.

Anthony, K., Wiencek, C., Bauer, C., Daly, B., & Anthony, M. K. (2010). No interruptions please: Impact of a no interruption zone on medication safety in intensive care units. *Critical Care Nurse, 30*(3), 21–28.

Armitage, G., & Knapman, H. (2003). Adverse events in drug administration: A literature review. *Journal of Nursing Management, 11*, 130–140.

Biron, A. D., Lavole-Tremblay, M., & Loiselle, C. G. (2009). Characteristics of work interruptions during medication administration. *Journal of Nursing Scholarship, 21*(4), 330–336.

Bliss-Holtz, J. (2007). Evidence-based practice: A primer for action. *Issues in Comprehensive Pediatric Nursing, 30*, 165–182.

Brown, C. E., & Ecoff, L. (2011). A systematic approach to the inclusion of evidence in healthcare design. *Health Environments Research and Design Journal, 4*(2), 7–16.

Cama, R. (2009). *Evidence-based healthcare design*. Hoboken, NJ: John Wiley & Sons, Inc.

Carey, R. G., & Lloyd, R. C. (2001). *Measuring quality improvement in healthcare: A guide to statistical process control applications*. Milwaukee, WI: American Society for Quality.

Chaudhury, H., Mahmood, A., & Valente, M. (2009). The effect of environmental design on reducing nursing errors and increasing efficiency in acute care settings: A review and analysis of the literature. *Environment and Behavior, 41*(6), 755–786.

Dijkstra, K., Pieterse, M., & Pruyn, A. (2006). Physical environmental stimuli that turn healthcare facilities into healing environments through psychologically mediated effects: Systematic review. *Journal of Advanced Nursing, 56*(2), 166–181.

Ecoff, L., & Brown, C. E. (2010). Evidence-based architectural and space design supports magnet empirical outcomes. *Journal of Nursing Administration, 40*(12), 505–507.

Edvardsson, J. D., Sandman, P., & Rasmussen, B. H. (2005). Sensing an atmosphere of ease: A tentative theory of supportive care settings. *Scandinavian Journal of Caring Science, 19,* 344–353.

Gillis, D. (2010). The art & science of evidence-based design. *UX Magazine, 523,* 1–6. Retrieved from http://uxmag.com/articles/the-art-and-science-of-evidence-based-design

Groccia, J. E. (1997). The student as customer versus the student as learner. *About Campus, 2,* 2.

Hendrich, A., Chow, M., Skierczynski, B. A., & Zhenqiang, L. (2008). A 36 hospital time and motion study: How do medical-surgical nurses spend their time? *The Permanente Journal, 12*(3), 25–34.

Hodgkinson, B., Nay, R., & Nichols, K. (2006). Strategies to reduce medication errors with reference to older adults. *International Journal of Evidence-Based Health*care, *4*(1), 2–41.

Interruptions to nurses during medication administration: Are there implications for the quality of patient care? (2010). *Policy,* (22). Retrieved from http://www.kcl.ac.uk/nursing/research/nnru/policy/Policy-Plus-Issues-by-Theme/hownursingcareisdelivered/PolicyIssue22.pdf

The Joanna Briggs Institute. (2009). Strategies to reduce medication errors in older adults. *Australian Nursing Journal, 17*(3), 30–33.

Leape, L. L. (1994). Error in medicine. *The Journal of the American Medical Association, 272*(23), 1851–1857.

Melnyk, B. M. & Fineout-Overholt, E. (2011). *Evidence-based practice in nursing and healthcare: A guide to best practice.* Philadelphia: Lippincott, Williams & Wilkins.

Moore, K. D., & Geboy, L. (2010). The question of evidence: Current worldviews in environmental design research and practice. *Cambridge Journals, 14*(2), 105–114.

Moore, K. D., & Geboy, L. (2011). Regarding the question of evidence: Worldviews in environmental design research. In M. Bonaiuto, M. Bonnes, A.M. Nenci and G. Carrus (Eds.) *Urban Diversity-Environmental and Social Issues.* Gottinger, Germany: Hostefe.

Morrill, P., Taege, K., & Slater, K. (2010). Lessons learned: A systems approach to lean and evidence-based design. *ASQ Healthcare Update.* Retrieved from http://www.kahlerslater.com/content/pdf/ASQ-Guest-Essay-August-2010.pdf

Pape, T. M. (2003). Applying airline safety practices to medication administration. *Medsurg Nursing, 12*(2), 77–93.

Patel, V. L., Cohen, T., Murarka, T., Olsen, J., Kagita, S., Myneni, S., Ghaemmaghami, V. (2011). Recovery at the edge of error: Debunking the myth of the infallible expert. *Journal of Biomedical Informatics, 44*(3), 413–424.

Safe practice environment chapter proposed by USP. (2008). *Medication Safety Alert.* Retrieved from http://www.ismp.org/newsletters/acutecare/archives/Dec08.asp

Stichler, J. F. (2010). Evaluating the evidence in evidence-based design. *Journal of Nursing Administration, 40*(9), 348–351.

Tucker, A., & Spear, S. (2006). Operational failures and interruptions in hospital nursing. *Health Services Research, 41*(3, Pt 1), 643–662.

Ulrich, R. S., Zimring, C., Zhu, X., Dubose, J., Seo, H., Choi, Y., . . . Joseph, A. (2008). *Evidence-based design resources for healthcare executives* [white paper]. Retrieved from https://www.healthdesign.org/sites/default/files/LitReviewWP_FINAL.pdf

Westbrook, J., Woods, A., Rob, M. I., Dunsmuir, W. T., & Day, R. O. (2010). Association of interruptions with an increased risk and severity of medication administration errors. *Archives of Internal Medicine, 170*(8), 683–690.

Evidence Analysis Grid

Article (APA Citation) Level of Evidence of Article (1–6)	Purpose of Study or Review	Design and Methods, Sampling Method, Population, Sample Size, Description of Interventions (if Any), Instruments Used, and Outcomes Measured	Major Findings/Findings Relevant to the Project	Critique of Study/Review for the Project (What Makes It Strong or Weak Evidence to Use)
Dijkstra, K., Pieterse, M., & Pruyn, A. (2006). Physical environmental stimuli that turn healthcare facilities into healing environments through psychologically mediated effects: Systematic review. *Journal of Advanced Nursing* 56(2), 166–181. doi:10.1111/j.1365-2648.2006.03990.x This is a level 1 study.	The review question is not clearly stated until the results section. The authors wanted to determine, based on research, if the design of a healthcare setting impacted the patients, and if so, what elements affected the patients and in what way. The authors wanted to gather evidence that could serve for the design of healthcare environments and research. They sought to collect conclusive evidence to formulate practice guidelines with evidence-based design.	This is a systematic review of 30 studies. A summary of findings is in the section heading, *Results of the Review* (p. 178). In the multiple stimuli studies, conflicting results were noted. Specific effects of single design elements appeared to be based on patient population.	Unfortunately, because no clinical guideline was determined, there is not a specific implementation that can be addressed. This review supports the idea that the physical environment affects patient health, and awareness of the impact of the environment is important. However, without further conclusive evidence, implementation into practice should be approached with caution. Additionally, in acknowledgement of this study, a systematic review of studies concerning the physical environment on patient safety is warranted.	Without review of individual studies, the consideration of the full extent of clinical outcomes cannot be determined. However, each study was evaluated in the table and in the narrative portion of the review. The table addresses outcome measures; it did not address individual study outcomes. The review mentions methodological flaws and gives one example, but it does not describe in detail evident flaws within each study. The authors make a clear recommendation that further clinical trials are necessary. The authors note that studies with less rigorous methodology have more positive conclusions. The authors sought to collect conclusive evidence to formulate practice guidelines with evidence-based design.

(continues)

Article (APA Citation) Level of Evidence of Article (1–7)	Purpose of Study or Review	Design and Methods, Sampling Method, Population, Sample Size, Description of Interventions (if Any), Instruments Used, and Outcomes Measured	Major Findings/Findings Relevant to the Project	Critique of Study/Review for the Project (What Makes It Strong or Weak Evidence to Use)
Hendrich, A., Chow, M., Skierczynski, B. A., & Zhenqiang, L. (2008). A 36 hospital time and motion study: How do medical-surgical nurses spend their time? *The Permanente Journal, 12*(3), 25–34. This is a level 4 study.	The purpose of this study was to identify the causes of nurse inefficiency and determine if the design of the hospital environment impacted nurse efficiency. The study aimed to reveal how nurses spend their time within their nursing functions, nonclinical activities, and waste. The study also looked at the nurses' movement efficiency. Finally, the study looked at the physiologic impact of the work environment on clinical nurses.	This was a quantitative descriptive time and motion study to identify how nurses spend their time. The time and motion study was conducted at 36 hospital medical-surgical units within 17 healthcare systems and 15 states. There were four protocols; A, B, C, and D to obtain baseline data for EHR, implement nursing activities, observe nursing movement, and record the nurse physiologic response. Nurses were randomly selected for A or B protocols. Then, all nurses were asked to participate in the C protocol, which automatically put them also into the D protocol. Nurses in the A and B group carried PDAs to document activities. Nurses in the C group wore radiofrequency identification (RFID) tags. Nurses in the D group utilized armbands to measure the physiologic metrics. A total of 763 nurses completed the study.	The study revealed the main location areas of nurses during their shifts. In order of frequency, the nursing station (38.6%), the patient room (30.8), somewhere on the unit (23.7%), and off of the unit (6.9%) were the locations. Nursing activity was also revealed. In order of time, nurses spent their day in nursing practice (77.7%), nonclinical functions (12.6%), waste (6.6%), and unrelated functions (2.8%). The study uncovered that more than 75% of nursing time was devoted to clinical practice, which included documentation, medication, and care coordination. These three areas of clinical practice were identified as targets for improving nursing efficiency.	Weaknesses: This study had a self-reporting methodology. Because nurses categorized their own activities during the study, there could have been some debatable category selections. Also, because nurses were concentrating on their clinical practice duties, they may have pressed incorrect buttons on their PDAs or forgotten to turn off their PDAs. Strengths: This was a fairly large study across several different hospitals in different states. Highly technological equipment was utilized to ensure quality results. Significance: The study recognizes three main ideas for improving efficiency: documentation, medication administration, and care coordination.

Citation	Purpose	Methods	Results	Strengths/Weaknesses
Tucker, A., & Spear, S. (2006). Operational failures and interruptions in hospital nursing. *Health Services Research, 41*(3, Pt 1), 643–662. This is a level 4 study.	The purpose of this article was to examine the work environment of nurses and the effects of the environment on patient care. Two sources were identified as causes for negative effects. First, as new information becomes available about the patient, the care plan is changed. Second, a glitch or an error occurs, which causes the caregiver to adjust to the operational failure. This study examines potential operational failures, their interference with nursing care, and what adaptations nurses make to compensate for the failures.	Direct observation, interviews, and surveys were utilized to collect data. First, 11 experienced nurses in complete and different shifts were observed at 6 different hospitals. Work activities were recorded. Next, 6 of the nurses were interviewed with a standard questionnaire. In the third phase, nurses and nurse managers from 48 different units and 21 different hospitals were surveyed.	There was an average of 8.4 operational failures per shift. The categories included: medication problems, medical orders, supply issues, and staffing issues. Observational findings concluded that the average task time for the nurse was 3.1 minutes. Nurses switched patient care every 11 minutes, and nurses were interrupted at least 8 times per shift. Nurses performed an average of 84 different types of tasks within a shift. This was defined in the study as *interweaving*. The term *partitioning* was defined as the separation of tasks for each patient. *Reprioritizing* was necessary when the plan of care was changed due to inherent clinical factors or to operational failures. All three tactics increase the likelihood of error.	Weaknesses: (1) This study only measured inpatients. (2) Observation may have changed the behavior of the nurses. A correlation between work tactics and medical errors could not be made because of the design of the study. Strengths: (1) The study concluded that 5% of interruptions were related to operational failures inferring that addressing these failures could lessen interruptions. (2) The study identifies coping mechanisms for operational failures.

(continues)

Article (APA Citation) Level of Evidence of Article (1–7)	Purpose of Study or Review	Design and Methods, Sampling Method, Population, Sample Size, Description of Interventions (if Any), Instruments Used, and Outcomes Measured	Major Findings/Findings Relevant to the Project	Critique of Study/Review for the Project (What Makes It Strong or Weak Evidence to Use)
Armitage, G., & Knapman, H. (2003). Adverse events in drug administration: A literature review. *Journal of Nursing Management, 11,* 130–140. This is a literature review with a low level of evidence; level 7.	This study was a literature review to explore the causes of medication errors.	This is a literature review with a low level of evidence (7). However, it provides a thorough overview of potential reasons for medication administration errors. This study adds an important angle to this proposal. It also helps as a comparison with other higher evidenced studies.	This is a literature review with a low level of evidence. However, the most important finding is the discussion of a system failure as opposed to an individual failure in a medication error. The study acknowledges the importance of changing the system as opposed to blaming individuals for medication errors. "Human error is a consequence rather than a cause" (p. 133).	This is a literature review, which makes it a low level of evidence. However, this study adds an important dimension to this proposal. The study does not acknowledge how many studies were reviewed for this literature review. The study identifies several causes for medication errors, and it identifies interruptions as a contributor to medication errors.
Biron, A. D., Lavole-Tremblay, M., & Loiselle, C. G. (2009). Characteristics of work interruptions during medication administration. *Journal of Nursing Scholarship, 21*(4), 330–336. This is a level 4 study.	The purpose of this study was to observe the work interruptions of clinical nurses during medication administration.	This is a descriptive observations study design. A better understanding of work interruptions is necessary to tackle medication safety issues. This study followed 102 medication administration rounds. This study found that nurse colleagues and system failures were the most frequent sources of interruptions. The article proposes that system failures should be targeted to maximize medication administration safety. Furthermore, the process of medication administration needs to be protected against work interruptions.	The study discovered 6.3 interruptions per hour that lasted about 1 minute and 32 seconds. Nurse colleagues and system failures were the primary interruption.	Medication administration is a frequent activity of nurses; and therefore, subject to the most frequent interruptions. Weaknesses: The direct observational study could have impacted the participants' activity. There is a generalization of data to inpatient healthcare settings. This was one setting. Strengths: Observation concluded that nurses' colleagues were the primary reason for interruptions. This indicates that eliminating this potential safety risk would have an impact on interruptions.

Westbrook, J., Woods, A., Rob, M. I., Dunsmuir, W. T., & Day, R. O. (2010). Association of interruptions with an increased risk and severity of medication administration errors. *Archives of Internal Medicine, 170*(8), 683–690. This is a level 4 study.	This study tested the impact of interruptions on errors in medication administration.	This is an observation study in 6 wards at 2 teaching hospitals. Clinical errors were identified by observation and charting. The study took place over 6 months with 98 nurses and 4,271 medications to 720 patients. This study determined that the occurrence of interruptions is associated with procedural failures and clinical errors. Each interruption caused a 12.1% increase in procedural failures. Each interruption caused a 12.7% increase in clinical errors. Nurse experience did not impact failures. Error severity increased with more interruptions. The risk of a major error doubled with interruptions.	Each interruption produced a 12.1 percent increase in failures and a 12.7 percent increase in clinical failures. Interruptions occurred in 53.1 percent of administrations. Error severity increased with interruption. The more interruptions, the greater the number of errors.	Weaknesses: Because this is an observational study, observed behavior could have changed. However, this study was performed over 6 months; so, sustained changes would have been difficult. Strengths: The study found that part-time nurses and nurses with less experience had fewer errors. It appears that more seasoned nurses become more comfortable with patients and patient care, undermining the need for safety structure. This study indicates that there is indeed a significant relationship between interruption and medication preparation and delivery.

(continues)

Article (APA Citation) Level of Evidence of Article (1–7)	Purpose of Study or Review	Design and Methods, Sampling Method, Population, Sample Size, Description of Interventions (if Any), Instruments Used, and Outcomes Measured	Major Findings/Findings Relevant to the Project	Critique of Study/Review for the Project (What Makes It Strong or Weak Evidence to Use)
Anthony, K., Wiencek, C., Bauer, C., Daly, B., & Anthony, M. K. (2010). No interruptions please: Impact of a no interruption zone on medication safety in intensive care units. *Critical Care Nurse, 30*(3), 21–28. This is a level 3 study.	This article described the implementation of a no interruption zone to limit interruptions and distractions encountered by nurses during medication preparation.	This is a quasi-experimental pilot study using methods of observations. The PICO question was: Does the implementation of a no interruption zone decrease the number of interruptions during medication preparation?	The no interruption zone decreased interruptions by 40.9 percent.	One concern about this study is the importance of communication between staff and between preceptors and nurses. Communication with coordination cannot be overlooked in patient safety. Strengths: Although the study did not count pharmacy rounds as interruptions, the authors noted that this could be disruptive to the nurse. Weaknesses: This study was performed in two ICUs only over 1 week. The study could not completely eliminate disruptions. The no interruption zone was not extended to the medication refrigerator. Also, there was not a final analysis on reduction of medication errors—only a reduction of interruptions. The study is significant because it directly addresses the reduction of interruptions.

Pape, T. M. (2003). Applying airline safety practices to medication administration. *Medsurg Nursing*, 12(2), 77–93. This is a level 3 study.	The purpose of this paper is to discuss the complexity in the nursing role and in the administration of medication. The author utilizes aviation science as a comparison to the standards and safety of medicine. Two interventions were tested. The PICO(T) is "Which distracters are more predictive of nurses being distracted during medication administration cycles?" (p. 83).	This is a quasi-experimental, three-group design that tested two interventions. The focused protocol and the Medsafe protocol were tested with education interventions. A medication administration distraction observation sheet (MADOS) was used to count distractions during medication administration.	In all three groups, distractions decreased. The Medsafe protocol had the greatest decrease in distractions. The study noted that visual cues and teamwork played a significant role in the reduction of distractions.	Weaknesses: Only one nurse was observed at a time. The nurses were observed during the day shift at busy times. There was no medication room in the unit where the study was conducted. Medication rooms may decrease distractions. The Hawthorne effect may have provided limitation to the study. Strengths: There was a clear relationship to the interventions and a decrease in interruptions. Further investigation of medical errors would be prudent.
	This is a review of evidence on the impact of interruptions on medication errors and methods for the reduction of interruptions.	The article reviews 12 pieces of literature. The author defined interruptions, reviewed the literature available, uncovered contributions to nurse interruptions, and reviewed interventions to reduce interruptions. Systematic reviews and primary research studies were included in the review.	There were three major findings within this review. Nursing interruptions contribute to medication errors. Interruptions interfere with cognitive abilities. There are multiple interventions available to minimize nursing interruptions.	This article combines several articles included in this grid to form clear conclusions and implications. This is an important addition to the grid because of the compilation of evidence. The weakness is in the length of the article, which is two pages. More insight would have been interesting.

Small Test of Change Timeline

IMPLEMENTATION PLAN AND TIMELINE

Project: The Impact of Evidence-Based Design

Project Leader (Student): Heather Hardin

	Activities Planned	Date
12/1–1/15	• Meet with pharmacy, clinical effectiveness, and submit IRB to project hospital for approval.	12.2011 completed
	• Submit letter of approval from project hospital to university IRB.	1.2012 completed
Checkpoint No. 1 1/16–1/27	• Submit timeline	1.16.2012
	• Get university IRB approval	1.31.2012
	• Meet with unit manager and PCC to discuss project implementation	1.16.2012
	• Collect preeducation interruption data and administer assessment	2.2.2012
	• Final Excel spreadsheet and code due	1.23.2012
	• Log No. 1 due	1.27.2012
Checkpoint No. 2 1/30–2/10	• Creation of implementation poster	1.30.2012
	• Hold educational session	TBD
	• Poster implementation on the unit	1.30.2012
	• Wimba	2.2.2012
	• Abstract completed	2.6.2012
	• Collect postimplementation data	2.9.2012
	• Log No. 2 due	2.10.2012

	Activities Planned	Date
Checkpoint No. 3 2/13–2/24	• Analyze data	2.17.2012
	• Log No. 3 due	2.24.2012
Checkpoint No. 4 2/27–3/9	• Wimba	3.1.2012
	• Develop poster and presentation	3.8.2012
	• Log No. 4 due	3.9.2012
Checkpoint No. 5 3/19–3/30	• Electronic poster presentation	3.19.2012
	• Wimba	3.22.2012
	• Present findings to unit manager and pharmacy clinical manager	3.23.2012
	• Log No. 5 due	3.30.2012
4/1–4/16/12	• Research week presentation	4.2.2012
	• Final paper	4.16.2012

Assessment for Quality Improvement Project

This is the five-question assessment to be administered before and after education to assess learning and compliance readiness.

This is a voluntary, confidential questionnaire intended for educational use only.

1. How many medication errors do you think occur in the United States every year?

2. To what degree do you believe that distractions during medication preparation cause medication errors?

Strongly disagree	Disagree	Neutral	Agree	Strongly agree
O	O	O	O	O

3. What is the most common source of interuptions on this unit during medication preparation?

4. How effective do you think the red carpet is in reducing distractions/interruptions on a scale of 1–5, with 5 being the most effective?

Not at all effective	Somewhat not effective	Neutral	Effective	Very effective
O	O	O	O	O

5. Describe how distractions affect you when you are preparing medications.

Evidence-Based Design Project Budget

Intervention	Projected Cost/Unit	Projected Unit Number	Cost	Cost Center	Approval Needed
Questionnaire	0.10	30	3.00	Personal	No
Poster	15.00	2	30.00	Personal	No
Additional flyers	0.10	6	0.60	Personal	No

The Timeline for the Red Zone Project

Action Item	Owner	Date of Completion	Comments
Obtain hospital IRB approval	Name	12/2011	Submit 11/2011 and discuss with (names)
Preliminary meeting with pharmacy director/clinical manager/patient safety director	Name	11/18/2012	Secure administrative support and discuss needs assessment. Present preliminary information. Get feedback.
Obtain university IRB approval	Name	1/2012	Submit 12/2011
Conduct kick-off meeting with nurse manager, pharmacy director, patient safety management	Name	1/2012	Discussed with (names)
Collect preeducation data and administer assessment	Name	1/2012	Begin discussing project with staff
Education session	Name	By 1/31/2012	Discuss with pharmacy and possibly coeducate
Poster implementation	Name	By 1/31/2012	Obtain approval for poster implementation prior to installation
Collect posteducation data	Name	By 2/15/2012	

Action Item	Owner	Date of Completion	Comments
Analyze data	Name	2/28/2012	Meeting with professor
Development of presentation	Name	3/14/2012	Final approval of presentation from professor
Present findings to manager and pharmacy clinical manager	Name	3/30/2012	Obtain feedback from stakeholders
Develop final paper for dissemination and publication	Name	4/20/2012	

Outline of Needs Assessment, Implementation, and Process Outcomes

Case	Making the Case	Necessary Data	Measurable Outcomes	Comments
Strategic case	This is a low-cost project with high impact. This is one aspect of the strategic plan of the hospital to increase patient safety. Medication errors impact patent safety, reimbursement, length of stay, and possibly accreditation.	Pharmacy strategic goals for 2012 Strategic goals for 2012 Patient safety management strategic goals Hospital-wide strategic goals	The number of interruptions before and after the education session and the implementation of posters. Employee buy-in of the red zone. After education, will they be more willing to comply with the red zone.	Strategic goals for the department may be difficult to obtain. These are largely kept confidential. Must have IRB approval. Because department head bonuses are dependent on strategic goals and plans, they will be interested in this project.
Business case	With a project cost of $34, the net return on this investment will be positive. Medication errors are rated from 1 to 4 with 4 resulting in significant harm or death. Potential savings will result from the avoidance of error.	There were not any level 4 errors in 2011 at the hospital. Costs are measured in dollars, and outcomes are measured in the decrease in the number of interruptions.	While this project primarily focuses on the number of interruptions, the total number of medication errors will be reviewed by patient safety and the education department.	Because of the timeline of this project, a reduction in medication errors cannot be observed. Immediate cost savings would be related to a decreased waste and returns of medications as a result of decreasing distractions and interruptions.

(continues)

Case	Making the Case	Necessary Data	Measurable Outcomes	Comments
Resources case	Infrastructure resources are minor. Approval for poster creation and installation is necessary.	There are no additional resources necessary for this project.	After completion of the project, there will be a need for ongoing education about medication errors. A report card of medication errors could be developed for employee communication.	This project is the beginning of what should be a continuum. The need for assessment and reassessment of medication errors should evolve over time.
Process outcomes	Because this is a process change, the evaluation portion of this project is pivotal to success. Feedback from staff and stakeholders should be encouraged.	The necessary data for the process change includes preeducation interruptions and employee compliance and posteducation interruptions and employee compliance.	The outcome measures for this project include the reduction in the number of interruptions and the increase in staff willingness to comply with the red zone.	Upper management support will be necessary in the implementation portion of this project. According to lean processes and the Center for Healthcare Designs, senior management has the ability to encourage changes within the organizational culture. Ultimately, this project requires a behavioral and therefore cultural change.

The Lived Experience of Chronic Pain in Nurse Educators

Moniaree Parker Jones

After reviewing the material, the reader will be able to:
1. Verbalize the importance of the interview as a data-gathering technique.
2. Describe how themes may be derived from interviews used in phenomenological research.
3. Verbalize the benefits of purposive sampling.

Abstract

Pain is associated with a wide range of disease and injury and is sometimes the disease itself. Millions suffer from chronic pain every year, and the effects of pain lead to tremendous costs for health care, rehabilitation, and lost worker productivity, as well as the emotional, psychological, and financial burden it places on patients and their families. The nurse has a key role in effective pain management with the need for accurate assessment, prompt intervention, and evaluation of pain relief measures for positive patient outcomes. The purpose of the study was to explore the lived experience of chronic pain in nurse educators in order to determine a better understanding for discovery in nursing curriculum. An interpretive phenomenological approach was used to frame this research study. The study employed a purposive sample of two associate degree nurse (ADN) educators and one baccalaureate (BSN) educator having personally experienced chronic pain.

Semistructured, three-part interviews were conducted using an interview guide. The participants of the study offered a depiction of the lived experience, and the researcher sought commonalities in meanings, situations, practices, and bodily experiences. Themes emerged, which aligned with and assisted in answering the research questions. Five essential themes from the study emerged: vulnerability, physician/provider trust, fear of disability, coping, and need for pedagogical discourse. Two subthemes—*stoic* and *alien*—also emerged. Understanding the lived experience of nurse educators with chronic pain is important and valuable to health care. Nurse educators are responsible and challenged in their daily work with the need to teach about chronic pain in the best way possible, assuring the best care possible. Implications for nursing curriculum and practice relate to preparing nurse educators and students, addressing psychosocial issues, and incorporating how to do better chronic pain assessments and better manage chronic pain.

Introduction

To grasp the issues involved in a greater understanding of chronic pain and what this understanding can offer to nursing pedagogy, it is essential to look into the lived experiences of nurse educators who have been personally affected by chronic pain. In listening carefully to the many accounts and stories of those with lived experiences, it is possible to direct more attention to those aspects that nursing has tended to overlook: namely the life phenomena. The phenomenology of every life occurrence that is described empirically and theoretically benefits the world because it allows for the study of the person in each unique situation, offers a way of studying the realms of health and illness, and allows for discovery in understanding the problems of subjectivity or objectivity. The phenomenology of life can be used to understand everyday practices, meanings, and knowledge embedded in skills, stress, and coping (Benner, 1985b).

Studies of life phenomena can contribute to the enlightenment of something central and forgotten in the world in which we live because research into the lived experience can be an example of how what is present and meaningful in the daily life of an illness or disease obtains a voice through the research. It opens up further conversation about what can be relevant research questions in the nursing of the future, of empirical, theoretical, and philosophical character. The phenomena of life need to be understood broadly, not only as an articulated philosophy of life, but also as something produced in clinical practice and in research as interpretations of life in the concrete lived experience (Benner, 2000).

A major reason individuals seek health care is the presence of pain. Pain is a complex, subjective experience that is difficult to evaluate with no objective measure existing, despite decades of research on the subject. A lack of knowledge concerning pain assessment and management is a consistent theme in the literature (Al-Shaer, Hill, & Anderson, 2011). The quality of pain care delivery in the United States continues to fall remarkably short of the potential for optimal care. Pain medicine remains fragmented and without a unified organizational pain model. These consequences of fragmented care threaten patient safety and well-being. Effective pain treatment requires the highest level of clinical reasoning, coordination of medical skills, and strategic use of resources using medical expertise (American Academy of Pain Medicine, 2011).

Research studies concerning pain management and nursing practice have focused mostly on cancer pain and staff nurses in general. Most studies highlight nurses' lack of knowledge related to pain and analgesics, the persistence of misconceptions related to opioid use, fear of addiction, and the frequent underestimation of patients' pain (Briggs, 2010; Clark, French, Bilodeau, & Capasso, 1996; Fontana, 2008). In a study by Fontana (2008), critical analysis of data revealed that decisions made by advanced practice nurses for patients with chronic pain are characterized by a conflict of interest in which the patients' best interests are given a low priority. This conflict, which is socially and politically created and maintained, renders nurses unlikely to fulfill their ethical responsibility to patients. Nurses did not see prescribing decisions as ethical ones and, as a result, did not recognize the conflicts that were at work in their decision making. Factors that included the best interests of patients consisted of nurses wanting to make the right clinical decision from a desire to identify the etiology of the pain as well as the use of their personal experience and education related to pain management. Clinicians talked extensively about their own best interests to reduce the burden of practice inherent in prescribing opioids. Their perceptions of controlled substance laws resulted in fear of Drug Enforcement Administration (DEA) scrutiny; as a result, they modified their practice to reduce this risk. The heavy influence by a desire to protect society from the illegal abuse and diversion of drugs resulted in conditional treatment and the creation of mechanisms of control to ensure compliance, taking away from the patient's welfare and pain relief.

Individuals experiencing chronic pain also deal with significant psychological, spiritual, and physiological side effects. Psychological issues of depression, anxiety, and anger can interfere with adequate pain assessment by nurses and result in loss of work, loss of independence, and interference with relationships and important life events (Duke, Haas, Yarbrough, & Northam, 2010).

Nurses play a vital role in the assessment and management of patients' pain across the life span and in diverse clinical settings. Research has shown, however, that knowledge deficits, especially in the areas of pain assessment and titration of dosages, may contribute to the undertreatment of pain (McCaffery, Grimm, Pasero, Ferrell, & Unman, 2005). Historically, nurses have been at the forefront of initiatives to improve quality of life for patients experiencing pain; however, many nurses maintain myths and beliefs about pain, and they lack up-to-date knowledge on pain techniques affecting their ability to provide good pain management to patients and families (Linkewich et al., 2007). In examining the barriers to effective pain management and positive pain relief outcomes, obstacles spring up at the level of patient, the healthcare professional, and the healthcare system itself. A nurse may have preconceived notions about a topic, and that belief will direct behavior, often in a way that is detrimental to patient care (Ashley, 2008). Education regarding pain assessment and pain management needs to be a high priority, because accurate knowledge and application of pain management principles are essential to clinical nursing practice as they directly and positively influence patient outcomes (Al-Shaer et al., 2011).

Pain is associated with a wide range of disease and injury and is sometimes the disease itself. Millions suffer from acute or chronic pain every year, and the effects of pain lead to tremendous costs for health care, rehabilitation, and lost worker productivity, as well as the emotional and financial burden it places on patients and their families. Pain affects around 116 million Americans—more than diabetes, heart disease, and cancer combined. The total annual incremental cost of health care due to pain ranges from $560 billion to $635 billion (in 2010 dollars) in the United States, which combines the costs related to disability days and lost wages and productivity (American Academy of Pain Medicine, 2011).

The nurse has a key role in effective pain management with the need for accurate assessment, prompt intervention, and evaluation of pain relief measures for positive patient outcomes (Plaisance & Logan, 2006). In the assessment of pain, the nurse depends partly on the message the patient can communicate to the nurse and partly on how the nurse perceives, interprets, and responds to the content of the pain message (Bergh & Sjostrom, 2007). These are the skills in nursing education that are some of the most important in chronic pain assessment, yet are lacking in the curriculum. A study by Goodrich (2006) to determine the knowledge and attitudes of nursing students and faculty about the science of pain management looked at the content of pain management material as well as the extent to which it is integrated into the nursing curriculum. Students were found to have gained knowledge in certain areas of pain management, but many gaps remained. The study revealed that pain management is not addressed consistently throughout the curriculum, and, as a result, there is a need to develop pain knowledge and skills into the plan of study.

The importance of addressing pain in curriculum is not new. The International Association for the Study of Pain (IASP), a leading professional forum for science, practice, and education in the field of pain, appointed an ad hoc committee challenged with preparing an outline for pain curriculum in basic nursing education. The committee, consisting of registered nurses and doctorate-prepared individuals, outlined minimal competencies in order to assess and manage pain. Entry-level nursing education varies among countries. The IASP curriculum represents the optimal level of pain education for nursing within the scope of what is possible considering the existence of some resource-poor countries. The publication addresses chronic pain as a multidimensional and complex phenomenon, requiring effective assessment and management based on current knowledge. The multidimensional nature of pain requires the involvement of working toward the effective management of pain experienced by patients in a variety of settings (IASP, 2006).

Every practitioner is involved in serving as an advocate for the person experiencing pain and ensuring that the chronic pain care adheres to ethical principles and standards of quality. The nurse has frequent contact with patients receiving care in the community, at home, or in inpatient or outpatient settings. This frequent contact places the nurse in a unique position because the nurse is usually the healthcare provider spending the most time with the patient, allowing for a more thorough assessment. In addition, the nurse is often the first person to assess pain or pain changes in a patient. The central role and responsibility in assessment and management of pain means that nurses are required to be knowledgeable about pain mechanisms, the epidemiology of pain, barriers to effective pain control, and the frequently encountered chronic pain syndromes (International Association for the Study of Pain, 2006).

Pain assessment involves a skillful process negating the assumption that all nurses have the same baseline knowledge about pain, because nurses have varied experiences in education and pain management (Michaels, Hubbart, Carroll, & Hudson-Barr, 2007). Recognizing that increased education fosters greater knowledge, nurse educators need to critically assess current curricula on pain assessment and management. The amount of time, the depth, the breadth, and the methods used to teach students about pain should be included in the assessment (Plaisance & Logan, 2006).

Several life phenomena (facts or situations being observed to exist or happen) have been described philosophically, but there is a lack of empirical nursing professional research. It is important to study life phenomena in nursing because often the most elementary phenomena of our existence are the ones we are least aware of in our daily lives as we go about caring for our patients. In nursing, there is the risk that life phenomena become invisible to those whose task it is to help the ill person adjust to life situations. The phenomenology of life's observances must therefore be understood broadly, not only as an articulated philosophy of life, but also as something produced in clinical practice and in research as interpretations of life in the concrete lived experience (Delmar, 2006). Studies about life phenomena can contribute something central and forgotten in the world in which we live. Dysvik, Sommerseth, and Jacobensen (2011), in a study, pointed out the important aspects of living with chronic pain. By listening to patients' narratives, chronic pain can be investigated, which might aid nurses in the quest to reduce pain and strengthen those areas that can lead to a meaningful life (Delmar, 2006). Chronic pain presents lifelong demands in coping with health changes and an unforeseen life course. There is often a profound change in people's ideas about themselves, and many people experience a sense of loss (Dysvik et al., 2011).

The reality of clinical practice in nursing is complex, multifaceted, confusing, and, in many ways, unpredictable. Pain, for example, can be physical and spiritual. Pain can be physical as a bodily lesion or the nervous system's reaction to an infection. Pain also generates the opening of feelings and moods, experiences of meaning, or meaninglessness. It means that the nurse looks beyond the immediate needs and sees the unique in the situation and then acts accordingly. Experience-based knowledge is then possible to be transferred to the concrete and unique situation (Delmar, 2006).

Pain that is not visible to others, yet felt and experienced by the individual, is viewed as subjective pain. Further highlighting the subjectivity of pain, according to Keyte and Richardson (2011), barriers to successful pain management for nurses are not simply related to knowledge, but are linked to factors such as the complexity (pain originating from multiple organ sources) and subjectivity of pain (pain experienced by the individual but not obvious to others), lack of accountability (healthcare providers who do not understand pain management), organizational issues (promotion of pain relief as a legal right or training issues within the system), and culture (such as fear of addiction or being seen as weak). The numbers of people who must live with multiple chronic illnesses and chronic pain will increase as the population ages. Through our personal stories, the intangible can become tangible, and the artfulness of good nursing practice can be rescued from the margins. Nursing as a practice is a socially organized body of knowledge with sets of skills and styles of relating to other practices and to science and technology. Socially organized in the world of nursing means learning or the actual practice of nursing is never achieved by isolated individuals. A socially embedded practice such as nursing holds more than its requisite science and technology. Caring in the practice of nursing is often described as artistic or intangible. It may be more accurate to say that the intangible and artistic caring is the core of nursing practice, because it renders technical, curative procedures, helping patients and families weather illnesses and sustain or regain familiar lifeworlds. *Lifeworld* means the particular social and historical world of the person, complete with culture, community, and networks of sustenance (Benner, 2000, p. 101).

A search of the literature for peer-reviewed articles using CINAHL, PubMed, ProQuest, Nursing Academic Search Premier, Google Scholar, and Allied Health Source to gain a better understanding of the phenomenology of the personally lived chronic pain experience of nurse educators and its relatedness to how they might articulate the lived experience to nursing education resulted in few findings. Nurses must tell their personal stories so that the hidden bedrock of caring practices for a healthy and good society will become more apparent to all. This means that experiential learning in the practice of nursing leads to the development of better practice environments so that the apparent intangibility does not lead to its dismissal. Healing relationships should not be reduced to propositional statements, yet we know them when we experience them, and we recognize them when they are missing. This differs from medical practice involving the objective sciences of pathophysiology, biochemistry, and genomics, among others. Each of these disciplines passes over the patients' lifeworlds and their lived, embodied experience in order to treat the physical, biochemical aspects of the disease or injury (Benner, 2000).

The subjectivity for this study may best be understood from the voices of nurse educators who have personally experienced chronic pain. The participants of this study offered a depiction of the lived experience, and the interpreter sought commonalities in meanings, situations, practices, and bodily experiences. The interpreter used distance and perspective to understand the immediacy of the lived situation. The experience-distant perspective must take into account the person in the situation. Nurse educators need to be the holders of knowledge. By engaging with others in shared inquiries, we come to understand how this insightful information forms professional knowledge that shapes our lives and stories, thereby illuminating our personal practical knowledge development (Benner, 1985b). Understanding the lived experience of nurse educators with chronic pain is important and extremely valuable to health care. Nurse educators are responsible and challenged in their daily work with the need to teach about chronic pain in the best way possible to assure the best care possible.

RESEARCHER'S POSITIONALITY

My previous experience from years ago as a young graduate nurse working in a small community emergency room plays an important role in the context of the study. Working toward a doctoral degree with a major in instructional leadership has changed how I view teaching and learning. I often misjudged and poorly assessed chronic migraine pain patients seen in the emergency room where I worked full time. The patients were viewed as drug seekers, and their pain experiences were viewed as not genuine, based on what I had learned in nursing school. In fact, I was never taught the different variances of migraine pain. Years later, when I experienced my first personal migraine headaches, which became chronic in duration, I began to gain insight into my personal lived experience. I found myself waking up each day and wondering if I could function normally with the pain. I wondered if I would be able to give that presentation scheduled for the day, interact with coworkers, and think clearly with the pain, and I wondered if the pain episodes would ever end. I was scared, and for the first time in my life unsure of my future. No one in my family has migraines. I began to question, "why me?" I felt that few truly believed or understood my pain experience. I felt shortchanged in my undergraduate curriculum regarding the understanding of chronic pain, which, in turn, led me to shortchange the patients committed to my care. As I started to teach in undergraduate nursing programs, it became apparent to me that many ways of teaching about pain in nursing programs exist, and that the quality of what I observed being taught was lacking. Although many organizations have given guidelines for pain assessment, the way in which these guidelines are articulated differs with each school. Most of the pain instruction taught is interspersed within the different nursing courses and for only a short and limited amount of time. This is disconcerting to me as nurse educator because I know that pain is one of the main reasons people seek health care. I believe it is essential for students to gain the best knowledge and skills possible, because this essential knowledge impacts significantly on patient care.

My personal experience with chronic migraine pain changed my life. I now understand the fear, the frustration, and the lack of understanding by practitioners about chronic pain. I know what it is like to finally find a practitioner (by the way who was a physician who personally suffered from migraine headaches) who truly understands your dilemma, who is nonjudgmental, and who will take the extra time to fully assess and treat you. I know the wonder of finding a practitioner who will not just prescribe you a pill and be frustrated if the pill does not cure your condition.

Deficits in teaching about chronic pain in nursing curriculum exist globally, as gleaned from the literature review. I am now challenged with trying to make sure the students entrusted to my service know about proper pain assessment and treatment. I tell my story when teaching students about chronic pain in hopes of making a difference in future nurses.

I do not want this same mistake to be repeated by other practitioners. I want to know if there is a better way for nurse educators to present chronic pain curricula to nursing students, to improve nursing education, and to impact nursing curriculum. Competent and knowledgeable practitioners are the key to excellent patient outcomes. Improving nursing students' knowledge by what we can learn from nurse educators who have personally experienced chronic pain seems important to explore. This is necessary in order to evaluate our methods of curriculum design and promote patient care. It is with this in mind that I began my journey to discover what can be learned about the lived experience of nurse educators who have personally experienced chronic pain with the attempt to gain understanding from their unique perspective.

PURPOSE OF THE STUDY

The purpose of this study is to explore the meanings and interpret as closely as possible the lived experiences of nurse educators who have personally experienced chronic pain or cared for another individual with chronic pain, in an attempt to better understand how these educators articulate and shape how they teach about chronic pain. Understanding the lived experiences of nurse educators can assist in determining how the lived experience links and gives voice to the way they teach about chronic pain assessment and management and determine if implications exist for reform in undergraduate nursing curriculum. For the purposes of this study, nursing faculty will be defined as any graduate-prepared instructor of nursing with a master's degree or higher, who has experienced chronic pain and who is employed by an Alabama Board of Nursing–approved registered nurse program.

RESEARCH QUESTIONS

There was one broad research question for this baseline study and additional focused questions. In what ways does the lived experience with chronic pain shape how a nurse educator understands and engages with pain assessment? Additional focused questions I attempted to answer are as follows:

1. How do nurse educators who have lived experience with chronic pain theorize or understand chronic pain?

2. How can the lived experience relate to how pain is taught by these individuals?
3. What are the prescribed methods of teaching chronic pain assessment where nurse educators teach, and how does it fit into the nursing curriculum?

SIGNIFICANCE OF THE STUDY

Pain is a subjective experience in which nurses must refrain from basing their assessment, management, and interventions on personal beliefs and judgments. Sensitivity and empathy are critical components of nursing education. Accurate knowledge and application of pain management principles are essential to clinical nursing practice as they directly and positively impact patient outcomes (Al-Shaer et al., 2010). Nurses may have a preconceived notion about a topic, and that belief will direct behavior, often in a way that is detrimental to patient care (Ashley, 2008). Despite some progress in research on physiological processes involved in chronic pain, it is still among the least well understood phenomena in medicine and nursing. Chronic pain changes lives because it is a multifaceted problem consisting of both physical and psychological components, in many cases, such as anxiety and depression (Fisher, Emerson, et al., 2007).

Several studies have investigated many aspects of chronic pain. These studies include: nursing students' knowledge and attitudes regarding pain (Plaisance & Logan, 2006), women in chronic pain (Skuladottir & Halldorsdottir, 2008), and living a meaningful life with chronic pain from a nursing perspective (Dysvik et al., 2011). Despite these studies, a literature search failed to reveal any present research focusing on how the lived chronic pain experiences of nurse educators may contribute to greater understanding about chronic pain assessment and nursing care, the amount of time that is devoted to teaching chronic pain management in nursing curricula, and the methods of nursing student instruction about chronic pain.

PHILOSOPHICAL PERSPECTIVE

Phenomenology was both the philosophical perspective and the methodology of this study. An understanding of what the lived experience of chronic pain is like for nurse educators contributes to the body of nursing knowledge. Exploration of the lived experience is best suited by a phenomenological approach such as Benner's (1994) *Interpretive Phenomenology: Embodiment, Caring, and Ethics in Health and Illness* and van Manen's (1990) hermeneutical phenomenological reflection in *Researching Lived Experience: Human Science for an Action Sensitive Pedagogy.* The nursing literature lacks studies that explore the qualitative aspects of nurse educators' experiences as they relate to chronic pain and how nurse educators with personal lived experience with chronic pain might articulate or shape pain assessment.

Phenomenology is descriptive in the sense of aiming to describe rather than explain why. A number of researchers and scholars distinguish between descriptive and hermeneutic or interpretive variants. Interpretive versions have emerged from the work of hermeneutic philosophers such as Heidegger (1962), who argued that people are embedded in the world of language and social relationships. Any understandings gained are founded on our experience and depend on our perspective. These understandings necessarily involve interpretation. In hermeneutic phenomenology, meanings can never be fixed. They are always emergent, contextual, and historical. These meanings shape our understandings and must be taken into account. The central concern of phenomenological research is a return to embodied, experiential meaning, to seek fresh, complex, vivid descriptions of a phenomenon (a human experience in all its complexity) as it is concretely lived (Finlay, 2009).

THEORETICAL FRAMEWORKS

Patricia Benner

Nurses encounter daily the lived experiences of patients, nurses, and other healthcare workers. Patricia Benner (1994) devoted much of her professional life studying nurses and their lived experiences to add to the body of nursing knowledge. Benner offered a different approach from the cognitive rationalist quantitative paradigm. It constitutes an interpretive movement away from epistemological linear, analytic, and quantitative methods toward a new direction of ontological, hermeneutic, holistic, and qualitative approaches. This approach is highlighted by the capacity to uncover, articulate, and bring recognition to embedded qualitative aspects of practice that are not apparent from the quantitative perspective. Benner notes that this research methodology constitutes a situation-based interpretive approach of describing nursing practice that overcomes some reductionism problems. It begins to critique Cartesian epistemology and focuses on the study of human beings from within their lifeworlds and projects embodiment, and their skilled know-how embedded in practice situations such as coping with chronic illness and health promotion (Chan, Brykczynski, Malone, & Benner, 2010).

Benner explained that articulation research describes, illustrates, and gives language to "taken-for-granted areas of practical wisdom, skilled know-how, and notions of good practice" (Benner, Hooper-Kyriakidis, & Hooper, 1999, p. 5). Interpretive phenomenology as a philosophy and a qualitative research methodology has its origins in the work of several philosophers such as Heideggar (1927/1962), Benner (1984, 1994), and van Manen (1990).

Phenomenology uses interpretation to uncover patterns, concerns, and meanings. Benner used three narrative strategies to assist in uncovering meanings of socially embedded knowledge: (1) paradigm cases (known as marker cases that stand out with a particular pattern of meaning), (2) thematic analysis (identification of common themes in interviews or observations), and (3) exemplars (smaller than paradigm cases but hold strong meaning as in a vignette or story of particular meaning). Understanding another person's subjective experiences and feelings by study is important to know how nurse educators perceive their role in nursing education. Benner (1994) believed that "the interpretive researcher creates a dialogue between practical concerns and lived experience through engaged reasoning and imaginative dwelling in the immediacy of the participants' worlds" (p. 99). There is no stepwise formula to follow in conducting interpretive phenomenological study. However, Benner, Tanner, and Chesla (2009) provided a clear delineation of the interpretive phenomenological method. Certain research practices typical of this approach can be

- Participant observations and interviews for data collection.
- Interviews that provide narrative access to the person's particular experience, capture the temporal progression of situations, and elicit stories in everyday language.
- Using three interrelated interpretive strategies (identification of paradigm cases, exemplars and thematic analysis) for analyzing the narrative and observation data.

Nursing theory using a phenomenological approach reflects the reality of nursing practice that is complex and situational. Small-group interviews and first-person experience used in interpretive phenomenology differ from participant reports of opinions or generalizations about practice. Experience-near narratives are stories that require the storyteller to dwell in the story as experienced, including thoughts and concerns, providing accounts of actual events, including dialog, all with as much detail as possible. The interviewer listens carefully to the story without interrupting unless understanding breaks down and clarification is needed. The philosophical underpinning accounts for the person's perceptions and meanings or at the very least, how the world presents itself to the storyteller in practice and is uncovered (Chan et al., 2010). Such knowledge generated from practice has great relevance for nurses. Benner is the author and past project director of a federally funded grant titled, Achieving Methods of Intra-professional Consensus, Assessment and Evaluation project (the AMICAE project). The research attempted to discover and describe knowledge embedded in the practice of nursing. The Dreyfus model of skill acquisition (originally developed with pilots) considers the advancement in skilled performance, based upon experience, as well as education, clinical knowledge development, and career progression in nursing (Altmann, 2007). The model posits that individuals, while acquiring and developing skills, pass through five levels of proficiency: novice/beginner, advanced beginner, competent, proficient, and expert. The five different levels reflect changes in the three general aspects of skilled performance:

1. A move from a reliance on abstract principles to the use of past concrete experiences;
2. A change from viewing a situation as multiple fragments, to seeing a more holistic picture with a few relevant factors; and
3. A movement from detached observer to active performer.

A move from novice to expert is characterized by transition from explicit, rule-governed behavior to intuitive, contextually determinate behavior. Progression from novice to expert is not guaranteed; not every nurse becomes an expert. "The Dreyfus model provides the concepts needed to differentiate between what can be taught by precept and what must be learned experientially from comparison of similar and dissimilar cases" (Benner 1984, p. 186).

Understanding the work of Dreyfus and Benner gives one a viable alternative to traditional ways of understanding practice, theory, and knowledge; not to devalue science. Benner believed that skilled pattern recognition can be taught and will lead to advancement through stages. The teaching is facilitated by a holistic assessment of the situation and not by breaking the situation down into individual parts. Benner believed that nurses develop and accrue global sets of paradigms about patients. These paradigms develop expert intuition and sets not readily apparent to the outside observer. Expert nurses use empirics, ethics, and personal knowledge. Individuals interpret their own concerns, practices, and life experiences that are always situated. They are engaged meaningfully within the context of the situation. Benner's work uses a Heideggerian phenomenological interpretive approach of synthesis. The Heideggerian approach (Heidegger, 1962) is an interpretive approach where synthesis and conclusions are derived from interviews, experience, and/or observations. Experience leads to intuition, ethical/moral reasoning, and personal knowledge. Benner's model uses practical reasoning, looks at what effects underlie reality, and proposes a guide to shape nursing practice. It provides a framework that supports lifelong learning for nurses; thus it is applicable to nursing practice, research, and education (Altmann, 2007).

Interpretive research is a systematic approach to interpreting text. Interview material and observations are turned into text through transcription. The interpretation entails a systematic analysis of the whole text, an analysis of parts of text, and a comparison of the interpretations for conflicts and for understanding the whole in relation to the parts and vice versa. This shifting back and forth reveals new themes, new issues, and new questions that are generated in the process of understanding the text itself. The participants offer depictions of the lived experience, and the interpreter seeks commonalities in meanings, situations, practices, and bodily experiences. Interpreters use their distance and perspectives to understand the lived situation. The interpreter enters into a dialogue with the text. For example, the interpreter must consider the experience-distant perspectives as possible points for interpretation: (1) the changing experience of the body; (2) changing social relationships as a result of illness; (3) changing demands and tasks of different stages in the disease process or illness trajectory; (4) predictable responses and effective coping strategies for treatment side effects and sequelae; and

(5) the particular of what the illness interrupts, threatens, and means to the individual. These provide a starting point for the interpretation without setting limits on what can be discovered in the process. The hermeneutic, or interpretive methodology described, is a holistic strategy because it seeks to study the person in the situation rather than isolating person variables and situation variables and then trying to put them back together (Benner, 1985b).

Max van Manen

The hermeneutic phenomenological method and human science approach of Max van Manen (1990) offers much to nursing research, as does that of Benner (1985a). Van Manen's phenomenology is commonly used in conjunction with other contemporary influences like Benner to explore and interpret the lived experience (Dowling, 2007). Common to Benner, van Manen views phenomenology as a philosophy of being as well as practice. This perspective allows a view of experiential understanding by questioning lived experience through reflective writing. In this way, meaning can be understood, and we can become practitioners of ever-fragile phenomenological wisdom (Munhall, 2007a). Benner shares the view, as does van Manen (2007, p. 11), that phenomenology is a project of sober reflection on the lived experience of human existence. It is sober in the sense that reflecting on experience must be thoughtful and as much as possible free from theoretical, prejudicial, and suppositional intoxications. A respect for the habitual, skilled body of the patient with a chronic illness causes the nurse to respect the patient's knowledge and develop lines of clinical inquiry that go beyond mere mapping of symptoms onto preexisting explanations. The patient's learning about his or her own illness becomes a source of clinical discovery and inquiry.

According to van Manen (1990), "'methodology' means the 'pursuit' of knowledge" (p. 28). The essence of this inquiry lies in the pursuit of knowledge to come to know the humanistic experience as presented by the lived experience of nurse educators and chronic pain. This method of inquiry supports the humanistic science that "aims at explicating the meaning of the human phenomena and at understanding the lived structures of meanings" (van Manen, 1990, p. 4). The interest of this study was in gaining a deeper understanding of the lived experience of nurse educators with chronic pain and "interpreting these meanings to a certain degree of depth and richness" (van Manen, 1990, p. 11). Van Manen's (1990) six research activities were used to identify, understand, and interpret the experience in question. These activities included:

- Turning to a phenomenon which seriously interests us and commits us to the world.
- Investigating experience as we live it rather than as we conceptualize it.
- Reflecting on the essential themes which characterize the phenomenon.
- Describing the phenomenon through the art of writing and rewriting.
- Maintaining a strong and oriented pedagogical relation to the phenomenon.
- Balancing the research context by considering parts and whole. (p. 30)

Van Manen (1990) recognized that the person cannot reflect on the lived experience at the time it is occurring; therefore, reflection is not immediate, but retrospective. A person lives in the moment and experiences specific emotions within the moment. The exact meaning derived from the moment's experience does not become known until reflection occurs. Cultural influences, memories, age, gender, one's upbringing, and the like influence the individual's experience. These meanings are different to different individuals. Some commonalities exist, however, and the identification is useful to understanding the phenomena. In phenomenology, questions relate to the search for meaning and significance. The meaning is derived from the interpretations applied to observed descriptions. Phenomenological research is the study of lived experience, the study of essences, the explication of phenomena, and the describing of experiential meanings as they are found in living (van Manen). Phenomenologically inspired research aims at describing essence of experiential phenomena; for example, the essence of living with a chronically painful body.

Phenomenology is essentially the study of the lifeworld in which we live. It aims at gaining a deeper understanding of the nature or meaning of everyday experiences. It differs from almost every other science in that it attempts to gain insightful descriptions of the way we experience the world without abstracting it. Consciousness is the only access human beings have to the world. It is by being conscious that we are aware of the world in some aspect. From a phenomenological point of view, to do research is always to question the way we experience the world and to want to understand the world in which we live as human beings. To understand it is to profoundly be in the world in a certain way, the act of researching, questioning, and theorizing. In doing research, we question the world's very secrets and intimacies that make up the world. Phenomenology is interested in the significant world of the human being. Phenomenology, not unlike poetry, is a poetizing project that tries a primal telling wherein the aim is to involve the voice in the world (van Manen, 1990). We must discover what lies at the core of our being so that we better find meaning in an attempt to improve our world.

Review of the Literature

In reviewing the literature, this researcher conducted searches in CINAHL, PubMed, ProQuest, Nursing Academic Search Premier, Google Scholar, and Allied Health Source for articles to gain a better understanding of the phenomenology of lived pain experiences and its relatedness to nursing curriculum. Search terms were *pain, chronic pain and lived experience, chronic pain and curriculum, pain/chronic pain and teaching nurses, pain and self-knowing, pain/chronic pain and phenomenology,* and *pain and nursing education.* The primary time frame for this search was 2006–2011. Some classic articles outside of this time frame were identified and included in the literature review. The thematic focus areas for this literature review included embodied or lived experience, chronic pain assessment, and curriculum and education of undergraduate nursing students regarding chronic pain. Each of these themes was explored further in the following literature review. As a result of this review, an identifiable gap was found related to the study of the lived experiences of nurse educators and any influencing factors congruent to the amount of information and time spent teaching nursing students about pain assessment.

CHRONIC PAIN AND THE EMBODIED OR LIVED EXPERIENCE: WHAT IS IT?

Despite substantial progress in the study of physiological processes involved in chronic pain, it continues to be among the least well-understood phenomena in medicine (Raheim & Haland, 2006). Phenomenology operates in the space of the relationship of who we are and who we may become, between how we think or feel, and how we act. These relationships have pedagogical consequences for professional and everyday practical life. Phenomenological reflection can contribute to the formative dimensions of a phenomenology of practice. Studying the lived experience makes possible thoughtful advice and consultation. In some sense, it is the practice of living and the exploration of how it relates to our personal and professional lives (van Manen, 2007). Phenomenology of the lived experience offers the moments of seeing-meaning or "in seeing" into "the heart of things." The phenomenologist gazes toward the regions where meaning originates (van Manen, 2007, p. 11).

EVOLUTION OF THE CONCEPT OF PAIN

The word *pain* comes from the Latin word *peona*, which means punishment. Even though the idea of pain as punishment has to a large extent disappeared, it is of interest to note how this early belief about the origin of pain reflected society's perception of the ultimate nature of reality, a pattern repeated over time. History offers early understandings that pain was often attributed to the presence of evil spirits that inhabited the sufferer. During the time of Aristotle (384–322 BC), and in keeping with Greek emphasis on the mind, attribution for pain shifted from the external spiritual forces to the mind (The Ancient Library, 2005, p. 929). The medical reform movement of the late 19th century gave way to the notion of psychogenic pain for pain that could not be objectively documented and therefore had no status in reality. This belief was consistent with the dominant conceptualizations held by the science of the day to be an objective undertaking characterized by empiricism, the belief that only that which could be experienced by the senses could qualify as reality. Any subjective expression of pain that could not be empirically verified was not real, except in the mind of the sufferer (Overgaard, 2010). During the mid-1900s, the positivistic, empirical approach to science began to be challenged. Thomas Kuhn's groundbreaking work in the philosophy of science explained how scientific understandings are always shaped by human values, understandings, and choices (Kuhn, 1996).

A key shift in understandings of pain 40 years ago is credited to Melzack and Wall (1965), who proposed the gate control theory. This theory asserted the existence of mechanisms in the body for altering pain signals before they reach the brain. The belief about an integration and interplay of mind and body in pain experience replaced Descartes's notion of a mind–body split. Thus was the view that the mind's interpretation is paramount to all pain, and thus the mutual exclusivity or clear distinction between physical and psychogenic pain was no longer valid. Pain became a subjective notion where the physical aspects of pain were subordinated to the authority of the experience constructed by the patient. If pain could not be empirically verified, then it was considered psychogenic, having social implications (Melzack, 1986).

What Makes Chronic Pain Problematic?

The ineffective management of pain leads to additional health issues. Pain that is not treated appropriately and promptly results in persistent pain that eventually causes irreversible changes in the nervous system. This cycle translates into progressive bio-psycho-social findings leading to further pain and disability. The functional human being becomes transformed into the dysfunctional individual seen as a burden to family, to society, and to oneself. Considering that we live in a country where there is adequate medical science, adequate technical skills, and adequate resources, delayed pain care is paradoxical, leading us to the need for effective remediation (Lippe, Brock, David, Crossno, & Gitlow, 2010).

Pain has been shown to have a significant adverse effect on work and productivity. A major study published in the *Journal of the American Medical Association* found that 13% of the total workforce in the United States experienced a loss in productive time (a mean of 4.6 hours per week) during a 2-week time period due to a chronic pain condition. Headaches, back pain, and arthritis were the most common conditions. The loss in production time among active workers had an estimated cost of $61.2 billion every year. A greater understanding of the lived experiences of nurse educators who have personally experienced chronic pain is needed in order to maximize patient care and nurse understanding. The goal of studying the lived experience is to fully describe the lived experience stressing that only those who have experienced the phenomena can best communicate them to the outside world (Mapp, 2008). This philosophical method of inquiry lends to the exploration of what shapes how nurse educators who experience chronic pain teach about pain, in an attempt to improve nursing curriculum from information learned from the lived experience.

CHALLENGES IN CHRONIC PAIN ASSESSMENT

Pain assessment is one of the most complex issues in nursing, and deficiencies in pain assessment may explain the high prevalence of unrelieved pain. People often ascribe different quantitative meanings to words used to describe pain, further complicating assessment (Bergh & Sjostrom, 2007). In the assessment of pain, nurses must realize that patients may refer to pain using different terms such as discomfort, hurt, ache, or pain all over meaning total pain, including physical and emotional dimensions. Assessment is dependent upon recognition of the barriers to pain assessment and pain relief. Patient barriers include the reluctance to report pain, concern that reporting pain will distract the practitioner from treating the underlying disease, fear that the pain means worsening disease, a desire to be viewed as a good patient, fear of addiction, concern over medication costs, and reluctance to take pain medications (Sherman, Matzo, Paice, McLaughlin, & Virani, 2004).

According to Hall-Lord and Larsson (2006), the assessment of chronic pain may be improved through self-reflection and awareness of attitudes in the assessment of pain. Nurses must continuously increase their awareness of personal biases when assessing and managing chronic pain. There is an element of moral agency (based on experience-based moral perception in practical situations to a nurse's response) involved in the treatment of chronic pain (Benner et al., 2009). Many hospital and hospice nurses have significant moral obligations to patients. The traditional approach of American healthcare ethics has evolved out of principles. The nurse often has to interface with the caregiver, who must be trained about chronic pain care. Understanding the beliefs, values, and other influences that give rise to caring behavior becomes important to the nurse. The patient has a right to pain relief or the best death possible. Nurses often encounter caregivers who are reluctant to give pain medications because of fear. These fears include respiratory depression of the loved one or addiction (Kirk, 2007).

According to the The Joint Commission (2011), it is estimated that in the United States, more than 76 million people suffer from pain. Pain can be chronic or acute. The importance of understanding the difficult issues found in pain assessment and management has been addressed by The Joint Commission and further justifies the importance of the nurse educator's responsibility for teaching about chronic pain. On January 1, 2001, pain management standards went into effect for JCAHO-accredited[1] ambulatory care facilities, behavioral healthcare organizations, critical access hospitals, home care providers, hospitals, office-based practices, and long-term care providers. These pain standards require organizations to do the following:

- Recognize the right of patients to appropriate assessment and management of pain
- Screen patients for pain during the initial assessment and when clinically required during ongoing periodic reassessments
- Educate patients suffering from pain, and their families, about pain management

The pain management standards were developed in collaboration with the University of Wisconsin–Madison Medical School, and were part of a project funded by the Robert Wood Johnson Foundation. These pain management standards appear in the "Provision of Care, Treatment and Service (PC)" and the "Rights and Responsibilities of the Individual (RI)" chapters of The Joint Commission's accreditation manuals (Joint Commission, 2011).

Pain crosses cultural and social lines, making assessment and pain management a high priority. Deficits in this area of practice may be attributed to inadequate knowledge (Al-Shaer et al., 2011). Patient perceptions may manifest in a reticence to report pain because of misconceptions about treatment and side effects. This reluctance to seek pain control may be exacerbated by the desire to be good and not wanting to bother the clinician (Duke et al., 2010). In a study by Yu and Petrini (2007), as a vulnerable group, older people are more likely to have serious side effects of medication therapy. They often present with serious side effects of medication therapy. Many have multiple medical problems and are more susceptible to inadequate pain assessment and management. Some people hold beliefs that older people are less sensitive to pain and hold beliefs that pain is normal and expected due to aging. Older people may be more reluctant to report painful symptoms than other adults (Yu & Petrini, 2007).

---

[1] The Joint Commission, as it is currently known, was using its previous name, the Joint Commission on Accreditation of Healthcare Organizations, or JCAHO, in 2001.

How Is Pain Measured?

Planning effective pain measurement and management is a crucial part of the nurses' profession. To achieve this, it is necessary to assess and measure what level of pain a patient may be having and to identify a potential course of action. Pain is multidimensional. Nurses' assessments of patients' pain may not be in accordance with what the patient is experiencing (Hall-Lord & Larsson, 2006).

The idea that pain is "whatever the patient says it is" has been a popular term since McCaffery (1972) first introduced the definition of pain to nursing. McCaffery's definition was mostly a response to a belief that pain was being undertreated in health care. McCaffery suggested that this undertreatment was due to healthcare workers' beliefs about how pain should manifest and fear of opioid addiction risks. She emphasized that pain, particularly chronic pain, will not always manifest through the classic signs of grimacing, restlessness, and vital sign changes. She believed that patients may distract themselves to mask the pain. There may be unfounded concerns over potential patient addiction to opioids, and she emphasized the difference between physical and psychological addiction. McCaffery's definition of pain was aimed at helping nurses to more fully embrace the patients' subjective experiences to pain and treat that pain liberally to provide relief.

Pain assessment includes identifying the location of the pain, realizing that many patients have multiple pain sites or have referred pain. In 1981, Donna Wong, a pediatric nurse consultant, and Connie Morain Baker, a child life specialist, worked together in a burn center in Tulsa, Oklahoma. Wong and Baker believed that with the proper tools, young patients could participate in assessing their pain, leading to development of the Wong-Baker FACES scale (Wong-Baker FACES Foundation, 2009). The method is a visual analogue scale to identify the degree of pain the individual is having. Initially, the numbers of 0–5 were used to quantify pain in children in order for staff to communicate effectively with the child, staff, and parents. This was updated using the numbers 0–10 to be more consistent with the numeric scale where 0 is no pain and 10 is the worst pain imaginable. The Wong-Baker FACES Pain Rating Scale may also be used to correlate the facial expression selected by the patient with the degree of pain he or she is experiencing The Wong-Baker FACES Pain Rating Scale is used with children and those with cognitive impairment.

According to Bozimowski (2010), assessing pain of any kind is traditionally grounded in outcomes management. This refers to the patient's report after an intervention, usually using a visual acuity scale such as the Wong-Baker FACES Pain Rating Scale. An obvious problem in this approach is not only the subjective nature of the pain interpretation, but also with the variables associated with the use of the pain scale. Because it is common practice for nurses to ask their patients to rate their pain on a scale of 0 to 10, it is more accurate to state that the practitioners use a pain numeric scale (PNS) more often than a true (VAS) visual assessment scale. The use of a scale such as the Wong-Baker FACES Pain Rating Scale has been generally accepted; however, it has been shown to be a poor indicator of clinically significant pain (pain that is outside of the range of normal) in primary care patients, in a study by Krebs, Carey, and Weinberger (2007). Krebs et al., using a pain numeric rating scale (NRS) with 275 adult clinic patients, found only moderate accuracy for identifying patients with clinically significant pain. It is possible that this simple measure cannot be expected to identify all clinically important pain in primary care. Pain is a multidimensional experience, and this dimensionality has important implications for its measurement. In settings where pain is chronic and complex, the simple pain NRS scale may fail to identify patients with pain-related suffering driven by functional limitations, illness, worry, or other factors (Krebs et al., 2007).

Stigma and Delegitimation of Chronic Pain

The noted anthropologist, Arthur Kleinman, defined delegitimation as "the experience of having one's perceptions of an illness systematically disconfirmed" (Kleinman, 1992, p. 347). For an individual to be legitimately ill in the eyes of others, the individual often needs to have a credible explanation for his or her illness. There is a belief that real and legitimate diseases have organic causes (Chang et al., 2006). In chronic pain, it is not always possible to have a credible explanation, especially when there is a lack of evidence to demonstrate physical pathology (Newton, Southall, Raphael, Ashford, & LeMarchand, 2010, p. 4). Patients for whom the pain stimulus does not appear to match the pain experience are often labeled as malingerers or as having mental health issues. The idea that "pain is whatever the patient says it is" may have contributed to moving nursing away from psychogenic labeling towards credibility of the patient experience. The concept of chronic pain over a 30-year period (1970s–1990s) changed from the perceived role of psychological problem to that which might be seen as having a relationship to the consequence of chronic pain. The centrality of the psychogenic component remained, but patients were likely to be blamed for their pain. This change in emphasis on subjectivity of pain helped to overcome some of the psychological consequences of "invisible pain" (Pesut & McDonald, 2007).

Jordan, Eccleston, and Osborn (2007), using an interpretative phenomenological analysis approach, reported on distress and pressures of parenting children with chronic pain. The authors described the guilt of parents in desiring something wrong to be found with their child. The elation of parents obtaining a medical label for their child's pain could be seen and understood in the face of feeling societal disbelief toward the reality of the pain. Holloway, Sofaer-Bennett, & Walker (2007) gave detailed accounts of enacted stigma experienced by those with chronic back pain. Individual interviews with 17 participants in narrative format regarding pain offered insight into loss experiences of being in various systems (i.e., healthcare and Social Security systems), and stigmatization was a main theme. Stigmas were socially wide ranging to include medical professionals, employers, the general public, and even spouses. One participant reported having her medication thrown at her by a nurse and was told she was "costing the NHS [National Health Services] far too much money" (Holloway et al., 2007, pp. 1, 459). Another participant reported being told his pain was due to lack of fitness. Another reported receiving letters accusing him of falsely claiming benefits following the receipt of his mobility car. These experiences display enacted stigma in contrast to felt stigma where there is no outright disbelief expressed toward the individual (Newton et al., 2010).

In a study by McCaffery et al. (2005), nurses' comments and suggestions were solicited in a survey developed to identify behaviors that may cause nurses to refer to a patient as drug seeking. The purpose was to identify what nurses think the term *drug seeking* means, to explore how nurses regard the use of the term *drug seeking* in health care, and to identify differences between general nurses, emergency nurses, and pain management nurses with regard to those items. Identified behaviors that would cause the majority of all three nurse groups to refer to a patient as a drug seeker were as follows: going to different emergency departments to get opioids, telling inconsistent stories about pain or medical history, or asking for a refill because the prescription was lost or stolen. All three groups of nurses agreed that when the term *drug seeking* was used, it was likely to mean the patient was addicted to opioids and that the patient was abusing pain medicine, or that the patient was manipulative. One half or more of the nurses indicated they had used the term *drug seeking* in talking about patients, but fewer than 10% said they used it in charting. After taking the survey, one half or more of the nurses in each group were less inclined to use the term. The use of stigmatizing terms in clinical practice exists (McCaffery et al., 2005). Healthcare professionals need to be aware of the tension patients face between being able to adequately describe their pain and to be understood so as not to risk the accusation of complaining about their pain. A more structured assessment of the patient's pain might help to overcome this tension (Newton et al., 2010).

Culture and Chronic Pain

The United States of America is a racially and ethnically diverse country with non-Caucasian minority groups now composing around one third of the U.S. population. By the year 2042, minorities are expected to become the majority. In 2050, the United States is projected to be 54% minority, yielding a multiethnic, multiracial, and multilingual society (U.S. Census Bureau, Origin, 2000–2050). Race is a complex, multifaceted term with different conceptualizations. Some investigators have defined race primarily by ancestry and combinations of physical characteristics. Others claim race is largely a social or sociopolitical construct that includes self-identity and culture (Fisher, Burnet, Huang, Chin, & Cagney, 2007).

A higher prevalence of risk factors for illness, such as lower socioeconomic status, poor health habits, and inadequate access to healthcare services, predisposes minority groups to suffer a higher burden of pain (Anderson, Green, & Payne, 2009). The literature on disparities in pain has suffered from inconsistent and discrepant uses of the terms *race* and *ethnicity* (Ezenwa, Ameringer, Ward, & Serlin, 2006). Because there are no universally accepted definitions of race and ethnicity, investigators must be careful in the definitions used. Barriers to optimal pain assessment and treatment for racial and ethnic minority patients include factors related to the healthcare provider and the healthcare system. Provider barriers often include the lack of knowledge and training related to pain treatment, inadequate assessment and treatment of pain, and beliefs and expectations regarding minority and culturally different patients. Limited access to care, lack of insurance, or underinsurance, and limited availability of resources add to the system barriers (Anderson et al., 2009). The significance of cultural influences on nurses' pain assessment attitudes is important as it is culture that guides its members' thinking, decision making, and actions. No culture is homogeneous, and there are distinct groups of people who have different expectations and attitudes. Each culture has its own system of attitudes and behaviors that shape how the members respond to their patients' pain (Harper, Ersser, & Gobbi, 2007). Cultural differences become important in the assessment of chronic pain and in bringing significance to understanding possible underlying pain behaviors.

Jimenez, Garroutte, Kundu, and Morales (2011) searched 109 peer-reviewed journal articles focused on pain in the populations of American Indian (AI), Alaska Native (AN), and Aboriginal Canadian Peoples (ACP) focusing on pain, pain assessment and treatment, and healthcare utilization. A key finding was that the AI/ANs have higher prevalence of pain symptoms and painful conditions than the U.S. general populations. They also found evidence in the articles for problems in provider–patient interactions that affect clinical assessment of pain, as well as indications that AI/AN patients frequently use alternative modalities to manage pain. Further study is needed to focus on all types of pain and comorbid conditions for understanding these problems. They concluded that studies about the lived experience of pain in these groups are needed because particular tribal populations can bring distinctive communication patterns to the medical encounter, including specific metaphors, disease models, and word usage, further complicating chronic pain assessment.

EDUCATION AND NURSING PAIN CURRICULUM

Teaching nurses and other healthcare professionals regarding chronic pain and its management presents several challenges. Responsibility comes about through a nurse's connectedness to the patient and family. Empirical qualitative research on the lived experience aligns itself well with the requirement of nurses' empathetic commitment toward patients and their family members. It unfolds what it means to individuals and their family to have to go through the experience of ill health and/or treatments and uncovers how these experiences are rooted in patients' lives and existence. Listening to the lived experience of healthcare workers and healthcare teachers can help us to understand what it means to provide care in a specific situation or under particular conditions (de Casterle et al., 2011).

According to a study by Duke et al. (2010), although pain management has been targeted as a top priority, it continues to be inadequately addressed. This descriptive study done in Texas included 162 junior and senior baccalaureate nursing students and 16 faculty members and looked at determining the knowledge and attitudes toward pain to establish a foundation for a systematic and comprehensive integration of pain content in nursing curricula. Significant differences were found in the assessment of pain through case scenarios. The study indicated the need for reevaluation of the way pain assessment and treatment is taught across the nursing curriculum. Despite the fact that pain content is covered in every semester of the program, understanding and retention were not evident in the study.

In a qualitative study by Briggs (2010), three questions were addressed to nursing students who were given treatment choices for patients in a case vignette. The vignette contained patients who were experiencing pain in which the student would determine the thought processes underlying their decisions. Data were collected from junior and senior nursing students to provide insight for nurse educators and to point to areas where curricula and instruction may be enhanced with the hope to reduce patient pain and improve comfort and satisfaction. The three questions asked were as follows: (1) To what extent do nursing students correctly rate patients' verbal reports of pain intensity in two case vignettes? (2) To what extent do nursing students who correctly rate patient pain also correctly administer the recommended dosage of analgesic under the conditions provided in the vignette? and (3) What rationales do students identify for their ratings of pain intensity and medication administration in the vignettes? The analysis of the quantitative data revealed that more than half of the students in the sample tended to assess pain accurately; however, rather than documenting verbal ratings provided by the patient, many were swayed by behavioral factors. It is misleading for educators to believe that students who accurately assess pain will also administer adequate amounts of analgesics. In this study, a theme emerged where students documented a middle ground or average by looking at the number between the patient's self-report and the number they believed to be correct, based on the patient's behavior. When 2 mg of medication was ineffective in controlling the patient's pain at the previous administration, students were reluctant to increase the dosage. Although this study was based on a hypothetical patient situation, there is concern for the need for additional study (Briggs, 2010). New qualitative data are needed to further assess the influence of the knowledge and beliefs that many students hold about pain management in outpatient and inpatient healthcare settings.

A phenomenological study done by Izumi (2006) demonstrates how listening to the voices of nurses in their own context can assist in further understanding ethical concerns about their connectedness to patients, as well as bridge the gap between the abstract universal ethics of health care and practical and local ethics. Izumi studied the lived experiences of families being approached for organ donation, parents facing imminent death of their children, and patients being treated using stem cell transplantations. The project investigated how people experience their lives when characterized by the presence of a specific condition such as a demanding health-related situation. Qualitative research into lived experience aligns itself to a phenomenological view of human existence. The researcher tries to uncover messages to benefit knowledge (de Casterle et al., 2011).

The Ineffectiveness of Current Nursing Pain Curriculum

Nurses have a key role in effective pain management. The nurse's accurate assessment, prompt intervention, and evaluation of pain relief measures are necessary for positive patient outcomes, yet acute and chronic pain continues to be poorly managed in many settings despite the introduction of pain management standards by The Joint Commission (Plaisance & Logan, 2006). Although many of the nurses in those studies rated their knowledge as adequate, their mean scores on knowledge and attitude surveys did not reflect current knowledge of pain management practices. Ineffective care of people experiencing chronic pain has been linked within the studies of the knowledge and attitudes of nurses (Fontana, 2008).

It is during the process of undergraduate education that students develop skills, knowledge, and attitudes that will accompany them into their professional practice. Attitudes are conveyed to students as they interact with one another, educators, and patients during their education. The findings in a cross-sectional study taking place between 2001 and 2005 with third-year students due to graduate from nursing school between 2002 and 2005 reported a gap in the existing research exploring the misconceptions (inaccurate knowledge and inadequate attitudes) student nurses have of adults experiencing chronic nonmalignant pain. These findings indicate that, like qualified and practicing nurses, students hold misconceptions about adults with chronic pain, representing inaccurate knowledge and inappropriate attitudes that appear not to be addressed to a substantial degree during the course of undergraduate education. It appears that chronicity and disability need to be obvious in the curriculum, and those educational processes that enable students to explore their own attitudes and engage in the perspectives of colleagues and patients should be encouraged. These findings are compelling because, even though the data were collected between 2001 and 2003, there is no evidence in the literature of substantial curriculum developments since that time (Shaw & Lee, 2010).

To test the hypothesis that educational deficits are in part responsible for the low priority given to pain management by nurses, a study conducted by Twycross (2000) was carried out to ascertain the pain content in the common foundation program (CFP) and the four branches of preregistration diploma nursing courses in England. Results indicated that while child and adult programs cover a broad number of topics, there is minimal pain content. These results suggest that there is superficial coverage of pain as a topic and there is a need to reevaluate the teaching of pain in preregistration nursing courses. The amount of time teaching pain is considered (on average less than 10 hours), making it apparent that the teaching of pain may not be in any depth. This superficial coverage of pain content makes it hardly surprising that nurses appear ill equipped to manage pain (Twycross, 2000).

Teaching about a subject (such as chronic pain) does not mean that the student has learned it. It is possible to engage in nonreflective learning such as memorization of facts, skills learning, and preconscious learning. This is learning that does not involve reflection. Reflective learning involves contemplation, reflective skills learning, and experiential learning. For learning to take place, reflection is needed (Twycross, 2002).

Despite the importance of pain, there is a relative lack of pain management curricula in health professionals' training and a lack of new studies reporting on pain curriculum. This is especially noted with respect to behavioral techniques as noted by Zalon (1995), who conducted a study to evaluate the nature of pain management training provided to nursing students in associate and bachelor degree programs. Results indicated that a relatively small amount of nursing curriculum was devoted to such training. Programs in the study reported, on average, only 9.6 clock hours of instruction dedicated to pain, with a large portion dedicated to nonpharmacologic techniques. Of the 9.6 hours, an average of 2.9 hours was devoted to coverage of such techniques. Nonpharmacologic strategies receiving coverage were both behavioral and nonbehavioral to include massage, application of heat or cold, relaxation, distraction, and recall of pleasant images techniques. Some programs reported the use of both theoretical and practical information on these techniques; however, the majority of program respondents reported these strategies were just mentioned. Unfortunately, the authors did not provide an estimate of total clock hours in nursing curricula reviewed. It appears, however, that the coverage of pain in nursing curricula is not proportionate to the incidence of pain or the impairment caused by the condition (Zalon, 1995).

Ferrell, McCaffery, and Rhiner (1992) conducted a content analysis of 50 of the most frequently used nursing textbooks and evaluated their coverage of pain-related material. Of the 45,683 pages reviewed, 249 of the pages included pain content. Results examining the coverage of the textbooks provided nonpharmacologic interventions with a total of 61 pages dedicated to behavioral and physical interventions. This number doubles the 31 pages dedicated to pharmacologic interventions. The authors noted that nonpharmacologic interventions were presented in a positive manner, but that the level of detail provided on these strategies was inadequate to prepare nursing students to use them effectively (MacLaren & Cohen, 2005).

In a more recent qualitative study using content analysis to describe pain management clinical judgment of senior nursing students (Samuels & Leveille, 2010), students reported their experiences of patients who ranged from 6 to 86 years old, including 2 pediatric patients. Forty-six of the patients were male. The 37 cases generated 178 clinical judgments from which 4 judgment themes emerged: intention to treat pain, making sense of assessment data, intervening for comfort, and communicating with others. The results of this study offer educators examples of pain management judgments that occur in practice. The findings highlight a need to present assessment and pharmacological knowledge in an integrated, contextual, and comprehensive manner well before the senior immersion experience. The need to help students delve further into patient assessments was identified, which suggested the use of role play or using paradoxes identified in practice to challenge student thinking. Studying the lived experience of nurse educators with personal chronic pain will help direct faculty in teaching and curriculum development in pain management practice realities.

Goodrich (2007) conducted a study to determine the baseline knowledge and attitudes of nursing students and faculty about the science of pain management and to evaluate the content of pain management material and the extent to which it is integrated into curriculum. In this descriptive study, students were found to have gained knowledge in certain areas of pain management from the beginning of their nursing program until graduation, but many gaps remained. Faculty members who tested satisfactorily on the pain knowledge and attitude survey did not address pain management consistently throughout their nursing courses. Survey results revealed gaps in the understanding of the use of pain medications, pain experienced during sleep, and believing patients' self-reports of pain. Other areas needing improvement included knowledge about the incidence of respiratory depression; equianalgesic conversions; use of placebos; ceiling effects of opioids; use of nausea medications; and the definitions of addiction, tolerance, and physical dependence. Faculty surveys identified strengths in the area of patient assessment and drug therapy. Areas needing improvement included knowledge about the ceiling effects of drugs and differentiating addiction from tolerance and physical dependence. The open-ended questions addressed how the science of pain management was incorporated into individual class content. Out of 10 faculty members, 7 indicated they included pain information within the course content. Pain concepts were presented in lectures and reinforced in student presentation topics, discussion in the clinical setting, and case study review. Six faculty members indicated they tested students on pain material, and 6 described themselves as being current in their knowledge of pain and related issues. As a result, there is a need to develop comprehensive plans to integrate pain knowledge and skills into nursing study. Despite the growing professional awareness of pain science, the study found gaps in nursing knowledge and attitudes incorporating pain interventions into patients' plans of care (Goodrich, 2007).

The American Medical Association (AMA), faced with the reality of the need to improve pain care, held its first Pain Medicine Summit in June of 2008. Resolution 321 (A-08) set into motion a process to bring together a diverse group of stakeholders[2] to discuss the future status of pain care in America. This process included a broad-based coalition of physicians and organizations dedicated to improving pain care. The First National Pain Medicine Summit final report (Lippe et al., 2010, pp. 1447–1448) identified the five most pressing issues:

1. Inadequate and fragmented medical education in the field of pain medicine, which needs to be fortified in scope, content, and duration.
2. Variable, diverse, and deficient credentialing and certification processes in pain medicine.
3. Suboptimal and fragmented pain care having a negative impact on direct patient care and public health.
4. Effective and prompt remediation in order to achieve the goal of high quality pain care.
5. Barriers inhibiting or retarding progress toward the common good.

Knowledge deficits and attitudinal barriers to pain management remain and challenge us to determine why these deficits exist. Nursing faculty need to critically review current curricula to determine the presence of the in-depth and up-to-date pain management instruction for evidence-based research and quality nursing standards of care. Educators should recognize the powerful influence of feelings and attitudes on pain management behaviors among nursing students (McCaffrey et al., 2005). Educators and healthcare providers need to understand the complexity of the pain management process. They must move beyond assessment

---

[2] The stakeholders included the American Association of Medical Colleges, the Accreditation Council for Continuing Medical Education, the Accreditation Council for Graduate Medical Education, the American Board of Internal Medicine Foundation, the American Board of Medical Specialties, the American Medical Association, the American Osteopathic Association, the American Osteopathic Board of Emergency Medicine, the Association of American Medical Colleges, the Association for Hospital Medical Education, the Blue Cross/Blue Shield Association, Christiana Care, the Council of Medical Specialty Societies, Crozer-Keystone Health System, the Educational Commission for Foreign Medical Graduates, the Federation of State Medical Boards, the Iowa Board of Medical Examiners, the Michigan Board of Medicine, the National Board of Medical Examiners, the National Board of Osteopathic Medical Examiners, the Robert Wood Johnson Foundation, and the Texas A&M Health Science Center.

and communication to implementation and evaluation of improvements in pain management (Michaels et al., 2007). Inconsistencies exist in the nursing process based on variables such as educational preparation, specialty area, and personal experience caring for others. It is important for faculty to assess students' knowledge and attitudes about the treatment of pain. The nursing curriculum and instruction should not only include pathology and the management of pain, but current research on common misconceptions held by nurses regarding pain control (Briggs, 2010). Preparing new graduates to manage pain and to be advocates for their patients experiencing chronic pain requires action so that these nurses can be mentors to others. The following quote from Benner and Wrubel (1989) clearly incorporates a view of the influence of habits, thoughts, practice, and illness that we have dogmatically rejected concerning the mind's influence in the chronic pain or other illness experience:

> We have much to learn from expert patients who have developed habitual skilled bodies in response to a chronic illness. A respect for the habitual, skilled body of the patient with a chronic illness causes the clinician to respect the patient's knowledge and develop lines of clinical inquiry that go beyond a mere mapping of symptoms onto pre-existing explanations. The patient's learning about his or her own illness becomes a source of clinical discovery and inquiry in its own right. (Benner & Wrubel, 1989, p. 74)

Patients with pain have the right to optimal pain management and should be able to expect that healthcare providers will adequately assess, inform, implement, and evaluate treatments for their pain. Given the psychological, spiritual, and physical costs of unrelieved pain, nurse educators have an ethical obligation to improve current practice through addressing curricular pain content, policy initiatives, and research (Duke et al., 2010). Phenomenologically inspired research aims at describing the essence of experiential phenomena, for instance the essence of living with a chronically painful body. This means descriptions must be able to capture the ambiguity and complexity of the chronic pain, the immediate and subjectively experienced phenomena, as well as the deeper meanings (Raheim & Haland, 2006). Meanings of the lived experience provide guidance for curricula that otherwise would be left unexplored. The investigation of one's own pain experience lends to knowledge about the world and others with similar experiences. From a phenomenological point of view, to do research is to always question the way we experience the world, to want to know the world in which we live as human beings. Then research becomes a caring act of wanting to know that which is essential to being. To care is to serve and to share our being with others (van Manen, 1990). The literature review reflects that no current research has been done related to how nurse educators articulate their personal lived experiences. There is a need for phenomenological studies to give richer data to address better ways of teaching pain assessment to nursing students. The hermeneutical method of interpretation can be used for research with the aim to affect people's perception of reality and help them to become aware of possibilities (i.e., alternative ways of being in the world). It is the interpretation integrated into the world that allows knowledge gained to be productive in human life and used to improve care (Lindseth & Norberg, 2004).

Phenomenology attempts to study the human experience as it is lived. It is not just a research method, but it is also a philosophy and an approach. This study is needed to identify themes, patterns, essences, and insight within the personal lived experience of nurse educators that may contribute to education, nursing practice improvement, and the promotion of patient care.

Research Design and Methodology

CONCEPTUAL FRAMEWORK

Qualitative Design

The purpose of this study was to interpret as closely as possible and explore the meanings of lived experiences of nurse educators who have personally experienced chronic pain, in an attempt to better understand how these educators articulate and shape how they teach about chronic pain. A qualitative approach was chosen for this study. This approach is chosen by researchers who are interested in understanding or seeking to change a social phenomenon. Creswell (2009) stated, "Qualitative research is a means for exploring and understanding the meaning individuals or groups ascribe to a social or human problem" (p. 4).

In qualitative research, questions and procedures change and evolve, data are collected from participants in the setting where the phenomena occurred; data are analyzed inductively using general details to broad themes. Meaning is derived from the data by the researcher (Creswell, 2009). In qualitative research, a phenomenological approach to inquiry is often used to explore the lived experience of individuals with a common phenomenon, focusing on what the participants have experienced as individuals and how meaning is ascribed (Creswell, 2007).

Phenomenology

Using a phenomenological approach frames research and allows the researcher a path for finding meaning in the lived experiences of individuals. Researchers using a phenomenological approach explore phenomena for meaning and understanding gleaned from individuals who have lived it and are willing to describe through communication their experience (Mapp, 2008).

Lived experiences do not manifest themselves immediately but are grasped by reflection on the past presence. Reflection does not occur while living through it; therefore, phenomenological reflection is retrospective (van Manen, 1990). When exploring lived experience, one must look with reflection based on past experience to glean present meaning.

METHODOLOGY

The central guiding question is, "In what ways does the lived experience with chronic pain shape how a nurse educator understands and engages with pain assessment?" Additional questions will focus on the following: (1) How do nurse educators who have lived experience with chronic pain theorize or understand chronic pain? (2) How can the lived experience relate to how pain is taught by these individuals? and (3) What are the prescribed methods of teaching chronic pain assessment where nurse educators teach, and how does it fit into the nursing curriculum? These questions were explored with a qualitative design consisting of three-part interviews and field notes.

The specific methodology that guided the data collection, analysis, and report writing was interpretive using the phenomenological works of Benner (1994) and van Manen (1990). Exploration of the lived experience is best suited by a phenomenological approach and point of view because to do research is always to question the way we experience the world, to want to know the world in which we live as human beings (van Manen, 1990, p. 5). Through phenomenology, we discover new ways of describing and understanding what it means to be a human being, who is finite and always situated in a world with a history and concerns. In exchange, nursing may draw on a mixture of natural and medical sciences that assist in understanding human beings in their physical and cultural diversity and in caring practices. A qualitative design is the most appropriate approach for answering the proposed questions because qualitative designs have been encouraged in areas of study where the voice of the group has been unexplored (Benner, 1994).

Recruitment and Selection

This qualitative study included purposeful interviews with three nurse educators who had personally experienced chronic pain or who had cared for someone with chronic pain. The participants met the inclusion-exclusion criteria. Additional criteria for participation was nursing faculty with a master's degree in nursing and who may also have possessed a degree in nursing or a related field beyond the master's degree, who taught full-time, and who lived in the United States. Only full-time nursing faculty were selected to participate in the study. Most phenomenological studies engage in a relatively small number of participants for a relatively long period of time (at least 2 to 3 hours), which is reflective of this study with the three-interview process. The participants were the experiential experts on the phenomenon being studied (Rudestam & Newton, 2007). A sample size was projected at the beginning of this study as being not less than three, but could have been adjusted depending on the quality of the text, the amount of the intensity, and until saturation was reached. The researcher knew that saturation has been reached when each additional interviewee added little to nothing to what was learned (Benner, 1994). According to Polit and Beck (2008), there are no rules for sample size in qualitative research. Sample size is largely a function of the purpose of the inquiry, the quality of the informants, and the type of sampling strategy used. Qualitative study sample sizes should be determined based on informational needs; hence a guiding principle in sampling is data saturation that is to the point at which no new information is obtained and redundancy is achieved.

DEFINITIONS

Nurse faculty are nurses licensed as professional nurses with a minimum of master's degrees in nursing and may possess further graduate degrees in nursing or a related field, and who are current instructors in schools of nursing either accredited by the National League for Nursing Accrediting Commission or the Commission on Collegiate Nursing Education. The participants used in this study had personally experienced chronic pain or had personally cared for someone with chronic pain.

Graduate degree refers to any master's degree in nursing and a higher degree in nursing or a related field, which meets the requirements for a faculty position within an accredited school of nursing.

Full-time faculty refers to those faculty members in academic or clinical positions within an accredited school of nursing for either a 9- or 12-month contract as required by the institution.

Chronic pain refers to persistent pain where pain signals keep firing in the nervous system for weeks, months, even years. There may have been an initial mishap such as a sprained back or serious infection, or there may be an ongoing cause of pain such as arthritis, cancer, ear infection, or other problem. Some people may suffer chronic pain in the absences of any past injury or evidence of body damage. Common chronic pain complaints include headache, low back pain, cancer pain, arthritis pain, neurogenic pain (pain resulting from damage to the peripheral nerves or to the central nervous system itself), psychogenic pain (pain not due to past disease or injury or any visible sign of damage inside or outside the nervous system). A person may have two or more coexisting chronic pain conditions. Such conditions include chronic fatigue syndrome, endometriosis, fibromyalgia, inflammatory bowel disease, interstitial cystitis, temporomandibular joint dysfunction, and vulvodynia. It is not known if these disorders share a common cause (National Institute of Neurological Disorders and Stroke [NINDS], 2011). The International Association for the Study of Pain defines chronic pain as an unpleasant sensory and emotional experience associated with actual or potential tissue damage. The precise definition of chronic pain is debatable; however, sources agree that chronic pain typically lasts 6 or more months and can be classified according to its origin (International Association for the Study of Pain, 2006).

Lived experience refers to the phenomena and essence of experience of living with a chronically painful body. The essence of lived experience as described by van Manen (2003) dwells in the tension between particularity and universality. This particularity refers to the subjectively experienced and concretely "lived through meanings" of being in the world, whereas universality is connected to essential structures within which our experienced world is enclosed. Rich descriptions of the lived experience of chronic pain must then be understood in this context.

SAMPLE SIZE, SETTING, AND ACCESS

A purposive sampling was sought to ensure the lived pain experience. Purposive sampling involves selecting volunteer cases that will most benefit the study. In qualitative studies, sample size is determined based on informational needs and data saturation. Data saturation is sampling to the point that no new information is obtained from the participants. The guiding principle in selecting the sample is that all participants must have experienced the phenomenon and must be able to articulate what it is like to have lived that experience. "The purposive sample method is one in which the researcher selects participants based on personal judgment about which ones will be most informative" (Polit & Beck, 2008, p. 763). Participants for this study were full-time educators of baccalaureate degree or associate degree nursing programs who taught about chronic pain to senior level student nurses and who had personally experienced chronic pain. These educators were recruited by sending a formal letter to the President of the Alabama League for Nursing. The Alabama League for Nursing is a professional organization that supports nursing educators and quality nursing education at all levels. The president distributed the request for participants by asking interested individuals to reply directly to the researcher via a confidential e-mail address, which was provided. Four individuals responded to the request for participants. One individual did not meet the inclusion criteria because she taught in a vocational school and not in a college or university setting.

PROTECTION OF PARTICIPANTS

Institutional review board approval was sought from, and approved by, the University of Alabama Institutional Review Board prior to beginning the study.

DATA COLLECTION

The methodology was based on the philosophical framework in which fundamental assumptions and characteristics of human science perspectives are made (van Manen, 1990). Within the methodology, techniques and procedures are applied in an approach that tries to avoid "constructing a predetermined set of fixed procedures, techniques, and concepts" (van Manen, 1990, p. 29). In phenomenology, the natural attitude is one in which there is a tendency to judge and to have already made judgments about existing phenomena. We already know, we conclude, we state the facts, and we take for granted what is meant. To shift to the phenomenological attitude, the researcher must refrain from making judgments about the factual. This is accomplished through bracketing. "Bracketing is the act of suspending one's various beliefs in the reality of the natural world in order to study the essential structures of the world" (van Manen, 1990, p. 175). The easiest way to do this is to narrate from lived experience. In narrating, we refrain from judging or concluding. We are not interested in stating facts, but in relating what we have experienced. We do not judge what is said as right or wrong, but rather participate in the story with comments such as, "so this is what you have experienced" or "so that is what you thought." The researcher brackets personal judgments about the factual and about what is the case in order to become open to our own experience. Data analysis was ongoing where data were analyzed throughout the process between interviews, allowing for the analysis to impact subsequent interviews.

Van Manen (1990) listed six activities that occur in gathering phenomenological research: (1) focusing on the phenomenon of interest, (2) investigating experience as we live it rather than as we conceptualize it, (3) reflecting on the essential themes that characterize the phenomenon, (4) describing the phenomenon through the art of writing and rewriting, (5) maintaining a strong and oriented relation to the phenomenon, and (6) balancing the research context by considering parts and whole. Lived experience is something recognized in retrospect (van Manen, pp. 30–31).

According to Seidman (1991), the purpose of in-depth interviewing is not to get answers to questions, nor to test hypotheses, and not to "evaluate" as the term is normally used. At the root of interviewing is an interest in understanding the experience of other people and the meaning they make of that experience. Van Manen's six activities for phenomenological inquiry assisted the researcher in understanding the interview process described by Seidman (1991), because from a phenomenological point of view, to do research is always to question the way an individual experiences the world and to want to know the world in which human beings live. Humans question the world's very secrets and intimacies, which bring the world as a world into being for us and in us. Research is a caring act; we want to know that which is most essential to being. The procedure to capture this inquiry was a three-part interview process based on Seidman's (1991) qualitative guide. The analytical work for this phenomenological study was field notes, transcription, and qualitative data analysis. Discoveries gleaned in interviews (meanings, the emerging themes, and the valid comments) were documented. The researcher looked at the discourses of life experiences in a social context. A scholarly approach was used with careful listening and hearing of the participants' voices.

PROCEDURE/SETTING

Three-part, face-to-face interviews were conducted. Each interview was audio recorded by the researcher in a mutually agreed upon location and later confidentially transcribed by the researcher for coding. Informed consent was obtained from all participants prior to the interviews. Information regarding the study's follow-up procedures and participant rights were given to the participant in writing before the interview. The participants were given a chance to ask questions prior to the start of the interviews. The study participants were contacted by the researcher to schedule a time to meet for the initial private interview. Subsequent private interviews were scheduled at times and places in mutual agreement with the researcher and the participant. The researcher asked a series of questions divided into three parts consisting of three interviews. The first interview focused on the life history of the participant. The second interview concentrated on the details of the participant's experience(s) with pain. The third interview asked participants to reflect on the meaning of their experience and to look at how factors in their lives interact to bring meaning. Ongoing data analysis occurred throughout the process of all three interviews allowing for impact on subsequent interviews. Responses of the participants in the study were kept only by the researcher in a password protected computer file and a locked file cabinet with key access only by the researcher.

DATA ANALYSIS

Data analysis was an ongoing process throughout the study. Research questions were used as a guide to review transcripts, and relevant data were identified to create meaningful units. The Colaizzi data analysis method for qualitative data analysis was utilized to help ensure validity

(Polit & Beck, 2008). The seven-step process was utilized to maintain uniformity. Information was transcribed verbatim from audio recordings of interviews. The text was analyzed for recurring ideas in the statements, phrases, and/or themes that captured the nature and core of the experiences described and was ongoing throughout the interview process based upon the process described by van Manen (1990). Each interview transcript was read several times, in order to identify lines of inquiry or meaningful statements. Each theme was allocated a color-matched number during coding of information. This part of the procedure required considerable time, as coding is an interactive process (i.e., the researcher coded and recoded as the scheme developed). Once the coding was matched to the transcripts, an attempt was made to interpret their meaning in the context in which they appeared. The interviewer asked the participants to confirm the right interpretation of what they said, which added credibility to the validity and reliability of the results (Guba & Lincoln, 1983). Paradigm cases were analyzed to distinguish between what van Manen (1990) terms incidental and essential themes (pp. 106–107). Van Manen argued that only some meanings that are gleaned from a given phenomenon are unique to it. These are the essential themes in which the phenomenon would not exist if this theme was not present. "Phenomenological themes may be understood as the structures of experience. When a phenomenon is analyzed, there is an attempt to try to determine what the themes are, the experiential structures that make up experience" (van Manen, 1990, p. 79). "Because our everyday lived experience is so taken for granted as to go unnoticed, it is often through breakdown that the researcher achieves flashes of insight into the lived world" (Benner, 1994, p. 59).

The data generally flowed into categories. The researcher moved back and forth making notes through journaling for an audit trail, color coding the text for common themes and essences, and utilizing Nvivo 10 software to assist in categorizing nodes found in the interview texts. The researcher began with excerpts of significant statements, which led back to the original transcripts and produced themes. After organizing categories, the researcher then searched for meaning among the categories in order to develop a meaningful interpretation of the data using the participants' words. The researcher then determined if the themes were essential or incidental by looking at the data as a whole. Credibility, dependability, confirmability, and transferability, as identified by Colaizzi (as cited in Polit & Beck, 2008, p. 520), were utilized to ensure trustworthiness. This method includes the following:

- Reading all protocols to acquire a feeling for them
- Reviewing each protocol to extract significant statements
- Spelling out the meaning of each significant statement (i.e., formatting meanings)
- Organizing the formulated meanings into clusters of themes. (A) Refer these clusters back to the original protocols to validate them. (B) Note discrepancies among or between the various clusters, avoiding the temptation of ignoring data or themes that do not fit
- Integrating results into an exhaustive description of the phenomenon under study
- Formulating an exhaustive description of the phenomenon under study with an unequivocal statement of identification as possible
- Asking participants about the findings thus far, as a final validating step

Interpretation required abstraction from the themes containing the participants' words to meanings so they could be looked at as a whole. The final abstraction yielded the true essence of the phenomenon of interest, lived experience. Through this process, the data were pushed to go beyond the words of the participants to a level of abstraction (van Manen, 1990). This level of abstraction, presented in the form of essences and known as member checking, is necessary in order to make the data meaningful to nursing and other disciplines.

SAMPLE DEMOGRAPHICS

Three out of four responding nurse educators met the inclusion criteria and were interviewed for the study. Two of the three nurse educators were nursing faculty with a master's degree in nursing working full time on two different campuses of an associate degree program (community college), and one of the nurse educators held a master's degree in nursing and a PhD in public administration and was employed full time as an assistant professor in a bachelor's degree university setting. All three nurse educators were female Caucasians over the 35-year-old age group. Faculty teaching years ranged from 16 to 18 years for the associate degree faculty and was 12 years for the bachelor's degree associate professor. Years of nursing practice ranged from 23 to 31 years as a registered nurse. Each nurse educator stated she worked 40-plus hours per week during the fall and spring semesters. All of the nurse educators were married. One educator had small children, one had grown children living out of the home with grandchildren, and one did not have any children. Subjects taught by the three participants included fundamentals, Medical Surgical Nursing I and II, leadership, obstetrics, pediatrics, and community health nursing. The average number of students per class ranged from 40 to 60 each semester. The types of chronic pain represented among the group consisted of rheumatoid arthritis, psoriatic arthritis (severe psoriatic dermatitis complication of feet and hands), and chronic back pain with history of severe pelvic pain. Each study participant's pain time of onset was 2–3 years from date of the initial interviews (see **Table 16-1**). The interviews were conducted during the months of May through July 2012 and were done at least one week apart for a total of three interviews each in person and one follow-up interview with one participant who was hospitalized related to her chronic pain, shortly after the course of her last interview. Each interview lasted about an hour.

TABLE 16-1   Demographic Data for Participants

	Participant A	Participant B	Participant C
Age group in years	> 35	> 35	> 35
Race	Caucasian	Caucasian	Caucasian
Highest degree	MSN	MSN	PhD
Number of years in nursing	23	31	25
Nurse educator years of teaching	16	18 yrs., 8 mos.	12
Courses taught	Fundamentals/med/surg	OB/med/surg Peds Leadership	Community health/med/surg
Type of chronic pain	Rheumatoid arthritis	Psoriatic arthritis with severe dermatitis	Chronic back pain Fibroid tumors
Years of chronic pain	3	2	2

Field notes and journals were used to connect the researcher's observations to the researcher's transcribed interviews and to continue the explorative process. The Colaizzi (Polit & Beck, 2008) method of interview material validation of data by the participant was used as a final step in the analytic method. Computerized copies of all data collected will be kept for 5 years, and a back-up copy will be kept on an external jump drive for 5 years. All data were collected on the personal laptop computer owned by the researcher and password protected. All equipment such as audio recorder and jump drive will be stored in a locked file cabinet for 5 years. Only the researcher will have access to the passwords used and the key. Pseudonyms were used during the private audio recordings to protect the identity of the participants. A reference code was assigned to each participant to facilitate confidentiality. All codes and contact information were kept in a locked file in the researcher's office. Only the researcher had access to stored information. Data analysis was ongoing throughout the study. An interpretive description of the lived experience was written and shared with the participants to verify the faithfulness of the descriptions and the interpretation of the experience as captured by the researcher. The participants were given a summary of the interviews and had the opportunity to clarify any misinterpretation of data.

TRUSTWORTHINESS AND VALIDITY OF THE STUDY

Trustworthiness and validity were established through triangulation, confirmability, and transferability. *Triangulation* refers to the use of multiple methods, sources, or referents to draw conclusions about what constitutes the truth. In qualitative research, this might involve trying to understand the full complexity of a poorly understood phenomenon by using multiple means of data collection to converge the truth (e.g., having in-depth discussions with study participants, as well as watching their behaviors in natural settings). It might also involve triangulating the ideas of multiple researchers working together as a team (Polit & Beck, 2008). Findings were clarified with each subsequent interview and through member checks to allow clarification and modification of the transcript and to establish credibility. *Credibility* refers to the truthfulness of the data (Polit & Beck, 2008). Credibility was maintained by keeping a journal-audit trail reviewed by committee members during the process detailing insights, content, and observations. Participants were invited to review their transcripts within a week after they were transcribed to add, change, or clarify their stories. This ensured that the researcher was building trustworthiness into each phase of the research and not just focusing on the end. *Transferability* refers to the extent to which qualitative findings can be transferred to other settings or groups (Polit & Beck, 2008). Transferability was maintained in that the findings of the research had meaning for nurses and nurse educators. *Confirmability* is the process of minimizing bias during the research process and in the final product (Polit & Beck 2008).

> A good description that constitutes the essence of something is construed so that the structure of a lived experience is revealed to us in such a fashion that we are now able to grasp the nature and significance of the experience in a hitherto unseen way. (van Manen, 1990, p. 39)

Bias is a major concern in designing a research study due to the study's ability to reveal the truth. *Bias* is an influence that produces a distortion or error in the study results. Biases can affect the quality of evidence in both qualitative and quantitative studies. It is the job of the researcher to prevent bias to the extent possible and to establish mechanisms to detect or measure it when it exists. Triangulation was used with multiple sources of information with points of view to counterbalance the biases or identify their existence.

Member checking is a process where feedback is provided to the research participants about emerging interpretations and to obtain the participants' reactions for clarity. Member checking is an important technique for establishing credibility and is an important process to represent the realities of the participants' statements of meaning (Polit & Beck, 2008). The researcher asked the participants at the beginning of each of the three interviews to reflect on what was talked about in the previous interview. The researcher provided written transcripts to each participant for input on meaning, feedback, and clarification.

Some limitations of the study were found in the possibility that participants could be inhibited by the presence of a tape recorder, and audio taping the interviews may have made them reluctant to share private thoughts and experiences. Including participants with a variety of different types of chronic pain may have caused some variation in scope. Conducting a set of narrative interviews is a delicate task in which the interviewer should create a permissive climate of comfort. As interviewees can only understand and narrate their lived experience in relation to their preunderstanding and the interviewers can only understand the narrative in relation, there is a risk of misunderstanding.

ETHICAL CONSIDERATIONS

There was minimal risk of psychological or physical harm to the participants in the study. Participants could withdraw from the study at any time without questions related to reasons for withdrawal. Confidentiality of interviews was assisted by using pseudonyms for the prevention of tracing. Each participant was assigned a reference code. All identifying information was kept locked in the researcher's office under lock and key. Only the researcher had access to the lock and key access. Participants were notified that the researcher was the only person who could match the names and data to the information obtained in the study. Confidentiality procedures were given to the participants at the time of the interview and when the informed consent was signed. Every effort to ensure a nonjudgmental perspective was made. The researcher attempted to identify and document personal biases in the interview process and utilize triangulation methods. Any opposing views to those of the researcher were kept private with a nonjudgmental attitude. The researcher's voice remained at an even tone to avoid any audible cues, and the researcher did not voice any personal beliefs, biases, or opinions that may have affected the integrity of the interview process. A faculty mentor was consulted as needed during the study to assist in avoiding potential research bias and to aid with any questions that arose during the study process.

Research Findings

This study used a phenomenological method to interpret as closely as possible the lived experiences of nurse educators who have personally experienced chronic pain. Using the broad and focused research question as a guide, the researcher carefully analyzed and reviewed the transcripts of three participants for emergent themes, totaling nine interviews. Initially, each interview transcript was read several times in order to identify lines of inquiry. Meaningful statements that described structures of experience emerged with some consistency describing the lived experience. Five

TABLE 16-2　Themes

Themes	Meaning
Vulnerability	Desperate, embarrassed, ashamed, crying, inferiority, hopelessness, loss of joy, disbelief, *Subtheme: stoic*
Physician/provider trust	Poor assessment, drug seeker mentality, questioning, not listening
Fear of disability	Desire to be normal, need for independence, betrayed by body, dependent, loss of socialization, disappointing family, difficulties with activities of daily living, *Subtheme: alien*
Coping	Self-realization, adaptation, understanding, reflection, accommodation
Need for pedagogical discourse	Lack of adequate teaching hours, poorly written texts, need for better chronic pain assessments, need for more psychosocial content

major themes emerged, paralleled, and assisted to answer the questions with two subthemes (see **Table 16-2**).

CHRONIC PAIN DEFINED

The definition of chronic pain used in this study refers to persistent pain where pain signals keep firing in the nervous system for weeks, months, or even years. Some people may suffer chronic pain due to a mishap such as a sprained back or serious infection, or there may be an ongoing cause of pain such as arthritis, cancer, or other problem. Some people suffer chronic pain in the absence of any past injury or evidence of body damage. Common chronic pain complaints include headache, low back pain, neurogenic pain, psychogenic pain, endometriosis, and more (NINDS, 2011). Nurse educators provided a description of their understanding of chronic pain at the beginning of the second interview.

The participants defined chronic pain in a variety of ways: Pain that you have off and on like a headache, pain that is not relieved, pain that is there but is never completely gone, unresolved pain, or pain lasting longer than 6 months. Throughout the literature, chronic pain is represented by a variety of definitions and the participants' representations were no different. During the analysis process, it also became apparent that there are similar viewpoints and understandings of how chronic pain is theorized among the group of participants. Each of the participants expressed that chronic pain is misunderstood by members of the healthcare system and by society in general.

RESEARCH QUESTIONS

There was one broad research question for this study. In what ways does the lived experience with chronic pain shape how a nurse educator understands and engages with pain assessment? Additional focused questions follow: (1) How do nurse educators who have the lived experience with chronic pain theorize or understand chronic pain? (2) How can the lived experience relate to how pain is taught by these individuals, and what are the prescribed methods of teaching assessment where nurse educators teach and how does it fit into the nursing curriculum?

In the initial interviews, all three participants were asked to tell a little about where they grew up, their earliest memory of hearing about or experiencing chronic pain, and to give some examples of life encounters with chronic pain. Two of the participants grew up in a rural area and one participant grew up in the city.

The first participant remembered learning initially about chronic pain at the age of 12 from an aunt who had pancreatic cancer. The aunt refused chemotherapy after it made her quite sick. Participant A reflected on her lack of understanding about genetic tendencies at such a young age. The participant said, "I don't know if I connected. I mean, I knew it was cancer. I knew she'd die, but I don't think I thought about that being genetic" (Participant A Interview I, ADN instructor).

The second participant remembered an uncle when she was about 5 years old who was one of her favorite people to go visit. She speaks of her intrigue with his illness. She expected him to be deformed and scary. She discovered something quite different. She stated,

> He had rheumatoid arthritis and was bedbound. He smoked a cigar and his hands were in a position where he could get his cigar in. He worked puzzles and had an aquarium by his bed. As a child, I was just intrigued by an adult doing puzzles and staying in the house all day long. Everyone came to his bedroom to visit him. I thought he would be scary, but he was not scary. Everybody loved him. (Participant B Interview I, ADN instructor)

The third participant remembers grandparents who had chronic pain related to degenerative arthritis and osteoarthritis. Her earliest memory is at about 8 years of age when she watched them struggle with their activities of daily living. Her early experience of observing chronic pain made a lasting impression that gave way to the career she chose in life. Watching relatives struggle stirred her compassion. She stated,

> I think that is what started making a lot of impressions on me that probably led to me wanting to be a nurse. Watching them struggle, I realized that because my mother was their only child, and not being in the same city that she was not going to be able to supply them with the resources that she would have liked for them to have. This was in the years before you had home health in a close proximity and all the support systems that could be put into place now. They were just in this tiny little town and just kind of struggling on their own. (Participant C, Interview I, BSN instructor)

During the first interviews, study participants were asked to describe if there is anything or things they believe shape how they view pain and to speak about any personal experiences that triggered anxiety or concern based on what they know about pain. One study participant talked about a patient she had cared for as a young nurse. She spoke about problems often encountered in the physician/provider trust relationship. Authenticity becomes an awareness of self by others that chronic pain may not exist in the absence of physical signs or the need for frequent pain medication. She said,

> She had a spinal injury and she was in a wheelchair. She had morphine in the house, which in the home . . . you try to have locked up. She had a guy come in and steal . . . she'd filed a police report where she tried to go after him and then she went to the hospital . . . and they treated her like a drug seeker at the hospital . . . and so I had to go through all kinds of avenues trying to get her more medication. The pain clinic refused to give her that. I called the patient advocate for her but they would not let me talk . . . so I said, fine, the patient is here, you talk. So, that's how . . . because she had such a hard time. I kind of got involved with her more than others. Just because

they were like, well, you know, you're just up here to get medication. Because that's who you go to, the drug clinics, and they will only provide a certain amount for the month. They refused to give her anything. I couldn't even talk the physician with the clinic into it. And so they said, well you know, you're just taking it. [The patient said:] "No, I didn't take it all, I actually had somebody break in." They did not believe her, but they gave her a shot and sent her home. Just a shot, they didn't give her anything else. Just a drug seeker is how they treat them in the ER. They just don't listen to them and the elderly on top of that. (Participant A, Interview I, ADN instructor)

A second participant voiced her thoughts about people who have chronic pain having a choice to make between what is considered adequate drug intake and what is considered too much. There seems to be a wisdom garnered and insight about the daily nuances of the disease and the lived knowledge about managing at arduous times. She said,

A choice to make . . . at a level they can tolerate. Some people become addicted, and then, they're seeking more with more drug-seeking behaviors. Where others will cope in other ways and not let it affect them as far as addiction in their family as much. So I've seen the difference in treatment with acute versus chronic that are already addicted. I believe there is a level they have every day . . . that they have learned to cope with, but once they go above that level, they've used all their coping ability to deal with it already, and they've exhausted it. I believe short-term management is fine. But you can't continue with short-term management. You've got to make it short-term and help them in different ways . . . maybe exercises, relaxation, but you can't continue medication. They have used up everything they have and they need some help . . . because the pain is real. (Participant B, Interview I, ADN instructor)

A third participant talked about how her most recent episode with pain has shaped how she views pain and how she has approached the assessment of pain in patients she has cared for in the past. The nurse may not realize that the patient who is hurting may not feel like answering so many questions until relief is obtained.

I remember thinking, Oh, gosh, I know exactly how my poor patients feel now. And . . . I remember the frustration of being in such severe pain and having nurses questioning me to death. And, that was my thought . . . you know, because literally you're lying there and you can't even open your eyes and you're thinking, Oh, don't keep asking me this because I am not in any shape to answer these kind of questions right . . . even though in the back of your mind you know they are having to ask you these things. They are having to try to get you to describe things. And, the more and more you feel like you can relate completely to your patient's frustration with feeling horrible and having us do these long detailed assessments on them, asking them these questions, over and over, and they're just thinking please just give me some relief, because I think I'm going to die today. (Participant C, Interview I, BSN instructor)

One other note made by this same participant about how pain has shaped her view has to do with stoicism. The culture of her family upbringing was to endure, as all would eventually be well. There is resistance to the disease nuances in order to prevent negative reactions by others. She said,

I tend to be sort of on the stoic side. Now I saw my grandmother had a lot of problems with chronic pain, in particular. Like I said, probably osteoarthritis related and a lot of surgeries. So, I'm sure she had a lot of scar tissue and adhesions. I always saw my mother being very stoic. She was never once a big one to complain you know? She was never sick with anything. She wouldn't be down for the count for long. And so, I think I tend to have that same kind of attitude. Because always my thing is, I'm the one who's saying, "I'm going to be alright. I'm going to be alright." You know, with the last episode with the pain from the fibroid, I kept telling them over and over . . . even though their thing was they wanted to take me to the ER, I said, "I am not going to the hospital, I am not going to the hospital." (Participant C, Interview I, BSN instructor)

Despite the stoicism of this participant she goes on to further comment about how her understanding and view of chronic pain changed when she took on work as a hospice (end-of-life care) nurse. She stated,

As far as my views of pain as a nurse, I worked for a long time with cancer patients and so, saw them in terrific pain. I think I have a lot more, probably liberal ideas on pain medicine for my patients than a lot of nurses do. Because I remember the days I gave cancer patients 18 mg of MS-Contin. You know, with a big glass of water . . . that's what it took to deal with it. And I remember when people used to not want to float to our cancer floor because their thing was, like, well, I can't give the medication y'all give and I am not going to do that. The doctor would prescribe MS-Contin way outside of the ordinary dose a nurse normally would give. You saw people that you knew were in the active dying process. I mean, you wanted them to be comfortable. These people would build up such a tolerance to it over the years of dealing with this. (Participant C, Interview I, BSN instructor)

THEMES

In the interviews, each of the three participants responded to open-ended questions with five essential themes emerging (see Table 16-2): *vulnerability, physician/provider trust, fear of disability, coping,* and *need for pedagogical discourse.* The subtheme *stoic* emerged related to the theme *vulnerability,* and the subtheme *alien* emerged related to *fear of disability.* The themes and meanings to follow reflect the experience of the participants as they expressed it.

Vulnerability

Vulnerability is an adjective defined as meaning exposed to the possibility of being attacked or harmed, either physically or emotionally, open to moral attack, criticism, or difficult to defend (Oxford English Dictionary, 2013). In the thematic breakdown, each of the participants indicated feeling on multiple occasions either desperate, embarrassed, ashamed, inferior, or hopeless, had cried on occasion, and displayed at times a loss of joy as well as disbelief. One of the participants illustrated this when she said,

It was honors night for the students and I had to wear a brace. I got home to get dressed and I could not get dressed. I could not zip my pants or anything. So I changed, put a dress on, and I put on the brace that just immobilizes so I could go because I had to speak at honors night. It bothered me because it was embarrassing to have to wear it. No big black brace is attractive. (Participant A, Interview II, ADN instructor)

Participant A further explained about her vulnerability when she spoke about the symptoms and embarrassing side effects related to dealing with the required treatment for her chronic pain. There is a fear that people in general, do not have a deep understanding of chronic pain and form their opinions, and often negative ones, based on what they see:

> Chronic pain is always there. It may be relieved up to like a level two or a three, but it's never completely gone. When I started with tendonitis, I could not do a lot because my joints would lock up and hurt. Now . . . my hands . . . when I wake up in the morning, I can't use my hands a lot because they feel like clubs, and it hurts to bend them, my fingers. This one was trying to lock up the other day so I started my methotrexate this week. It has been about five days now but it will go down with the methotrexate. It aches and mine is a weakness associated with it also. You can't do a lot with your hands because they hurt. I pay for a clinical day of twelve hours on the floor. I do clinical once a week. I had to stop taking it when I had my wisdom teeth taken out because it is an immunosuppressant. He [physician] gave me a new medication, and I can't even think of the name of it. It was for nausea. Hopefully, it will keep my hair from coming out. It thinned. It's really thin. It makes me feel old when you can't do things you feel like an idiot and old woman. It was more of a self-esteem issue too. (Participant A, Interview II, ADN instructor)

Participant B described her vulnerability manifested in tears, shame, and inferiority by telling about an encounter she had during a time when her hands were cracking and bleeding from the psoriasis.

> When I say things, I'm very calm with it. If I'm upset or anything, I don't let them see the emotion behind it. So particularly on one visit to the physician, I had some psychological issues to discuss because it was beginning to affect me when I would hand money to someone when I'm shopping. I have had them [store clerk] draw back when they see my hands and it had upset me. That had happened the day before. So when I went for my scheduled appointment I tried to tell her about it. It started out very well but then I lost my little composure in my front and I started crying. That was the first time I let her see my emotion. (Participant B, Interview I, ADN instructor)

She further spoke about her vulnerability and inferiority manifested in hiding her condition when dealing with students in the clinical setting. When asked if she shared her physical pain and difficulties with the students she said,

> The doctor had said not to wash my hands as much and to try to keep some type of gloves on to see if they would not sting so badly. So, um . . . telling a nurse not to wash her hands is like, oh sure! (Laughter). I think because I had my gloves on the students were seeing me wash my hands and the students were doing most of the touching at that point. I had a higher level group of students and so they knew how to do more things. I would try intentionally, not to have them where they could see my hands so well because I did fear that they were not going to want me touching them because I had blood under my gloves. I would keep my hands back and try to keep them out of the field of vision. If I had to do anything, I tried to hold them back away. (Participant B, Interview II, ADN instructor)

Participant B went on to say she would start having what she termed "pity parties" or feelings of hopelessness when she would sit at home and not do things with her family. This would depress her because she did not want to be left out of the activity. The negative feelings include fear, anger, frustration, self-consciousness, and depression. Anxiety and anger can be part of the emotional response to chronic pain and especially during very painful days of the illness or disease. It is often a normal response to the limitations imposed by the disease or illness. She stated that "good health equals joy in life."

> I have learned this about myself . . . that I have to be more guarded about my feelings because I tend to get more sensitive. Because I am hurting, I take things more personally than they are meant to be. I'm tending to overreact to a situation that I may not have even paid attention to before. It's not coming from outside, it's coming from within me. That's different because I've always trusted my feelings really well, and now I'm having to examine them. I think one of the things I have realized more this past week . . . and it may be because of thinking about it and answering questions, is that I don't want to be a burden. I don't want to be the person that somebody

says something about thinking I am lazy because I am not doing any-thing. Maybe I should try to get up and go do it. It's challenging me to examine my feelings. My daughter is getting married and came home this weekend. At showers, I'm worried about, are people think-ing that I am just lazy or not a good hostess? Do I need to tell them that I have a problem? Or do I need to just be quiet and smile and let this pass? This weekend we had a lot of people that didn't know me. I wondered, do they think that this is a grandmother who just comes and thinks she's privileged to not do anything? (Participant B, Interview III, ADN instructor)

Participant C was not expecting her disbelief behavior and feelings of hopelessness when she was caught off guard at a follow-up physician's phone call. The physician asked her to come back next week and he would do some more invasive testing. Because she is a nurse and knows the order of things, she thought about the kinds of tests that are usually completed prior to biopsies. This lived experience gives way to the notion that people in the medical profession have a fair understanding, but not an in-depth understanding of chronic pain. This insight leads to searching for the right provider until a satisfactory one is found. She said,

I wanted to sit down and look at the lab work from last week. I wanted to sit down and look at a biopsy report. I wanted to be able to read this on my own. And, um . . . and then, of course, you know I managed to get off the telephone with him and then just kind of sat there stunned. You know, sort of thinking, well, . . . what just happened? You know, basically at that point, life stopped. I started making telephone calls to everybody I knew that could give me some information on this. Could it be cancer? That's the only reason I could think of why the doctor himself would call me at home to tell me this. (Participant C, Interview III, BSN instructor)

Participant C revealed an emerging therapeutic occurrence, also found in the interview with participant B, and not expected by the researcher. Both participants voiced that these interviews were proving to be cathar-tic and helpful in allowing unvented reflection to appear. There is a ten-dency to see life in a different light, to take one day at a time, and to learn from the personal experience. There is almost a sense of, "I have a knowledge that not everyone has unless they have been down this road or participated in the journey. She stated,

> You are expected to deal with it. There's this thing, I really think as a woman you're expected to sort of just suck it up and take it because you don't want to inconvenience everybody else. And kind of, if at all possible, downplay it. I have found myself at least 20 times the last couple of weeks doing it with my family. You don't want anybody to know what it was really like. You don't want anybody to know. I have to say these interviews have been very helpful because I don't know that there is anybody that I've been able to let them really know just how scared I was this week when I saw the GYN physician and the pain hit. Because I was so scared and quite honestly, I'm so ashamed as a Christian that I was that afraid. I kept thinking to myself, this is not the way you're supposed to be as a Christian, to be so scared. But I was so afraid. I remember putting my make-up on to go to the doctor and my hand shook so bad I thought I was going to have my eyebrows drawn on upon my scalp! It's almost like you had too much knowledge as a nurse. Every crazy thing you've ever seen or heard about happening in a hospital was going through your mind. I am not going to say this to my parents. I don't want to make a spectacle in front of my students. So what do I do? I get in an elevator and ride all the way down and trot all the way across campus to the nursing building. I was determined I was going to get there before I passed out. It's so embarrassing when your boss has to help you across the hallway to the nursing care clinic. It makes you feel vulnerable. I'm not one of these. I don't like feeling vulnerable. That's one of my things. (Participant C, Interview II, BSN instructor)

Subtheme: Stoic. The subtheme *stoic* emerged meaning "a person who can endure pain or hardship without showing their feelings or complaining" (Oxford English Dictionary, 2013). For example, Participant A said, "And I guess it depends on your personality. I don't want to be told I can't do that, because I can do it." There is a resilience that seems to be cultivated from the chronic pain experience. Although participants recognized their physical limits, they did not exaggerate them and instead showed zealous perseverance in using their remaining abilities.

Participant B said,

So, I've gotten very good at blocking . . . the back pain. And I would find that I would hurt in my jaws because I would clinch. . . . Maybe this is something that I'm expected to have to just tolerate. You know, maybe other people deal with this and don't have to have pain medication. So maybe I'm just being a wuss, and I need to just toughen up.

Participant C reiterated her grandmother's pain, her mother's stoicism, and her own stoicism. "So unless you know, essentially, you are just doubled over in pain, you are almost better off if you just don't say anything" (Participant C, BSN instructor).

Physician/Provider Trust

Physician/provider trust contributed significantly to the data from the interviews and is talked about 52 times in the transcripts. The majority of the contributing statements have to do with failure to listen or hear the individual's needs, along with poor chronic pain assessment. Participant A told about her visits to the chiropractor, whom she felt attended to her muscle pain best compared to her physician. She has seen several physicians in an attempt to get pain relief. During Hurricane Katrina, a physician visited the town where Participant A lives to help with the storm victims who were living in shelters. Participant A volunteered and observed a particular physician assessing storm victims. She said,

Physicians, half the time, they don't listen to you. They don't believe . . . and that's when I chose a doctor here who is really nice. If there is ever a problem, they just push you off. So I chose Dr. [name omitted] because I knew she would listen. She listens to what you say. I know as my experience as a nurse that you can tell them stuff and they don't listen. Chiropractors are better at listening and they will treat you. There are a lot of things they can do that are nondrug, a lot of massage or the heat. They have this new thing called spinal stretching. I had to chase a physician down. I did home health and they sent a guy home with no pain medicine after he had surgery. It's the way hospitals run now. You have the internist and you have the guy outside. I chased one doctor. Called and he did not answer. He was a primary but the other physician didn't order it. He would not answer my pages. I finally called the operator and asked where he was. He was doing rounds. I found him and asked him what was going on. He said he did not have my number. Well, that is not an excuse. He told me he would not write the prescription for anybody but for me he wrote the script for the patient . . . and then I took it to the pharmacy. So, you know my experiences with physicians, they don't listen well. (Participant A, Interview I, ADN instructor)

Dissatisfaction with medical care included short visits, restricted medical model of care, and limited choices. Participants verbalized disappointment over the lack of progress or new knowledge about etiology and treatment. The participants changed providers frequently in order to gain satisfaction. There appeared to be a lack on the provider side of getting involved with the disease process. Participant B told about a situation she encountered with her family physician, who did not seem to be listening to her in the same way he was listening to her husband.

My husband had some sort of lesion on his chin, and it looked like a spider bite. He went to the same general practitioner and told him it "hurt like hell." The first thing he did was to start writing a prescription for pain and he never asked for any. A day later, I go to that same physician and am hardly able to walk into the office. I have a bite also on my abdomen that looks just like the one he has on his chin. We believe the spider got into the bed and bit both of us. I hurt so badly. My pants or anything touching against it, my underclothes hurt the spot. Not once! Not once did he give me anything for pain! I thought, is this a man/woman thing? They have treated me for a long time and never had me asking for pain medication. I did not ask for anything. So maybe I'm just being a wuss and I need to just toughen up. I haven't been back to that physician. I'm thinking of changing physicians. (Participant B Interview I, ADN instructor)

Participant B went on to talk about how difficult it was for her to get a definitive diagnosis. She could not get in to see a specialty dermatologist for 3 months. She called another physician group and scheduled an appointment. She kept as many as three appointments for assurance of a physician who would listen and get to the bottom of her problem. She was wrongly diagnosed three times before the final physician in a larger town gave her a definitive answer to her problem. There was a sense of relief that "there is this creature and that's what I've been dealing with all of these times."

Participant C spoke about having a lot of anger and lack of trust over the way her gynecologist treated her after presenting to his office with the primary problem of chronic pain. This conversation took place initially and was followed by an appointment to a different physician with whom she developed a greater trust. She later found that she did indeed have the diagnosis of ovarian cancer.

> There was no offer of any kind of pain medication while a biopsy was being done. In fact, the comment was made "that's what I like about you nurses, you're tough." I felt like once he found out I was a nurse, any kind of flow of information stopped. I had to be the one to bring up the subject of the possibility of cancer with him. He immediately brushed it off and said, Oh well, I'm not really thinking about that. But then we go directly into taking a biopsy! He really, really brushed over and discounted the whole idea. Then, I get this call and he is reading the biopsy results to me over the phone. Yet, he cannot give me any kind of details as to what size. Is this in fact cancerous? Pre-cancerous? Anything? No. Huh-uh, just kind of reading the results off to you. He just wanted me to come back for some more invasive things. Well, as I was listening to him reading this off, my thought was, I know exactly how all of my patients I've dealt with as a nurse have ever felt now because I literally could feel myself start to get hot and sweat to start rolling down inside my clothes. My first thought was . . . I really don't even know what he's saying, then it registers and you think, Oh dear God, is this man telling me I have cancer? Every-thing in the world is going through your mind from I should have gone sooner. I should have paid more attention to what was going on. How stupid of me not to realize that this pain was significant. I don't have time to have surgery. Who is going to tend to my fam-ily while I am off? Everything in the world goes through your head. (Participant C, Interview II, BSN instructor)

Later she reflected on her physician visit, her pain assessment, and her feelings of being almost invisible,

Combined with this last phone call, I am going to change GYN's because the more I got to thinking after I got home, you know, he did not offer me so much as a Tylenol! He did not explain to me he was doing a biopsy. I thought well, so much for that big explanation! And when he said oh, you nurses are so brave I thought . . . so you've had one of these done? I didn't appreciate that at all. (Participant C Interview II, BSN instructor)

Participant C continued with more about poor assessment saying,

You know it is kind of like the fifth vital sign and whatever your patient says it is. This really hit home with me. You know, trying to do all the classic things of trying to describe it appropriately. What was so interesting is trying to do all the right things and right ways you wish somebody would describe and he picked up on his one thing he wanted to know . . . who referred me? I said, well the clinic at the college where I work because there is where I presented with pain. So I'm going to describe my symptoms and he asks me what I do there. Oh well, I teach. And I thought, who cares? What difference does it make if I collect garbage there. So, that is how he found out I was a nurse. His main concern seemed after that that he might be giving too much information out to me. (Participant C, Interview II, BSN instructor)

Fear of Disability

All three participants universally experienced fear of disability at various times during the study interviews. Fear of disability is described as a desire to be normal, a need for independence, being betrayed by the body, being dependent, a loss of socialization, disappointing the family, and difficulties with the activities of daily living. Fear revolved around concerns related to adverse effects of medications, future outcome of the disease process over time, possible physical deformity and forced dependency, and inability to assume usual personal and professional responsibilities. A subtheme of *alien* emerged as well, and is discussed in the following section.

Participant A described her first encounters with feeling disabled when she said,

Sometimes I couldn't put my bra on. My husband had to help me. Then it would go away. After I had my last child . . . right before I had her, I got to where I had a knee, they said I pulled a tendon. They were not sure. I went ahead and got a cortisone injection because I was pretty far along. I couldn't walk, couldn't get off the commode, that kind of stuff. I couldn't raise my arms . . . you heard it pop and then one day I couldn't raise it. I thought, oh I pulled it but nothing that would lead you to it because it was on one side. And then it was my knees. I thought I pulled it going up and down the stairs in the auditorium. I didn't know what I'd done. You know, it's like you sit down on the commode, like I talk about in fundamentals class. You don't think about not being able to move and do simple things. I couldn't get off the commode. You had to pull yourself up. I couldn't squat; if I was on the floor wrapping presents, I'd have to roll to get up. Then I got the cortisone injection, I got a little bit better. (Participant A, Interview I ADN instructor)

She further explained,

And I had my baby. She was almost a year and I could not pick her up. It got further in that summer and she knew I couldn't pick her up. She had to pull up because I get tenosynovitis so easy. I had to put my hands under her shoulders and she'd turn on around and I'd pull her onto me . . . I can see patients one day a week and that's all I need to see. And I am getting true feelings that I'm too old to get on the floor because with RA and my back, eight hours into it, I have to sit down a lot more. (Participant A, Interview I, ADN instructor)

The lived experience with chronic pain is like the extraordinary transformation of a caterpillar to a butterfly. There is no conscious decision to become a butterfly, but instead the metamorphosis occurs through the forces of nature. The participants seem to face the challenges of chronic pain on a daily basis and to develop resilience while coping with the grief of their negative feelings brought on by the diminishing physical abilities. In speaking about the future Participant A said,

As far as the future or present, just the same thing, that I can continue to take the medicine. That I won't be able to do anything, I mean that's the fear. I won't be able to move because it's a different pain than acute pain. It just aches all the time. (Participant A, Interview 1, ADN instructor)

Participant B talked about her fear of job loss when she said,

When I am coming up for something I know is going to be very important for me to be able to walk and use my hands, I start getting anxiety about, am I going to have a flare? If I'm clear enough I could do it now, is it going to make it 'til I can accomplish this? Or, am I going to have a flare and then I'm going to have to figure out how I can do this or what I can do about it. So it's caused a lot of anxiety. Even when my hands will get to a point they feel, I'm thinking, oh please can you stay this way until I get this done? Or, you know as closer as it gets, I'm thinking, Oh no, is that going to pop open? So it causes me anxiety during clinical. I know that classroom and I'm okay and can manage in ways I have learned to manage. Parts of clinical I can manage. When my hands are really bad . . . I don't know that I can do it. And . . . that's scary, when you do this for your livelihood and because you love doing it. It's not just something you do but you love to do it. (Participant B, Interview II, ADN instructor)

Difficulties in the activities of daily living are described as she talks about them.

You know, sometimes I've caught myself just crying before I get up because I know how bad it's going to hurt. Can I do my hair today? Can I put on my jewelry today? I can get a shower and that feels good, but can I blow dry my hair with a dryer and use a curling iron? Am I gonna be able to present myself the way I want to today? And then the next step is . . . okay, now it's time to put your feet on the floor and that is very painful. My feet hurt worse in the morning time. My pain level on most those days is about a 7 out of 10. (Participant B, Interview II, ADN instructor)

There are accommodations to hide her condition related to her fear of disability. Adaptation to the accommodations needed become necessary. Developing new life skills such as alternative ways to succeed in a task, setting priorities, saying no, and using laughter to deal with difficulties become essential. There is also a need to deal with lost abilities and to reconcile.

> So, when I was doing clinical, my hands started to crack and bleed inside the gloves. So I would have to put some kind of dressing that could withstand water so I could wash my hands and then I would put on gloves and keep gloves in my pocket. The way the rooms were arranged, I could step outside the curtain, wash my hands, try to get them to stop bleeding, and put a new set of gloves back on. I don't want my students to miss out on something because of me. I want them to get that experience. (Participant B, Interview II, ADN instructor)

The desire to be normal and have independence in the simple things like dressing cause creativity on the part of the pain patient as explained when she said,

> If a callus comes next, it's going to split. And you know, to put my clothes on, I had to change the way I dress because I needed elastic. If I'm having a flare-up, I can't zip or button. So I'm looking at pullovers or elastic or I'm actually putting off going to the bathroom if you have worn something that day you are going to have to deal with. It's like, this is going to hurt but you've got to go to the bathroom. You can't call somebody in the bathroom to zip your pants and button your buttons. (Participant B Interview II, ADN instructor)

Participant C spoke about how the pain prevents her activities of daily living and mobility:

> I was thinking about it lately. It's very frustrating when you realize changes you find you are making in your ADLs to accommodate it. You find that after you have had one of these episodes you are trying to prevent yourself from going somewhere by yourself, in case you have an episode and you are stranded somewhere, and all of a sudden you can't drive because you are just incapacitated. You find that you don't go anywhere without your pain medicine. I mean, literally within arm's reach. Just in case. And there is always that thing of like, what if, what if, just in case I've you know, I don't want to be somewhere where there's nobody to help me, there's nobody, you

know, that I can't reach my pain medicine? And so that's the most frustrating thing for me, is you find that you are changing your activities of daily living to accommodate this. (Participant C Interview I, BSN instructor)

Participant C went on to explain her feelings of loss of control and concerns about disappointing others with any disability due to her illness. There is cognizance of the need for others. Despite the realization of the potential need for dependency, total dependency is resisted due to fear of disability and deformity that might lead to loss of stamina and fortitude or perhaps even her job.

It will be a real hardship on my job if I am to be out an extended period of time . . . um, you know, and there's just a lot of things and people that depend on me. For various things; whether it's your job or it's your parents or your husband or . . . whatever it is. You know? And I'm . . . nobody is indispensable, like the house might burn down while I was out of commission. (Participant C, Interview II, BSN instructor)

She further explained,

I think one of the biggest issues with me and the whole chronic pain thing is, I don't want it to ever be where it affects my job, where there's some doubt with my boss of things like, well, I don't know if she can do that. I don't know if she can handle that. Maybe this is too much for her. Because, I try to pride myself on being that one kind of like, I mean, if they give me something I'll take it I'm fine, I'm good with it, no problem, I can handle it. You don't complain. You don't act like this is too much and you don't want to seem like you are overwhelmed whether you are or whether you aren't. So that was a big thing. And I've actually thought about that, you know, a good bit that I don't want it to be something like this where it affects my job. (Participant C, Interview III, BSN instructor)

Subtheme: "Alien." Two of the three participants spoke about chronic pain and the feeling of a *creature* or *alien* living inside them. The other of the three participants did not describe her illness in the same way; however, she did refer to her hands as *clubs*, which is considered foreign to how one's limbs should feel. Participant A commented, "Now my hands . . . when I wake up in the morning, I can't use my hands a lot because they feel like clubs, and it hurts to bend them, my fingers" (Participant A, Interview II, ADN instructor).

Participant B stated, "I researched and found out that it was true. That there is this creature. And that's what I have been dealing with all the times" (Participant B, Interview I, ADN instructor).

Participant C stated,

> The helplessness, the feeling of, that initial feeling that your body has betrayed you, that thing, where that's your first thought. It's like it's almost somebody else's body. The thing of, what the heck is this that's going on in here? And why is this so difficult to figure out. What kinds of things are you going to have to do to accommodate this? Because it's almost like it's this whole separate little compartment that lives inside of you and you are having to do all this stuff to kind of accommodate this thing that has taken up residence there. It's sort of like having a little alien up in there. It's sort of like you are having to rest more, change the way you eat, and there are all kinds of things. (Participant C, Interview III, BSN instructor)

Coping

The coping theme describes the many feelings of the nurse educators with chronic pain who are placed in a situation of incredible responsibility with performance expectations in the life and work settings. The theme *coping* describes the many thoughts and feelings taken on by the individual dealing with chronic pain and how they deal with the chronic pain. The theme encompasses self-realization of the disease/illness itself, the seeking of understanding of the disease/illness process, the facing of reality, adaptation, accommodation, and reflection about the lived experience.

Participant A describes the difference the medication methotrexate makes in her life when she says,

> It has to get into your system so right now, it's still where I was. When I move and I'm busy, I'm not really conscious of it. But in the morning when I'm getting ready, I am. Plus, it's really numb. I don't even know the word. It's like they are clubs . . . my fingers are and they feel like you can't manipulate your fingers. I have to go back on

something. My doctor just told me it was a good vacation when I had to stop taking it for my wisdom teeth removal. (Participant A, Interview II, ADN instructor)

And she says, "I just want to stay the same way or better. But if I don't, I'll just accommodate for it however I have to . . . and continue to teach . . . the same things I've been doing with the pain and the ADL experiences" (Participant A, Interview III, ADN instructor).

Participant B explained about coping, accommodation, and adaptation when she said,

When we go on family trips, I don't want to be the one that causes the family not to get to do something or they feel bad because they had to leave me behind. So, many times, I will think, Okay, where are we going? Where could I sit and be a part of this but not have to walk as much? Because of the pain in my feet and my husband's had to take on a different role. Which is strange because I see myself as the caregiver and the helper. The one that, you know, makes things work smoothly. And now he's had to come around to thinking, Okay. I'm going to be out of town, what do I need to do for these days? Because he's not coming back and he will see that I haven't been able to do certain things or get things. One of the things that is funny is just drinks. To open the top of drinks. He will come back and I'll still have all the drinks in the refrigerator and he knows how much I enjoy them. He is, "why did you not, you know they're cold. I put them in there" and I'm . . . um, I couldn't open them. That's very frustrating. And you know to put my clothes on, I had to change the way I dressed because I needed elastic. Can't zip or button. (Participant B, Interview II, ADN instructor)

She further explained about additional ways she uses coping mechanisms when she stated,

And if I am going to an Alabama ballgame, I know it's going to hurt. I know once I get to my seat that I will feel some better, but I'm going to hurt. It's something I can tolerate to be with my family because we are big tailgaters. You know, things like that. I have found ways to use lidocaine. Putting it on my feet, I found it helped with my shoes. I have found that I can say, "I'd like to sit here a while. Y'all go on down and you know, I'll catch up with you later. I have just found ways to not feel left out or not try to focus the attention on, "Oh, mother's coming. I don't want that to be, Mother's coming down, now we can't do certain things" . . . because I want them around and to not dread it. (Participant B, Interview II, ADN instructor)

Participant C discussed her faith as a basis for self-reflection and understanding, saying,

I just, you know, literally talking about praying without ceasing, I did. Because I just thought—it was just panic at first, and I thought, "this is terrible." What kind of way is this for a Christian to act, you know? And of course, I'm praying that the Lord would actually heal everything completely. The thing is that he'll give me direction to the right way to go with the treatment when they suggest things. (Participant C, Interview III, BSN instructor)

Participant C reflected that pain is not always a negative thing. The description is one of personal inner strength in adapting to changes and reconciling losses. The self becomes changed or transformed by the lived experience of chronic pain despite any negative physical changes that might occur.

It could very well be in my case that this got me to a doctor before anything more significant could happen, maybe before cancer started or something like that. So, in the case with something like that, pain can be a really good thing if it's like a warning signal to you. In my case, I truly believe it is making me trust God more. It's putting me in a position I have to trust Him. There's nothing else I can do. And another good thing about that, if there's nothing I can do, there's nothing I have to do. So in a lot of ways, it is a freeing thing. It's okay for at least a little while to fall apart. Now, you know, there's a point where you have to get it all together or they'll institutionalize you, you know? (Participant C, Interview III, BSN instructor)

Need for Pedagogical Discourse

Each of the three participants indicated that pedagogical discourse exists in nursing education as identified by meanings of lack of adequate teaching hours, poorly written textbooks, poor chronic pain assessments of patients, and the need for more psychosocial content in nursing curricula. Many of the examples given by the participants related to their personal dealings with chronic pain and their insight into what is missing in the curricula.

Participant A spoke about time to teach about pain when she said,

> There's not adequate time to teach about pain. In the fall, I talk a little bit about it and in the spring when I teach medical-surgical class and GI symptoms. Over the course of three semesters, I guess I teach about 2 weeks total. I want to say 6 hours altogether if you are talking about three semesters. It's connected to everything else because everything has pain as a part of it. We are crammed full anyway. I just pull in a lot of pain scales and a lot of different ways that the student can identify pain. But pretty much, we use what we have in the textbook or the assessment sheet. I think because of what happened to me, I try to tie it into a lot more when we do talk about activities of daily living because I teach fundamentals. We go . . . about the pain and how it affects everything. How you know, they don't realize when you go to the restroom and you can't get up. Do you hurt, you know, how does it affect you? What can you do with your ADLs? I don't think, before I ever did that because it was just a segment in a book that you had to teach. So, I try to expound upon everything that kind of associates with me. Of course, like the GI stuff I teach, we talk about the pain and everything and what causes this. But I try to put it with what's happened to me. So . . . they don't understand it. They don't think about it. I think home health probably did that too. Because I would be in the houses and I would see when they were home . . . things they would have to do for pain with ADLs or how they walk. Does that make sense? (Participant A, Interview II, ADN instructor)

In the third interview, when asked what sense chronic pain makes to her, she said,

> I hope to be doing what I am doing right now and not debilitated. That was my biggest problem I guess, worrying about the future because of what I have leading to debilitation if you don't take the right medicine.

So, I just want to stay the same way or better. But, if I don't, I'll just accommodate for it however I have to and continue to teach the same things I've been doing with the pain and how it affects patients with ADLs and their experiences. I didn't spend a lot of time on chronic pain, even though I had the community health background and I've done tons of home care. Just because I have experienced it, I know how to teach them now, the patients and the students. Now I know what they are going through, as opposed to when I didn't beforehand. (Participant A, Interview III, ADN instructor)

When asked if there is anything she does different now in how she previously taught about pain she said,

Just that I make them do a good pain assessment . . . go in-depth with it, where before, you just kind of passed it off. The joke was that this county's worse with more people on drugs because of the doctors. Initially I thought that there were going to be more people wanting drugs, more people wanting pain medicine and you have to do the assessment. I don't think one gave credence to pain a lot unless it was surgical pain or cancer pain. That was the way I learned in school and it is just the whole mindset of people you work with here. I mean they didn't teach you to think that people were drug seekers. It's just pain was not a big thing you learned about. You did your assessment and you did ask about the pain, you learned your pain scale and I remember that picture (pain scale). You learned all that stuff, but they didn't do an in-depth assessment back then. You learned about surgical pain, cancer and childbirth pain. But, it wasn't what it is now where you do a better pain assessment. You still see nurses not assess it as well as they know they should and know what questions to ask. That's what I try to teach to students. In class and clinical . . . more in clinical I guess because we have patients right there. We talk about it in class because I have to grade their assessments. We put them on the computer and I make them go back and ask if they did not ask. I am trying to make them understand that the patient is a holistic entity, not just "that patient in that room." When the student is done assessing, I assess the patients and see what they were weak in and see that nothing is left out. When you teach patients to take medicine, you have to teach them that it is important to control chronic pain. All the aspects of pain . . . that I didn't do before because it didn't happen to me. So I think, after the fact, just knowing you couldn't go to the bathroom, you know . . . get off the commode . . . really sticks in my mind. You know, cause I did home health for so long and I did a housing assessment when you are in the house. I don't think I realized how important it is than what I gave credence to . . . taking it for granted. We used to talk about fibromyalgia or RA. I was like, God, I don't want fibromyalgia because you can't treat it. Really, you know, we used to kind of make fun of it as to whether it was a true illness or not? I was like, okay, I'm getting paid back for all those people I didn't believe, I guess when they were really hurting and you couldn't find anything wrong with them. So it makes you think, pain is the holistic part for the patient, you know. Pain controls everything . . . you can't learn if you are in pain. I hope that I teach the students how to do a better pain assessment and to realize that part of their role is to do that and not treat it like it's not their role. (Participant A, Interview III, ADN instructor)

When I asked Participant B how she teaches about pain and how often, she replied,

I teach pain in fundamentals in the fall and spring. In the summers, we don't really have a pain module but if we are covering arthritis or any of those issues, then I bring the pain element into it and about how they have to cope with the pain and what medications. As far as that, I bring that in but fall and spring have the larger pain modules that we do. I spend a total of about 45 minutes on pain in general. When we do clinical, of course, with care plans, then we address the client's needs and often times it will be pain or discomfort when they start trying to do their care plans. I do find myself staying longer on chronic pain to try to get an understanding for the students to develop that understanding of their clients and even their family that they may be experiencing. I think it is more getting them to get the concept in their mind that chronic pain is real. It's not everyone out there drug seeking and trying to get attention or loving the sick role. (Participant B, Interview II, ADN instructor)

Participant B also spoke about barriers that exist to teaching.

I think that there are barriers because, I've seen students go into clinical and hear other nurses at report talking about how much medication or pain medication that patient has taken. I know myself, that when I had my first baby, I would not ask for any pain medication in the postpartum area because I knew how they talked about someone that took medication. *"She had every dose she can have and she'll ask you for it before it's due."* So, yeah, I think that's been an issue. You know, the students get that when they go to report. They get a prejudice or a bias opinion about someone they've never seen because we nurses talk about it in report. (Participant B, Interview II, ADN instructor)

With the elderly and need for general compassion she commented,

If they are in the hospital setting, I see more. With the elderly, when we take [students] into the nursing home, I don't see them looking at the clients and going, *"Oh they're not having pain."* But in the hospitals, they will say you know, *"They've already had their pain medicine"* and then let it go. To me that is totally inappropriate. You know they are saying their pain scale is this and you've looked for the signs I have told you because we have learned that pain is subjective and what the patient says it is. Once they have looked and they have already had their pain medication, they dismiss it and think, you know well, they can't be hurting that bad! I think what's missing is realizing that there is more than just medications we can do to help pain. They have pain so let's put a pill in their mouth and then we are through. I think compassion and caring is missing and that is hard to teach someone. What is also missing in my view is that people are going into nursing for a job and financial security and don't really have the characteristics that we see in people who come because they want to help. I try to bring it home and make it personal with them. If we are talking about arthritis, because that's one of the ones we talk about a lot, I'll ask about sharing with their families, if they've had someone with chronic pain issues or arthritis or anything that comes in. What did they see? What did they do? How did they make them feel? I always say, you know, if this were your family member, if this were your mother, or if this were your child experiencing it what would you want done for them. You know would you want someone there that was caring and considerate, checking on them and letting them know somebody is there? (Participant B, Interview III, ADN instructor)

Participant B talked about poorly written textbooks and the need for more psychosocial content in textbooks. There are deficits in the understanding of chronic pain as a disease/illness. Understanding the nature of chronic pain and how chronic pain manifests itself in individuals will give insight into better nursing care.

I take more time talking about how to deal with chronic pain and how to understand what the person is going through, rather than just talk about chronic pain and what we can do. You know the textbook issues with it. I go more into the psychosocial rather than just the physiological and treatment modalities. I tend to stay more in the psychological. I teach those, but spend more time in the psychological and psychosocial. You really don't find that in the textbook a whole lot. Maybe it's a couple of sentences so I add more to it. (Participant B, Interview III, ADN instructor)

Participant C spoke about the amount of time she spends teaching and the psychosocial issues that need to be taught about pain. There is insufficient time to cover chronic pain in-depth with only about an hour devoted to chronic pain in lecture/classroom activities.

I teach about pain as part of health assessment. You know, what does it mean? What does it mean to your patient? Essentially, it's whatever your patient says it is. It is integrated into the curriculum and not a separate topic. I spend maybe about an hour on pain. The one thing I have picked up here lately is all the mental health issues that go along with that. You know? How . . . like I said, just how frustrating, how exhausting it is and the fear of what if it comes back? What am I going to do if it hits during graduation or somewhere that I literally cannot jump up and run out? (Participant C Interview II, BSN instructor)

Participant C was asked if her chronic pain has changed her as a teacher and she replied,

> Oh, absolutely because I want to bring in something about pain and I think you would call it the pain experience because it is not just a, can you rate it on a 1- to 10-scale kind of thing which they had me do. It is an overall complete experience of like, how does your life change with this? Not only is it truly, you know what the patient tells you it is. . . . but you need to ask more so you need to focus on things other than just well, is it sharp? Is it stabbing? It is more than the rate it from 1 to 10 kind of thing. You need to ask questions about how is your life changing as a result of this pain. What kind of things are you having to stop doing or start doing? What are you having to do to accommodate this? It is almost like it is a whole separate little compartment that lives inside of you and you are having to do all this stuff to accommodate this thing that has suddenly taken up residence there. You are having to change, rest more, change what you eat and all kinds of things. (Participant C, Interview III, BSN instructor)

SUMMARY

In this chapter, the researcher introduced the sample findings from the thematic breakdown of the data obtained while exploring the nurse educators' lived experience with chronic pain. The research questions and designated nodes or themes were aligned and used as a guide to make sense and describe the findings represented by the study participants. The researcher shared experiences from the participants' perspective to include emotional responses and findings of impact related to the lived experience of chronic pain in nurse educators.

Through the process of intuiting, the data were pushed to go beyond the words of the participants to a level of abstraction (van Manen, 1990). This level of abstraction, presented in the form of essences, is necessary to make the data meaningful to nursing and other disciplines. Each theme was reviewed for understanding of the impact of the shared experiences. The emergent themes of *vulnerability, physician/provider trust, fear of disability, coping,* and *need for pedagogical discourse,* as well as the two subthemes, *stoic* and *alien,* were examined in relationship to the research questions.

The stories of the nurse educators who have personally experienced chronic pain interviewed for this study demonstrate an inconsistency in the number of hours chronic pain is taught in the curricula as well as the need for better textbook materials dealing with chronic pain assessment and psychosocial issues dealing with chronic pain. The nurse educators in this study were relatively new to personally experiencing chronic pain. None of the nurse educators had more than 2 or 3 years of the lived experience with chronic pain. Through the findings, the researcher was able to better understand the meaning behind the lived experiences of nurse educators with chronic pain and how these lived experiences impact the way chronic pain is taught.

Discussion, Limitations, and Recommendations

The literature reviewed indicates a knowledge deficit in understanding chronic pain by healthcare providers and in nursing education. According to the research participants, a lack of understanding about chronic pain continues to be a concern in both patient care and in nursing education. These areas of concern have led the researcher to understand the significance of this research to further the literature and the implications for nursing education and healthcare practice.

At first, the researcher reviewed the literature and compared the data from the study with the data from the literature review. The researcher continued the exploration by looking at the data from an interpretive phenomenological standpoint, attempting to view what was there, what was not there, and to determine what insight could be gained from the phenomenological perspective. Finally, the researcher began the tedious process of interpretation of findings using the research questions, emergent themes, and essences gleaned from the participants to understand. The interpretation and analysis of the findings were also understood from the researcher's personal history and experience as a nurse educator impacted by the knowledge of chronic pain. The researcher attempted to look for the story under the story to determine meaning behind the experience from the participants. The thematic representations of the participants and the research questions were used to guide and interpret data. This understanding is important because, as previously stated in the literature, we have much to learn from expert patients who have developed habitual skilled bodies in response to chronic illness, and the patient's learning about his or her own illness becomes a source of clinical discovery and inquiry in its own right (Benner & Wrubel, 1989, p. 74).

The purpose of this study was to interpret as closely as possible and explore the meanings of lived experiences of nurse educators who have personally experienced chronic pain, in an attempt to better understand how these educators articulate and shape how they teach about chronic pain. This chapter discusses theoretical implications relevant to the results of the study; conclusions based on the findings; limitations of the study; and recommendations for practice, education, and research. Lived experience research from a phenomenological point of view is to question the way the world is experienced and to want to know the world in which we live as human beings (van Manen, 1990). Van Manen indicated that, "there is one word that most aptly characterizes phenomenology itself . . . thoughtfulness . . . in the words, or perhaps better, in spite of words, we find 'memories' that paradoxically we never thought or felt before" (pp. 12–13).

From the analysis of the study participants' responses, there emerged five major themes: *vulnerability* (mentioned 67 times), *coping* (mentioned 64 times), *physician/provider trust* (mentioned 52 times), *fear of disability* (mentioned 47 times), and *need for pedagogical discourse* (mentioned 34 times). Two subthemes also emerged: *stoic* (mentioned 17 times) and *alien* (mentioned in some form by each participant). The analysis process involved an immersion in the data consisting of multiple readings of the transcript interviews, the selection of significant statements the participants voiced in describing their lived experience, and color-coded grouping of nodes, statements, and essences to define meanings and themes. Nvivo software was utilized to assist in the node groupings. Defined themes and meanings were adjusted continuously until the final meanings and themes that were descriptive of the participants' lived experience with chronic pain emerged. The researcher explored the lived experiences of each participant from a phenomenological viewpoint in an attempt to identify the meaning behind the experiences and interpret for understanding. It is important to recognize that meaning for an individual is how we individualize nursing care. Meaning should be at the core of our nursing care and is what we do and plan with others.

DISCUSSION

The following section reviews the research questions. It is important to note that the perspectives of the participants of this research are their truth as interpreted by the researcher along with the analysis and interpretation of the findings. The key elements of the major themes of this study are aligned with the research questions. The analysis is the lived experience as perceived by the researcher looking in with knowledge and experience with chronic pain, while attempting to understand the meaning behind the experience from the participants. The thematic representations of the participants, along with the research questions, guided the interpretation of the data. Van Manen indicated that, "When a person shares with us a certain experience, then there will always be something there for us to gather" (van Manen, 1990, p. 92).

In phenomenology, "The human being is seen and studied as a 'person' in the full sense of that word, a person who is a flesh and blood sense maker" (van Manen, 1990, p. 14). For the researcher, using van Manen's approach to phenomenology does not stand before practice in order to inform it, but rather theory enlightens practice. He says, "Practice or life always comes first, and theory comes later with reflection" (van Manen, 1990, p. 15).

The interview process used in this study involved three separate interviews lasting approximately one hour, and separated by at least a week. The importance of the interview technique used by the researcher cannot be underestimated. Every attempt was made to honor the participant in the ways listed previously during the interview process, in order to have rich and quality data. According to Benner,

> Interviews are a familiar form of exchange in contemporary life. Several factors contribute to the success of the disclosive interview process. These include the attitude, or philosophical positioning of the interviewer, the interpersonal comfort of the researcher, maintaining a stance of curiosity and openness to unanticipated answers from the participant, and listening with a sensibility for the need to probe further in a specific direction. The researcher must have an appreciation that the interviews comprise access to disclosive spaces, as opposed to opportunities to interrogate participants, lending the researcher to a position of better understanding. (Chan et al., 2010, p. 18)

BROAD RESEARCH QUESTION

In what ways does the lived experience with chronic pain shape how a nurse educator understands and engages with pain assessment?

Participants linked their personal descriptions of the phenomenon of living with chronic pain in their conversations and synthesized with one another in the explanatory accounts of their lived reality. The participants gave definitions of chronic pain using descriptive words of the phenomenon representing their understanding of chronic pain. The descriptive definitions included the phrases "pain that does not go away," "pain that stops your activities of daily living," "unresolved pain that keeps coming back," "pain lasting longer than 6 months," "pain that stops you in your tracks daily," and "pain you can't truly describe to anyone." The participants' definitions line up with the chronic pain definition of the IASP (2006), which defines chronic pain as characterized by continuous pain that persists for at least three months and is unresponsive to available medical treatments. The theoretical understanding of these participants and how this understanding shapes their engagement of teaching about chronic pain is further discussed with each theme identified from the study.

Vulnerability

Each participant described significant vulnerable experiences encountered by healthcare professionals, some outsiders, and family members related to vulnerability such as feeling desperate, feeling embarrassed, feeling ashamed, crying, feelings of inferiority, hopelessness, loss of joy, and disbelief in their own illness. The subjective experience of being weakened mentally and emotionally regarding one's own level of individual and psychological well-being can lead to a kind of vulnerability or demoralization. In an article introducing an evolving theory on women's sense of control by Skuladottir and Halldorsdottir (2008), women who are demoralized because of their pain and disempowering encounters with health professionals and others can manage to regain a sense of control and be remoralized. Yeung, Arewasikporn, and Zautra (2012) presented a two-factor model to classify vulnerability and resilience that differentiate stable and modifiable indicators that influence adaptation to chronic pain. The framework underscores the importance of incorporating social resilience into the development of interventions that aim to promote adaptive and prevent maladaptive functioning in chronic pain patients. The ability to attune to others' emotions, to build social bonds, to improve communication, and to have mutual understanding and trust may promote resilient functioning.

Several common features such as vulnerability, coping, and fear of disability were found in other phenomenological studies of the lived experience. In a study by Yeung et al. (2012), two factors, vulnerability and resilience, were shown to influence adaptation to chronic pain. The ability to expand resilient capacities, such as staying attuned to others' emotions, building of social bonds, and improving communication and trust appeared to encourage or promote resilient functioning. In a study by Kindermans, Roelofs, Goossens, and Huijnen (2011), findings suggest the existence of several activity patterns related to disability and depressive symptomatology in patients with chronic pain. Activity patterns such as avoidance behavior and persistence behavior play an important role in disability outcomes. Patients who exhibit resilient behaviors tend to have better pain adaptation.

Through the words and phrases of the participants, it is evident that their understanding and sense of vulnerability is present as it relates to the chronic pain experience. Participants spoke about the fear of what they know as nurses concerning chronic pain and disease processes. Each one of the participants spoke about the adjustments that are required when dealing with the chronic condition of pain. Despite a lack of validation at times by others, resilience and the willingness to be open to vulnerability are clearly evident as they cultivate wisdom, fortitude, and insight into living with chronic pain. These rich descriptions capture the ambiguity and complexity of the chronic pain as discussed in the early literature (Raheim & Harland, 2006). These meanings give guidance for curricula that otherwise would be left unexplored. The investigation of pain experience lends to knowledge about the world of others with similar experiences.

Each of the participants in this study identified ways they incorporate social resilience to avoid some of the vulnerability they feel. Some of these ways included having a stoic attitude and handling things with prayer; trying to figure out ways to manage the pain, such as topical medication; the importance in staying positive; adapting to travel; and adapting to the activities of daily living such as wearing elastic pants because of the inability to zip or button. The information identified in this study mirrors that by Lindseth and Norberg (2004) who said it is the interpretation integrated into the world that allows knowledge gained to be productive in human life and used to improve care.

Subtheme: Stoic. The individuals in this study worried about the vulnerability of everyday life. Lundman and Jansson (2007) confirmed this in a study about the meaning of living with a long-term disease. The study showed that the main cause of worry in long-term disease was not the disease, but rather its consequences in everyday life. Study findings found that participants talked little about the disease while their narratives were permeated with expressions of worry about daily life, the people close to them, and the future. The hopelessness came from feelings of uncertainty about the future. The study showed a great need for fellowship and belonging to alleviate feelings of hopelessness and isolation. The results revealed a high priority given to values such as working, taking care of oneself, and independence. This is in keeping with the subtheme *stoic*. Each of the participants voiced the importance of doing what they love to do, which is to teach and give their best to the students they instruct. Like many individuals, having this stoic attitude helps with personal security that the chronic pain threatens.

Each of the study participants spoke about the importance of moving on with their chronic pain. This included the need to look for alternative ways to function, learning to deal with it, and not being a quitter. Challenges in pain assessment need to be acknowledged by healthcare professionals, as well as the need for empowerment in order to promote self-protection of the individual. There needs to be a true dialogue where individuals can tell their story in order for meaning to be found. Until these stories are heard, clinics will remain tense places and individuals will remain unheard. Pain is a subjective experience in which healthcare professionals must refrain from basing their assessment, management, and interventions on personal beliefs and judgments. Sensitivity and empathy are critical components of understanding and learning about chronic pain (Al-Shaer et al., 2010).

There is a tradition within nursing that sees stoicism as a virtue. Nurses are ready to put up with any hardship in order to ensure the well-being of patients (Scott, 2001). The nurse educators in this study spoke about the need to remain stoic, making comments such as, "learn to deal with it" or "suck it up (pain) and go on," "I have gotten good at hiding it," and "I have accepted the need to accommodate the pain." Personality features such as optimism are potential resilience resources. Optimism has been associated with lower ratings of pain. This underscores the importance of incorporating social resilience into the development of interventions to promote adaptive behaviors contributing to stoic type behaviors (Yeung et al., 2012).

Physician/Provider Trust

The accuracy of pain assessments has received considerable empirical attention. Across a wide range of conditions and settings, nurses often underestimate pain compared to patient self-report. Many reasons likely exist for these discrepancies, including provider bias and lack of insight into the decision-making processes. In a study by Hirsh, Jensen, and Robinson (2010), biases related to patient sex, race, and age appeared to be prominent in practitioner decision making about pain assessment and treatment. The providers in their study appeared to have minimal awareness of bias as indicated by the lack of correspondence between statistical and self-report data. Nurses can learn from these studies by becoming aware of the need for better insight into patient chronic pain assessment and management.

Despite the lack of validation by others, resilience is evident as individuals grow in wisdom, fortitude, and insight into living with chronic pain. The study participants indicated that healthcare providers do not always seem to have an in-depth understanding of chronic pain. The participants spoke of the need for the nurse to enter into the lifeworld of the patient through dialogue with an exploration of the lived experience. Empathetic listening to the chronic pain patient's concerns, including spirituality, is essential in promoting encouragement and resilience. Initial literature findings also indicate that provider–patient interactions affect clinical assessment of pain. Jimenez et al. (2011) identified that there is a need for distinctive communication patterns in patient encounters such as disease models, word usage, and metaphors, to avoid complicating chronic pain assessment. Pediaditaki, Antigoni, and Theofandis (2010) found that healthcare professionals' personal experiences of pain helped them gain insight into the complex issue of pain. It would be unethical and irrational for healthcare professionals to seek pain in order to improve their pain management skills; yet they can gain knowledge from those who have experienced pain and thereby improve their understanding of everyday clinical pain management and assessment.

All three participants in this study spoke about physician/provider trust issues of concern. One of the participants said she was treated differently for pain compared to her husband. Both of them had visited the same physician only a few days apart for what appeared to be a spider bite. Her husband was given pain medication and she was not, even though her bite was around her waist where her clothes touched the area and her husband's bite was on his chin. Another participant spoke about changing physicians several times because she did not feel she was being listened to concerning her condition. This participant had witnessed a treating physician being kind to other patients who were being seen in her town after hurricane Katrina. This witness to the kindness shown by the provider caused her to change over in order to receive the trust that she was going to get the care she deserved. A third participant felt her condition was not taken seriously and was being brushed aside as minor. This participant changed providers only to be hospitalized a few days later when she was found to have ovarian cancer. Listening and trust issues are found in the literature frequently. In a study by Cocksedge and May (2005), data emphasized the importance of spotting cues during patient interactions. Factors influencing judgments in assessment of patients included pressure of work, the healthcare provider's mood or feelings about the patient, and the context of the interaction. Methods of limiting, blocking, or resisting listening included reassuring, changing the subject, interrupting, or making a plan, reducing sympathy, and using body language. Pain has consequences on patient well-being and functional status, as well as health-related quality of life. Chronic pain is detrimental as it affects physical and psychological well-being in both adults and children. There is increasing recognition that pain as a distinct symptom is often poorly addressed in the setting of chronic illness, even with terminal disease. The reasons for poor pain control and assessment may be multiple, including inadequate control of disease, poor attention to a treatment plan, and barriers on the part of the patient or physician (Fitzcharles, Dacosta, Ware, & Shir, 2009).

All three of the study participants spoke about physician disbelief related to the need to prescribe pain medications and the emotional distress related to not being heard by the physician. The invisibility of pain is possibly the central problem that chronic pain patients face, and it is an aspect that affects the identity of the individual. Newton et al. (2010) explored the phenomenon that chronic pain patients and their experience of being believed is often alluded to in the literature. Key results from their study of a narrative review of the impact of disbelief in chronic pain noted three main themes: stigma, emotional distress, and isolation. There is strong evidence to suggest that the experience of being disbelieved by the healthcare provider is stigmatizing.

In the initial literature review, a study by Shaw and Lee (2010) found that student nurses demonstrated misconceptions about adults with chronic pain to a considerable degree. The specific knowledge deficits were apparent with between 59% and 79.6% believing that psychological impairment, stress, and depression have some causative role in the experience of chronic nonmalignant pain. Further deficits in knowledge were apparent with between 38.2% and 54.8% demonstrating inaccurate understandings about the treatment of pain. This was specifically the existence of tolerance among patients with chronic nonmalignant pain and the risk of addiction to opioids. Slightly more than 34.5% of the participants indicated they believed chronic pain patients were likely to be manipulative, and almost one half (47.9%) of the respondents indicated they believed that patients with chronic pain may exaggerate their pain to gain compensation. The misconceptions represented inaccurate knowledge and inappropriate attitudes that were not addressed, to a substantial degree, during the course of undergraduate education.

Fear of Disability

All three participants spoke about their fear of disability. All three participants said that the inability to perform the activities of daily living (ADLs) was a major concern. They expressed the need for independence. Fear of loss of the ability to function socially and fear of disappointing the family were anxiety-provoking factors. All three participants talked about the inability to function due to pain and implications for job loss. Fear of relapse during periods of remission was another concern. They spoke about the elevation of fear when a sudden onset or exacerbation with their chronic pain occurs, such as not being able to open a can or bottle top, dress oneself, walk in shoes due to friction, or being caught without pain medication. The participants suffer in silence regarding their inabilities and hold to secrecy for the most part. A study by Kindermans et al. (2011) provided support for the existence of several important activity patterns in participants with chronic pain. Results showed that pain avoidance, activity avoidance, excessive persistence, and pacing were all related to higher levels of disability. Increased understanding of the lived experience and activity patterns might help to improve tailored care for patients with chronic pain.

Pain-related fear leads to avoidance behaviors such that individuals defer activities they perceive as threatening (Perry & Francis, 2011). Evidence supporting the effects of significant symptom experience of people living with disability, especially for symptoms of pain and fatigue, was explored, in a study by Patterson, Doucett, Lindgren, and Chrischilles (2012). Symptom experience is found to partially mediate the effects of disability on self-reported general health status and physical functioning.

This suggests that symptoms serve as an important link to health outcomes in persons with disability. Further understanding of symptom experience may identify useful approaches to improving quality of life, associated costs, and the processes associated with being disabled.

The participants in this study experienced difficulty with symptom relief with the most difficult periods at the beginning of their diagnostic process. One participant could not get three out of four physicians to prescribe something for her pain. She suffers from severe psoriatic psoriasis with bleeding and cracking lesions of the hands and feet. Her job requires that she instruct students to draw up medication in a syringe using tactile hand movements and to wash her hands frequently. The participant found ways to do her job. She carried gloves and bandages in her lab coat pocket in order to cover her painful and bleeding fingers. This attempt to compensate for the results of her disease process offered her hope to continue to do her job duties. The healthcare provider had not given her options, so she developed her own methods for coping. Finding ways to compensate and improve symptoms offers hope to situations leading to fear of disability. Open communication and provider trust are necessary to deter the feelings of permanent disability or loss in cases where individuals suffer emotionally out of fear.

Subtheme: Alien (feeling as though something foreign has become housed in the body or that something has taken up residence). The chronic pain discussion of the three participants took on a personification role. Participant A stated that her arms and hands feel like clubs. Participant B referred to her pain as an organism or creature. Participant C said,

> It's like a separate compartment with an alien living inside you. It is almost like it's somebody else's body. The thing is, what the heck is this that's going on in here? And, why is this so difficult to figure out? It is the helplessness, the feeling that your body has betrayed you.

As we consider how we might communicate human experiences of pain, one of the most salient characteristics of our species is our embodiedness. Human beings are creatures of flesh. Primarily our experiences and how we make sense of what we experience is dependent upon the kinds of bodies we have and on the ways in which we interact with the environment we inhabit (Vakoch, 2011). Reflecting on the words of the participants leads to the belief that the terms *alien* and *creature* are the internal human reasoning of the participants speaking out to say, "I want you out or I am going to have to accept you!"

Coping

The meaning of coping expressed by the participants seems to be linked to self-realization, adaptation, understanding, reflection, and accommodation. Coping manifested with the participants in many ways, such as adaptation to the activities of daily living, understanding not to let pain get out of control, toleration of pain at times, understanding the importance of a positive attitude, finding ways to deal with the pain, acknowledging the pain, acceptance of the pain, and understanding that pain is a warning signal. Retaining a sense of control in chronic pain challenges the learning to live with pain and the ability to cope with the unpredictability and incurability of the pain. There is a challenge to find meaning in the suffering, create personal space, be self-protective, and keep a positive self-image and self-esteem while trying to live a normal life (Skuldottir & Halldorsdottir, 2008).

The statements made by the participants match a study by Park and Sonty (2010), who examined the role of positive versus negative emotion in the relationship between control and coping efficacy and pain-related interference in social activity in a sample of chronic pain patients. After controlling for level of education, income, and average pain intensity, positive emotion, but not negative emotion, was found to partially mediate the relationship between control and coping efficacy and pain-related interference in social activities. This suggests that positive emotions may play an important part in predicting the relationship between control and coping efficacy and social functioning in chronic pain patients.

Each of the participants in this study had a tremendous desire to continue to work and not become disabled. Each indicated that they saw themselves in the future teaching nursing. They represent examples of adapting to a new form of existence, living with chronic pain. Holding on to participation on important arenas seems to be an essential part of successful coping strategies and a caring attitude toward one's body (Raheim & Haland, 2006).

In a study by Fisher, Emerson, and colleagues (2007), chronic pain was found to elicit innovative adaptive responses to coping by making interesting temporal, lifestyle, and cognitive adaptations. Frequently used temporal changes included allocating more time to undertake a task or shortening the time devoted to a task. The participants in this study frequently attempted to alter schedules to lessen the pain debilitation time. One would ask her husband to open the soft drink caps before he left town so she could easily access them while he was gone, because her arthritic condition prevents her from being able to open soft drink cans and bottle caps. Another participant talked about coping by praying on a daily basis. She stated that her pain has actually caused her to trust her faith more.

Need for Pedagogical Discourse

In this study, nurse educators shared stories about their lived experiences with chronic pain and described how they teach about pain in the classroom and clinical setting. One educator recalled a time earlier in her career when she first learned about a chronic pain condition called fibromyalgia. She stated, "I didn't think as much about pain before. Now I realize the importance. I'm getting paid back for all those people I didn't believe" (Participant I, Interview III). She talked about how the utilization of additional pain assessment techniques and pain scales are now a part of her lesson plans. She also goes behind the student in clinical practice to do an assessment on the student's assigned patient in order to grade the student on how well the pain assessment was completed. She emphasized the importance of not letting chronic pain or any type pain get out of control. A frequent quote she used was, "It's not just that patient in that room" (Participant A, Interview III). Shaw and Lee (2010), studying misconceptions about chronic pain held by student nurses across 3 years of undergraduate education, found that student nurses hold misconceptions about adults with chronic pain. The study demonstrated inaccurate understandings in relation to the treatment of pain, specifically the existence of tolerance among patients with chronic nonmalignant pain and the risk of addiction to opioids. This represents inaccurate knowledge and inappropriate attitudes not addressed, to a substantial degree, during the course of undergraduate education. Chronicity and disability need to be obvious in the curriculum.

Another participant spoke about her desire to be thorough when teaching about pain assessment and management. She teaches students to understand that a pain patient may be more sensitive or frustrated, may feel inadequate, or even be angry. She frames these additions to her lectures based on her own actions and experience with chronic pain. She feels it is important to teach reassurance on behalf of the patient and to incorporate that the patient is not a burden. Validation of the pain is essential. Speaking about the family role in pain is important for the students to understand. She uses discussion frequently in her classroom and integrates more psychosocial content. She is quick to point out that there is a deficit in the psychosocial issues in nursing curricula. She believes that the psychosocial aspect is only touched on in the textbooks, leaving the necessity to teach this up to the nursing instructor. In a nursing curriculum study by Kantar and Alexander (2012), subordination of judgment skills was revealed with preceptors' responses helping to identify deficiencies in the skills. The multiple-case study was designed to better understand the influence of nursing curriculum on clinical judgment development in baccalaureate nursing students and the capacity to provide safe nursing practice in healthcare settings. Healthcare providers are responsible for assessing and treating pain based on a patient's verbal and nonverbal communication. Inconsistencies exist in the nursing process, based largely on such variables as a nurse's educational preparation, specialty area, and personal experience caring for others. These various factors may influence nurses' responses to and beliefs about pain (Al-Shaer et al., 2011; Briggs, 2010).

One of the participants stated, "I feel like I know every patient I have ever had now." She went on to say that teaching the pain scales is not enough. Additional teaching focus needs to be on things describing pain such as, "Is it sharp, is it stabbing, etc.?" We need more of "What have you had to stop or start doing?" "Do you have to accommodate this?" "Are you resting more?" (Participant III, Interview III). She believed pain is a warning signal and tried to bring these areas into her lecture and classroom experiences. The results of a study by Dysvik et al. (2011) shed light on important aspects of living with chronic pain. By listening to a patient narrative, the total situation can be investigated, which might aid nurses in the quest to reduce pain and strengthen those areas that can lead to a meaningful life. The extent to which living a meaningful life is possible depends on many factors, including a person's belief system and attitudes, early life experiences, illness, personal resources, the meaning of pain, and extent to which nurses understand the overall situation.

NARROW RESEARCH SUBQUESTION 1

How do nurse educators who have lived experience with chronic pain theorize or understand chronic pain?

The nurse educators interviewed in this study shared their personal knowledge about living with chronic pain. Personal knowledge is a powerful reminder that the life being lived is the life of the recipient of nursing care. Nurse educators who have personally experienced chronic pain are in the position to justify their actions and support an individual's agency when it comes to better understanding how pain is theorized. Personal knowledge is the theorized knowledge of the individual as a self with a personal biography who occupies a certain social space and acts according to his or her own desires and intentions for reasons that make sense to him or her (Dyck, 2002). This knowledge links to the patient as a person. Because this knowledge is linked to nursing work, insight is given to practicing nurses enabling them to think more theoretically about their work and to articulate it in the world.

Benner (1984) was the guiding theorist for this research study. Benner postulated that studying the person in the situation is required in nursing practice because nurses coach patients through their illness, injury, or birthing, or when facing death. An objectified, detached view of practice covers over the patient and nurse as well as the relational caring practices that allow the nurse to coach, accompany, bear witness, and empower patients and families. The nurse educators in this study allowed for insight into the connection between the body with chronic pain and its connection in biomedical discourse related to the lived experience. Discussions based on in-depth interviews about their daily lives emphasize the powerful influence of dominant social norms in the medical world and the social world. From these conversations, nurse educators need to theorize carefully about how the medical environment plays a major role in producing or magnifying unnecessary vulnerability, lack of provider trust, fear of disability, need for coping strategies, and the need for pedagogical changes. How these educators engaged with the environment and their provider encounters was mediated through both their diagnosis and with their activities of daily living. In many instances, through the lack of embodying insight on the part of providers and others, their care was lacking and their chronic pain assessment and management suffered. Benner explained that articulation research describes, illustrates, and gives language to "taken-for-granted areas of practical wisdom, skilled know-how, and notions of good practice" (Benner, Hooper-Kyriakidis, & Hooper, 1999, p. 5).

The participants of this study indicated that persons with pain have the right to optimal pain management and should be able to expect that healthcare providers will adequately assess, inform, and implement good pain care. Frustration was expressed by all of the participants and was related to chronic pain treatment and the disease itself. Specific issues included appointment response times, not receiving pain medications, ineffective results from physician visits, incorrect diagnoses, and believing they actually had a chronic pain diagnosis.

Feelings of self-consciousness were conveyed by all three participants with respect to physical body changes, attempts to hide their illness, and fear of being viewed as a drug seeker or lazy. Resultant of being physically ill or undiagnosed, all of the participants experienced sadness. Comments such as, "I knew I was going to have to learn to live with it," and "I need to learn to adapt to the pain," reflected the emotional intensity felt by the individuals.

The participants spoke about what they perceived to be the needed role of a healthcare provider or nurse who is caring for the patient with chronic pain. They expressed the desire for the healthcare provider or nurse to encourage the patient to talk about their pain, demonstrate compassion, listen as though they are truly interested in their problem, and offer possible choices in treatment plans. The participants expressed a lack of involvement by healthcare providers during the assessment phase of their chronic pain. The participants remarked, "There is a lack of personalization to the experience," "It's an uncaring attitude of the provider," and "There is a lack of communication." The nurses in this study theorized chronic pain by seeing the lived experience of chronic pain as complex and life changing. Living with chronic pain means understanding days of depression, anger, frustration, fear, and self-consciousness. It is, at times, an emotional roller coaster. There is need to retain a sense of control and not give up in spite of the pain. The inability to maintain a sense of control of self and pain and to avoid demoralization is a common chronic pain issue. Chronic pain patients are challenged to find meaning in their suffering, to create personal space, and to be self-protective while keeping a positive self-image to live a normal life. Health professionals are viewed as potentially powerful people in the lives of chronic pain patients. Empowerment and disempowerment from health professionals greatly influence whether the chronic pain is or is not demoralized (Skuladottir & Halldorsdottir, 2008).

The nurses in this study spoke about the importance of successful adaptation to chronic pain. Resilience plays an important role in adaptation to chronic pain and can be heard in the voices of the women interviewed. It is vital to acknowledge that an individual can be resilient in some ways and not in others. For example, one can learn from a challenging experience without fully recovering from it. Important purposes in life may be lost while, at the same time, new plans and goals are shaped by the learning and growth that has resulted from successful adaptation. Success in one area may often facilitate resilience in the other two (Yeung et al., 2012). The nurse educators in this study spoke about the importance of support systems to help with their chronic pain issues. Comments like, "I don't know what I would do if I did not have my husband to help me dress some mornings, especially when I am having a flare-up," "I have a fear of being 'needy' to others," "I debate to tell, or not to tell about my chronic pain in social situations," and "Sometimes I feel my family doesn't understand" are examples of the importance for resilient responses to stressful events like living with chronic pain. Life difficulties and struggles help to fuel an individual to develop resilience while learning to cope with grief, negative feelings, anger, fear, and depression. The ability to cultivate an inner strength to adapt to changes is necessary to find meaning and rise above personal suffering. There is evidence from a study by Park and Sonty (2010) that maintaining a satisfactory quality of life while living with a chronic pain condition could depend on mediators that result in decreasing the effects of stress (thus leading to an improved quality of life) or an increase of its effects (thus leading to a deterioration in the quality of life). A positive emotion appears to protect against increases in negative emotion during times of increased pain or stress, facilitating coping. The protective function of positive emotions is only beginning to be understood. The evidence thus far indicates a need to consider such resources as important clinical tools, strategies, and avenues for future research.

NARROW RESEARCH SUBQUESTION 2

How can the lived experience relate to how pain is taught by these individuals? What are the prescribed methods of teaching chronic pain assessment, and how does it fit into the nursing curriculum?

The diagnosis of acute pain and interventions are often simple, but this is not usually the case with chronic pain, as the processes of investigation, diagnosis, and management are often complex and lengthy. The American Association of Colleges of Nursing (AACN) is the national voice for baccalaureate and graduate nursing education. AACN's educational, research, federal advocacy, data collection, publications, and special programs work to establish quality standards for nursing education; assist deans and directors to implement those standards; influence the nursing profession to improve health care; and promote public support for professional nursing education, research, and practice curriculum. Using a national consensus-based process, AACN has led the development of a series of essentials documents that outline competency expectations for graduates of baccalaureate, master's, and doctor of nursing practice (DNP) programs. Using these documents, schools of nursing are able to ensure they adhere to the highest standards for their educational programs and meet accreditation guidelines. AACN also has published quality indicators for research-focused doctoral programs, a white paper on the clinical nurse leader, and guidelines defining the essential clinical resources for nursing education, research, and faculty practice (AACN, 2008). The essentials documents regarding baccalaureate nursing education do not specifically address pain assessment but are broad to include the ability to identify, assess, and evaluate patient care.

The National League for Nursing Accrediting Commission (NLNAC) supports the interests of nursing education, nursing practice, and the public by the functions of accreditation. Accreditation is voluntary and is a self-regulatory process by which nongovernmental associations recognize educational institutions or programs that are found to meet or exceed standards and criteria for educational quality. Accreditation assists in improving the institutions or programs as related to resources invested, processes followed, and results achieved. The NLNAC monitors certificate, diploma, and degree nursing programs and is tied closely to state examination and licensing rules and to the oversight of preparation for work in the profession. The mission of the nursing education unit reflects the core values and is congruent with its missions/goals. The organization has the administrative capacity resulting in effective delivery of the nursing program and achievement of identified program outcomes (NLNAC, 2013a).

Accreditation is important to nursing curriculum for strengthening educational quality and fostering educational equity, access, opportunity, mobility, and preparation for employment (NLNAC, 2013b). Although chronic pain is not specifically addressed in the accreditation curriculum guidelines for NLNAC or AACN, curriculum that includes educational courses to enhance professional nursing knowledge and practice as well as evidence-based clinical practice are core to the criteria needed to meet the program outcomes.

Each of the participants stated that they do teach about pain differently since experiencing chronic pain personally. The impact on their understanding has allowed them to reflect on how they want to be treated regarding their pain and what they need to add to their teaching plans. It is important to help the student to know that not every patient is a drug seeker and that most are simply trying to find an answer or find someone who will listen. Bias during clinical reporting time at change of shift is a problem. Nurses have been witnessed making judgmental remarks about patients seeking pain medications or patients appearing to hyperinflate their pain symptoms. The importance of teaching students about these types of judgments in the clinical setting is important in order to help them avoid negative mentoring.

The participants acknowledged that it is important to make the material personal in their lectures about chronic pain. When assessing pain it is important to ask things like, "What can you not do with the pain, and what can you do with the pain?" "Do you rest more, and are you eating?" Assessment is more than just a pain scale. Each participant stressed the importance of caring and compassion. It is debatable in their opinion about whether you can teach caring and compassion, but it is important to look for ways to assess that the student is caring and compassionate. It is also important to add the psychosocial aspects of pain assessment and pain management to curriculum content. These findings are consistent with a study by Shaw and Lee (2010) where qualified practicing nurses and students were found to hold misconceptions about adults with chronic nonmalignant pain. This represented inaccurate knowledge and inappropriate attitudes that are not addressed, to a substantial degree, during the course of undergraduate nursing education. Chronicity and disability need to be in the curriculum. Through listening to chronic pain patient narratives, situations can be investigated to aid the nurse in the quest to reduce pain and strengthen those areas that can lead to a meaningful life (Dysvik et al., 2011).

Participants indicated that their lived experience with chronic pain has affected how they teach about pain in diverse ways. Since their personal experience with chronic pain, each participant said they take more lecture time in class on the topic of chronic pain and on the topic of pain in general. Pain is integrated into the curriculum at all three of the schools represented in this study. Each of the participants expressed the need for more time to teach the subject of pain because they spend only about an hour each time it is taught. Each participant indicated that pain is covered over the course of three or more semesters ranging from fundamentals class to the gastrointestinal, hematology, and cardiac modules. There is some variance as to which modules are covering pain; however, the periods and subject matter appear to be similar. Scheduling does not allow for longer than the allotted time. This is because of the amount of material nurse educators are expected to cover prior to routine exams in preparation for students to be ready for the National Council Licensure Exam (NCLEX) upon graduation.

Understanding the prescribed methods of teaching nurses about chronic pain assessment is important for the future care of patients. Goodrich (2006) studied students' and faculty members' knowledge and attitudes regarding pain management. The majority of the faculty in her study perceived themselves as competent in pain management and believed their current practice to be maintained through reading professional journals and attending continuing education programs. Faculty appeared to have basic knowledge to build pain management skills into curriculum, yet integration of pain content is inconsistent.

Each of the three participants indicated that pedagogical discourse exists in nursing education as identified by lack of adequate teaching hours, poorly written textbooks, poor chronic pain assessments of patients, and the need for more psychosocial content in nursing curricula. Many of the examples given by the participants related to their personal dealings with chronic pain and their insight into what is missing in the curricula.

Chronic pain is a complex, dynamic disorder, impacting the individual in a multitude of ways. The purpose of this study was to better understand the ways in which the lived experience with chronic pain shapes how a nurse educator understands and engages in pain assessment. Through this study, the researcher also looked at how pain is theorized by the lived experience, how pain is taught, and the prescribed methods of teaching as well as how chronic pain fits into the curriculum. Through a living relationship with oneself, others, and the world, human beings assign meaning to experiences. In this living relationship, things such as self and others matter. When experiencing an illness or something like chronic pain, the habitual living in a homelike world is disrupted. During the illness or pain, the *I* becomes forced to confront the fact that this *I* is in the world as a lived body. So, if understanding life, meaning, and concerns fails, this renders into experiences of being desituated (learning ways outside the real world experience; Benner & Wrubel, 1989). Through the lived experience, we are led to think about the need to teach in a different way.

The participants talked about the importance of teaching students to collect accurate and complete information when doing a pain history. It is necessary to teach the importance of observing, recording the location of pain, the duration, the frequency, the degree of pain, and the characteristics that will help in making the correct choice of effective management of pain. The importance of observation in pain assessment is made clear by The Joint Commission, which defined pain assessment as part of the vital signs measurement (Joint Commission, 2011). Findings in a study by Pediaditaki et al. (2010) suggested that healthcare providers become more sensitive to patient pain after their own experience of pain. Statements such as, "I now think I know every pain patient I have ever had better," "Now I know fibromyalgia is real," and "I didn't think much about pain before my situation" confirm that pain can be the teacher who will help us to see the human being in a different light with concern, interest, and compassion for care.

The educators in this study pointed out that taking time to assess, looking the patient in the eye, having a caring tone in the voice, showing interest, being cognizant of body language, and being thorough in patient encounters are all things that should be included in teaching student nurses about chronic pain assessment and management. The educators also pointed out that it is important that the teacher assess the student's ability to carry out an assessment that includes these important components. The educator cannot properly assess the student for learning unless the educator can verify in some way that the student has reached the objectives for good pain assessment and management. The teaching objectives are assessed by these nurse educators through observing the patient assessment encounters by the students, going over a student's computerized pain assessment to check for completeness with feedback to the student on the day of clinical practice, and telling personal stories about the life lived with chronic pain. The participants also use classroom activities such as vignettes that stress the psychosocial aspects of chronic pain, classroom discussion about factors related to the activities of daily living, and the role of stress on chronic pain. The lived experience of chronic pain has provided the nurse educators in this study with valuable insight about how to approach teaching chronic pain in the classroom. The knowledge provided by their life experience of chronic pain serves as an important heuristic tool that can help healthcare professionals decipher what they see and hear, and to make well-informed decisions about what is most likely most appropriate or the best approach to helping the chronic pain patient. This knowledge can contribute considerably to the adequacy of ethical decisions attuned to a specific situation and to nursing curriculum change (de Casterle et al., 2011).

The educator's dilemma is how to include an ever-growing body of essential knowledge in the curriculum that is already full and in a manner that is pedagogically sound. Both the associate degree and baccalaureate nurse educators in this study said chronic pain is taught using an integrated model of curricula where pain is discussed throughout the semesters and included in several different modules of study. For example, pain is included in the fundamental, medical-surgical, and obstetrical nursing modules. The extent to which pain is covered depends upon several types of curriculum. These are the *operational curriculum* (includes knowledge, skills and attitudes emphasized by faculty in the classroom and clinical setting), the *illegitimate curriculum* (that which is actively taught by the teacher and how its importance is communicated to the student such as caring, compassion, and power), the *hidden curriculum* (consists of values and beliefs taught through verbal and nonverbal communication by the faculty who may not be aware of their expressions, priorities, and interactions with students), and the *null curriculum* (the curriculum that is not being taught, such as content or skills the faculty think are not critical to the design; Billings & Halstead, 2009). Each of the participants estimated that pain in general (including acute and chronic pain) is covered in about 10 hours or less total in the ADN and BSN nursing curricula. This is interesting, because the length of ADN and BSN programs differ in semester hours of preparation for graduation. To test the hypothesis that educational deficits are in part responsible for the low priority given to pain management by nurses, a study was conducted to ascertain the pain content in the common foundation program in four branches of nursing courses in England. Results indicate that while child and adult programs cover a wide breadth of topics, pain is covered in 10 hours or less. These results indicate superficial coverage of the pain topic. When the amount of time spent teaching pain is considered (on average less than 10 hours), it becomes apparent that the teaching may not be in any depth (Pediaditaki et al., 2010; Twycross, 2000, 2002). Further study is needed regarding the number of hours spent teaching about chronic pain in schools of nursing. Curriculum development is led by, and reflective of, the mission and philosophy of the institution and guided by the community and stakeholders.

Preparing new graduates to assess and manage pain and to be advocates for their patients with pain requires action so that these graduates can be mentors to others. Modeling this mentoring relationship puts emphasis on the importance of nurse faculty being adequately prepared to teach pain management across the curricula (Duke et al., 2010). Healthcare professionals have to keep in mind that chronicity of pain represents constant aggravation for the pain patient. Nurse educators and healthcare providers can help patients navigate through the difficulties of dealing with the persistent and invisible nature of chronic pain by understanding, validating, and teaching students about the lived experience of chronic pain. Treatment must take into account the context of each individual, emphasizing support, empowerment, and acknowledgement of the individuals' own resources (Skuladottir & Halldorsdottir, 2008).

IMPLICATIONS FOR NURSING

As evidenced by the thematic review from this study, there are implications for better instruction, nurse educator training, and nursing curriculum change regarding how chronic pain is taught. Nurse educators and teachers are eternal learners. Almost every day we learn something new about ourselves, about our students, and about our teaching. The unyielding commitment to help students reach their full potential leads us to question how we teach. Teaching is an embedded part of the teacher's identity. It is important to explore new ways to teach familiar and unfamiliar content. Sharing personal stories with students can be a powerful way to connect the student to the subject matter. Educators are works in progress, continuously evolving, seeking, and transforming. Nurse educators must consider how experiences influence the selection of content and pedagogy in the classroom (Cone, 2007).

In a study by Pediaditaki et al. (2010) designed to gain insight into the way the personal experience of pain affects the attitude of healthcare professionals toward pain management, participants recognized the insufficient knowledge of staff regarding pain management. They assessed that the personal experience of pain is a chance for self-criticism. They also noticed that after a personal experience of pain, there is an increased sensitivity to the problem of pain with more awareness of the patient's needs. Furthermore, they proposed educational interventions to focus on a holistic approach and to improve communication skills. Pain is experienced by all people through time and has no boundaries. Schools of nursing and other healthcare educational establishments should enrich their curriculum with pain education, using those who have had personal experience of pain to illustrate the importance of empathetic pain management. It would be advantageous to invite ex-patients who had substantial experiences of pain to illustrate where gaps in the system need improving.

Nurse educators in this study were asked about their thoughts, feelings, and knowledge related to chronic pain. Through this study, the researcher added to the body of knowledge about the lived experience of chronic pain and implications for how pain is taught in nursing schools. The research on the lived experience of nurse educators with chronic pain filled a gap in the literature regarding how pain is assessed and taught by individuals who have actually had chronic pain. This research is important for nursing education, because in order for the problem of poor chronic pain assessment to be remedied and for better nursing instruction to occur, chronic pain assessment must first be realized, studied, and brought forward for change. The resultant information is significant because it comes from first-person accounts of nurse educators who have personally had chronic pain. These nurse educators have insight that is evidenced by life itself giving meaning and understanding for education.

The researcher concluded that nurse educators believe chronic pain is underassessed, misunderstood, and poorly addressed by medical practitioners and nursing students. This presents a negative impact in patient care. The findings from this study support the need to challenge educational epistemologies that suggest there is a consistently corresponding relationship between pain scales, objective pain assessment, and preconceived judgments regarding chronic pain assessment and management. Deconstructing this way of thinking is important by using interpretive pedagogies, which change our preconceived notions. Subject matter presented in the classroom needs to focus on understanding the problem, which may not resemble the clinical situation in which nurses function. Instruction should be based on context and experience. Nurse educators who use only content-based instruction tend to underpin the gap between theory and practice (Kantar & Alexander, 2012).

Preparing new graduates to manage pain and to be advocates for their patients experiencing pain requires action through mentoring so that these graduates can be mentors to others. Modeling this mentoring relationship means emphasizing the importance of nursing faculty being adequately prepared to teach pain management across the curricula. Persons with pain have the right to optimal pain management and expect healthcare providers to adequately assess, inform, implement, and evaluate treatments for pain. Given the psychologic, spiritual, and physical costs of unrelieved pain, nurse educators have an ethical obligation to improve current practice through addressing curricular pain content, policy initiatives, and research (Duke et al., 2010).

According to the American Association of Colleges of Nursing (2008), learning opportunities for baccalaureate and associate degree nurses, including direct clinical experiences, must be sufficient in breadth and depth to ensure the nurse graduate attains practice-focused outcomes and integrates the delineated knowledge and skills into the graduate's professional nursing practice. The knowledge provided by qualitative studies can serve as an important heuristic tool to help nurse educators and healthcare professionals to decipher what they see and hear, and to make well-informed decisions about the most appropriate approach to nursing care. This knowledge can contribute considerably to ethical decisions regarding chronic pain assessment and management (de Casterle et al., 2011).

This study shows that the personal experience of chronic pain can enable nurse educators a better way to comprehend the complexity of chronic pain leading to improved holistic approaches to improvement in pain assessment and management. There is a need to ensure that nurses have the knowledge and skills to assess and manage pain effectively. Regular updates about chronic pain and changes in practice are necessary for nurse educators to use in teaching students. Teaching strategies that support adult learning and various other learning styles need to be incorporated in the classroom and clinical experiences of student nurses. There is a need for further research related to classroom teaching methods, learning retention, and transference to the clinical setting.

LIMITATIONS OF THE STUDY

The study participants were all Caucasian females from a middle-class perspective. Studying a broader range of ethnicities would be helpful, and it would be helpful to include male participants in the sample. The study represented two participants from a rural background and only one from a metropolitan area. It is noted that all three participants had been diagnosed with chronic pain for less than 3 years during the interview time frame. It would be interesting to know if the number of years each participant has suffered with the chronic pain would alter the results such as their willingness to talk about their pain more in front of students.

RECOMMENDATIONS FOR FUTURE RESEARCH

The discovery challenge of the lived experience of nurse educators with chronic pain answered many questions, just as it fostered additional questions. Further research that will focus on gender differences in chronic pain assessment and the lived experience is needed. Additional studies regarding provider gender in the assessment of pain might be helpful in eliminating gender bias on the part of the provider and the participant. Additional studies to see if age differences might skew the data would be beneficial. Research should be conducted on ways to implement the findings of the lived experience of nurse educators with chronic pain into the nursing curricula. The study's findings may assist with the development of other studies on the structure of nursing curriculum. This could assist in curricula that teach better chronic pain assessment and management, establishment of a curriculum framework, and the creation of strategies or tools for the classroom. The research revealed a deeper understanding; however, limitations were present and questions remain for further study.

References

Al-Shaer, D., Hill, P. D., & Anderson, M. A. (2011). Nurses' knowledge and attitudes regarding pain assessment and intervention. *Medsurg Nursing, 20*(1), 7–11.

Altmann, T. K. (2007). An evaluation of the seminal work of Patricia Benner: Theory or philosophy? *Contemporary Nurse, 25,* 114–123.

American Academy of Pain Medicine. (2011). *AAPM facts and figures on pain.* Retrieved from http://www.painmed.org/patientcenter/facts _on_pain.aspx

American Association of Colleges of Nursing. (2008). *The essentials of baccalaureate education for professional nursing practice.* Retrieved from http://www.aacn.nche.edu/education-resources/baccessentials08.pdf

Anderson, K. O., Green, C. R., & Payne, R. (2009). Racial and ethnic disparities in pain: Causes and consequences of unequal care. *Journal of Pain, 10,* 1187–1204.

Ashley, J. L. (2008). Pain management: Nurses in jeopardy. *Oncology Nursing Forum, 35*(5), E70–E75.

Benner, P. (1984). From novice to expert. *American Journal of Nursing, 82*(3), 402–407.

Benner, P. (1985a). The oncology clinical nurse specialist: An expert coach. *Oncology Nurse Forum, 12*(2), 40–44.

Benner, P. (1985b). Quality of life a phenomenological perspective on explanation, prediction, and understanding in nursing. *Advances in Nursing Science, 8*(8), 1–14.

Benner, P. (1994). *Interpretive phenomenology: Embodiment, caring and ethics in health and illness.* Thousand Oaks, CA: Sage Publications.

Benner, P. (2000). The wisdom of our practice. *The American Journal of Nursing, 100*(10), 99–105.

Benner, P., Hooper-Kyriakidis, P., & Stannard, D. (1999). *Clinical wisdom and interventions in critical care: A thinking in-action approach.* Philadelphia, PA: Saunders.

Benner, P., Tanner, C., & Chesla, C. (2009). Entering the field. In *Expertise in nursing practice: Caring, clinical judgment, and ethics,* 29–60. New York, NY: Springer Publishing.

Benner, P., & Wrubel, J. (1989). *The primacy of caring: Stress and coping in health and illness.* Reading, MA: Addison-Wesley.

Bergh, I., & Sjostrom, B. (2007). Quantification of the pain terms, hurt, ache, and pain among nursing students. *Scandinavian Journal of Caring Science, 21,* 163–168.

Billings, D. M., & Halstead, J. A. (2009). Curriculum development: An overview. In N. Dillard & L. Siktberg (Eds.), *Teaching in nursing: A guide for faculty* (pp. 79–80). St. Louis, MS: Saunders.

Briggs, C. L. (2010). What were they thinking? Nursing students' thought processes underlying pain management decisions. *Nursing Education Perspectives, 31*(2), 84–88.

Chan, G., Brykczynski, K., Malone, R., & Benner, P. (2010). The living tradition of interpretive phenomenology. In C. Hall, T. Artman, & C. Savor (Eds.), *Interpretive phenomenology in healthcare research* (pp. 113–137). Indianapolis, IN: Sigma Theta Tau International.

Chang, I., Toner, B. B., Fukudo, S., Guthrie, E., Locke, G. R., Norton, N. J., & Sperber, A. D. (2006). Gender, age, society, culture, and the patient's perspective in functional gastrointestinal disorders. *Gastroenterology, 130*(5), 1435–1446.

Clark, E. B., French, B., Bilodeau, M. L., & Capasso, M. L. (1996). Pain management knowledge, attitudes, and clinical practice: The impact of nurses' characteristics and education. *Journal of Pain and Symptom Management, 11*(1), 18–31.

Cocksedge, S., & May, C. (2005). The listening loop: A model of choice about cues within primary care consultations. *Medical Education, 39*, 999–1005.

Cone, T. C. (2007). In the moment: Honoring the teaching and learning lived experience. *Journal of Physical Education, Recreation & Dance, 78*(4), 35–54.

Creswell, J. (2007). *Qualitative inquiry & research design: Choosing among five approaches.* Thousand Oaks, CA: Sage.

Creswell, J. (2009). *Research design: Qualitative, quantitative, and mixed methods approaches.* Thousand Oaks, CA: Sage.

De Casterle, B., Verhaeghe, S., Kars, M., Coolbrandt, A., Stevens, M., Stubbe, M., & Grypdonck, M. (2011). Researching lived experience in healthcare: Significance for care ethics. *Nursing Ethics, 18*(2), 232–242.

Delmar, C. (2006). The phenomenology of life phenomena in a nursing context. *Nursing Philosophy, 7*, 235–246.

Dowling, M. (2007). From Husserl to van Manen: A review of different phenomenological approaches. *International Journal of Nursing Studies, 44*, 131–142.

Duke, G., Haas, B., Yarbrough, S., & Northam, S. (2010). Pain management knowledge and attitudes of baccalaureate nursing students and faculty. *Pain Management Nursing, 14*(1), 1–9.

Dyck, I. (2002). Beyond the clinic: Restructuring the environment in chronic illness experience. *The Occupational Therapy Journal of Research, 22*, 52S–60S.

Dysvik, E., Sommerseth, R., & Jacobensen, F. (2011). Living a meaningful life with chronic pain from a nursing perspective: Narrative approach to a case story. *International Journal of Nursing Practice, 17*, 36–42.

Ezenwa, M. O., Ameringer, S., Ward, S. E., & Serlin, R. C. (2006). Racial and ethnic disparities in pain management in the United States. *Journal of Nursing Scholarship, 38,* 225–233.

Ferrell, B. R., McCaffery, M., & Rhiner, M. (1992). Pain and addiction: An urgent need for change in nursing education. *Journal of Pain and Symptom Management, 7,* 117–124.

Finlay, L. (2009). Exploring lived experience: Principles and practice of phenomenological research. *International Journal of Therapy and Rehabilitation, 16*(9), 474–482.

Fisher, G. S., Emerson, L., Firpo, C., Ptak, J., Wonn, J., & Bartolacci, G. (2007). Chronic pain and occupation: An exploration of the lived experience. *American Journal of Occupational Therapy, 61,* 290–301.

Fisher, T. L., Burnet, D. L., Huang, E. S., Chin, M. H., & Cagney, K. A. (2007). Cultural leverage: Interventions using culture to narrow racial disparities in healthcare. *Medical Care Residency, 64,* 243S–282S.

Fitzcharles, M., DaCosta, D., Ware, M., & Shir, Y. (2009). Patient barriers to pain management may contribute to poor pain control in rheumatoid arthritis. *The Journal of Pain, 10*(3), 300–305.

Fontana, J. S. (2008). The social and political forces affecting prescribing practices for chronic pain. *Journal of Professional Nursing, 24*(1), 30–35.

Goodrich, C. (2006). Students' and faculty members' knowledge and attitudes regarding pain management: A descriptive survey. *Journal of Nursing Education, 45*(3), 140–142.

Guba, E., & Lincoln, Y. (1983). Epistemological and methodological bases of naturalistic enquiry. In G. Madaus, M. Scriven, & D. Stufflebeam (Eds.), *Evaluation models* (pp. 311–339). Boston, MA: Kluwer Nishoff.

Hall-Lord, M. L., & Larsson, B. W. (2006). Registered nurses' and student nurses' assessment of pain and distress related to specific patient and nurse characteristics. *Nurse Education Today, 26,* 377–387.

Harper, P., Ersser, S., & Gobbi, M. (2007). How military nurses rationalize their postoperative pain assessment decisions. *Journal of Advanced Nursing, 59*(6), 601–611.

Heideggar, M. (1962). *Being and time.* (J. MacQuarrie & E. Robinson, Trans.). New York, NY: Harper & Row (Original work published 1927).

Hirsh, A., Jensen, M., & Robinson, M. (2010). Evaluation of nurses' self-insight into their pain assessment and treatment decisions. *The Journal of Pain, 11*(5), 454–461.

Holloway, I., Sofaer-Bennett, B., & Walker, J. (2007). Stigmatization of people with chronic back pain. *Disability and Rehabilitation, 29*(18), 1456–1464.

Izumi, S. (2006). Bridging western ethics and Japanese local ethics by listening to nurses' concerns. *Nursing Ethics, 13*(3), 275–283.

Jimenez, N., Garroutte, E., Kundu, A., & Morales, L. (2011). A review of the experience, epidemiology, and management of pain among American Indian, Alaska Native, and aboriginal Canadian peoples. *American Pain Society, 12*(5), 511–522.

Joint Commission, The. (2011). *Facts about pain management.* Retrieved from http://www.jointcommission.org/pain_management/

Jordan, A. L., Eccleston, C., & Osborn, M. (2007). Being a parent of the adolescent with complex chronic pain: An interpretative phenomenological analysis. *European Journal of Pain, 11*(1), 49–56.

Kantar, L., & Alexander, R. (2012). Integration of clinical judgment in the nursing curriculum: Challenges and perspectives. *Journal of Nursing Education, 52*(8), 444–453.

Keyte, D., & Richardson, C. (2011). Re-thinking pain educational strategies: Pain a new model using e-learning and PBL. *Nurse Education Today, 31,* 117–121.

Kindermans, H., Roelofs, J., Goossens, M., & Huijnen, I. (2011). Activity patterns in chronic pain: Underlying dimensions and associations with disability and depressed mood. *The Journal of Pain, 12*(10), 1049–1058.

Kirk, T. W. (2007). Managing pain, managing ethics. *Pain Management Nursing, 8*(1), 25–34.

Kleinman, A. (1992). Pain and resistance: The delegitimation and relegitimation of local worlds. In M. D. Good, P. E. Brodwin, B. J. Good, & A. Kleinman (Eds.), *Pain as human experience: An anthropological perspective* (pp. 347–347). Los Angeles: University of California.

Krebs, E. E., Carey, T. S., & Weinberger, M. (2007). Accuracy of the pain numeric rating scale as a screening test in primary care. *Journal of General Internal Medicine, 22*(10), 1453–1458.

Kuhn, T. S. (1996). *The structure of scientific revolutions.* Chicago, IL: University of Chicago Press.

Lewis, C. S. (1940). *The problem with pain.* London, England: Harper Collins.

Lindseth, A., & Norberg, A. (2004). A phenomenological hermeneutical method for researching lived experience. *Scandinavian Journal of Caring Science, 18*, 145–153.

Linkewich, B., Patrica-Habjan, S., Poling, M., Bailey, S., Kortes-Miller, K. (2007). Educating for tomorrow: Enhancing nurses' pain management knowledge. *The Canadian Nurse, 103*(4), 24–28.

Lippe, P. M., Brock, C., David, J., Crossno, R., & Gitlow, S. (2010). Special article: The first national pain medicine summit final summary report. *Pain Medicine, 11*, 1447–1468.

Lundman, B., & Jansson, L. (2007). The meaning of living with a long-term disease: To revalue and be revalued. *Journal of Clinical Nursing, 16*(7b), 109–115.

MacLaren, J. E., & Cohen, L. L. (2005). Teaching behavioral pain management to healthcare professionals: A systematic review of research in training programs. *The Journal of Pain, 6*(9), 481–492.

Mapp, T. (2008). Understanding phenomenology: The lived experience. *British Journal of Midwifery, 16*(5), 308–311.

McCaffery, M. (1968). *Nursing practice theories related to cognition, bodily pain, and man–environment interactions.* Los Angeles: UCLA Students Store.

McCaffery, M. (1972). *Nursing management of the patient with pain.* Philadelphia, PA: JB Lippincott.

McCaffery, M., Grimm, M. A., Pasero, C., Ferrell, B., & Unman, G. C. (2005). On the meaning of "drug seeking." *Pain Management Nursing, 6*(4), 122–136.

Meleis, A. I. (2006). *Theoretical nursing: Development and progress* (4th ed.). Philadelphia, PA: Lippincott, Williams & Wilkins.

Melzack, R. (1986). Neurophysiological foundations of pain. In R. Sternback (Ed.), *The psychology of pain* (pp. 1–24). New York, NY: Raven Press.

Melzack, R., & Wall, P. (1965). Pain mechanisms: A new theory. *Science, 150*, 971–976.

Michaels, T. K., Hubbart, E., Carroll, S. A., & Hudson-Barr, D. (2007). Evaluating an educational approach to improve pain assessment in hospitalized patients. *Journal of Nursing Care Quality, 22*(3), 260–265.

Munhall, P. L. (2007a). Historical and philosophical foundations of qualitative research. In *Nursing research: A qualitative perspective* (pp. 99–126). Sudbury, MA: Jones and Bartlett.

Munhall, P. (2007b). Meanings in mothers' experience with infant death. In *Nursing research: A qualitative perspective* (pp. 211–238). Sudbury, MA: Jones and Bartlett.

National Institute of Neurological Disorders and Stroke (NINDS). (2011). NINDS Chronic Pain information page. Retrieved from http://www. ninds.nih.gov/disorders/chronic_pain/chronic_pain.htm

National League for Nursing Accreditation Commission (NLNAC). (2013a). *Standards and criteria for associate degree nursing.* Retrieved from http://www.nlnac.org/Manual%20&%20IG/2003_manual_TOC. htm

National League for Nursing Accreditation Commission (NLNAC). (2013b). *Standards and criteria for baccalaureate degree nursing.* Retrieved from http://www.nlnac.org/Manual%20&%20IG/2003_ manual_TOC.htm

Newton, B. J., Southall, J. L., Raphael, J. H., Ashford, R. L., & LeMarchand, K. (2010). A narrative review of the impact of disbelief in chronic pain. *Pain Management Nursing, 14*(3), 1–11.

Overgaard, S. (2010). Intersubjectivity: The problem of other minds. In S. Gallagher & D. Schmicking (Eds.), *Handbook of phenomenology and cognitive science* (pp. 230–261). New York, NY: Springer.

Park, S., & Sonty, N. (2010). Positive affect mediates the relationship between pain-related coping efficacy and interference in social functioning. *The Journal of Pain, 11*(12), 1267–1273.

Patterson, B., Doucette, W., Lindgren, S., & Chrischilles, E. (2012). Living with disability: Patterns of health problems and symptom mediation of health consequences. *Disability and Health Journal, 5,* 151–158.

Pediaditaki, O., Antigoni, F., & Theofandis, D. (2010). Research on the influence of healthcare professionals' personal experience of pain on the management of pain. *International Journal of Caring Sciences, 3*(1), 29–39.

Perry, E., & Francis, J. (2011). Self-efficacy, pain-related fear, and disability in a heterogeneous pain sample. *Pain Management Nursing.* Manuscript submitted for publication.

Pesut, B., & McDonald, H. (2007). Connecting philosophy and practice: Implications of two philosophic approaches to pain for nurses' expert clinical decision making. *Nursing Philosophy, 8*, 256–263.

Plaisance, L., & Logan, C. (2006). Nursing students' knowledge and attitudes regarding pain. *Pain Management Nursing, 7*(4), 167–175.

Polit, D. F., & Beck, C. T. (2008). Analyzing qualitative data. In H. Surrena & H. Kogut (Eds.), *Nursing research: Generating and assessing evidence for nursing practice.* Philadelphia, PA: Lippincott Williams & Wilkins.

Raheim, M., & Haland, W. (2006). Lived experience of chronic pain and fibromyalgia: Women's stories from daily life. *Qualitative Health Research, 16*(6), 741–761.

Rudestam, K. E., & Newton, R. R. (2007). The method chapter: Describing your research plan. In *Surviving your dissertation* (pp. 87–115). Thousand Oaks, CA: Sage Publications.

Samuels, J. G., & Leveille, D. M. (2010). Senior nursing students' clinical judgments in pain management. *Nurse Educator, 35*(5), 220–224.

Seidman, I. E. (1991). In *Interviewing as qualitative research: A guide for researchers in education and the social sciences* (pp. 1–19). New York, NY: Teachers College Press.

Shaw, S., & Lee, A. (2010). Student nurses' misconceptions of adults with chronic nonmalignant pain. *Pain Management Nursing, 11*(1), 2–14.

Sherman, D. W., Matzo, M. L., Paice, J. A., McLaughlin, M., & Virani, R. (2004). Learning pain assessment and management: A goal of the end-of-life nursing education consortium. *The Journal of Continuing Education in Nursing, 35*(3), 107–120.

Skuladottir, H., & Halldorsdottir, S. (2008). Women in chronic pain: Sense of control and encounters with health professionals. *Qualitative Health Research, 18*, 891–901.

Twycross, A. (2000). Education about pain: A neglected area? *Nurse Education Today, 20*(3), 244–253.

Twycross, A. (2002). Educating nurses about pain management: The way forward. *Journal of Clinical Nursing, 11*, 705–714.

Vakoch, D. A. (2011). What does it mean to be human? Reflections on the portrayal of pain in interstellar messages. *Asta Astronautica, 68*, 445–450.

van Manen, M. (1990). *Researching lived experience: Human science for an action sensitive pedagogy.* Albany State University of New York Press.

van Manen, M. (2003). Lived experience. In M. Lewis-Beck, A. Bryman, & T. F. Liano (Eds.), *Encyclopedia of social science research methods* (Vol. 2, pp. 579–580). Thousand Oaks, CA: Sage.

van Manen, M. (2007). Phenomenology of practice. *Phenomenology & Practice, 1*, 11–30.

Wong-Baker FACES Foundation. (2009). *FACES history*. Retrieved from http://www.wongbakerfaces.org/resources/faces-history

Yeung, E., Arewasikporn, A., & Zautra, A. (2012). Resilience and chronic pain. *Journal of Social and Clinical Psychology, 31*, 593–617.

Yu, H., & Petrini, M. A. (2007). A survey of Chinese nurses' current knowledge of pain in older people. *Journal of Clinical Nursing, 16*, 963–970.

Zalon, M. L. (1995). Pain management instruction in nursing curricula. *Journal of Nursing Education, 34*(6), 262–267.

Glossary

a priori codes Codes that were developed previously and did not require the researcher to develop them as part of the research project.

abstract Brief summary of the process of implementing a research study.

analysis of variance (ANOVA) Analysis that tests whether group means are different, but also considers the variation that will be present among all of the groups.

attrition Loss of research subjects that occurs during the course of the research study.

autonomy Ethical principle related to informed consent. This provides a person with the right to make an informed decision about whether to participate in a research study.

basic theme The lowest order theme that can be derived from text. It is a simple idea that is characteristic of the data.

beneficence Ethical principle that guides healthcare providers to act in the best interest of the research participant. It is the principle of beneficence that provides the participant with protection from harm.

bias Any influence that is capable of distorting the results of a research study.

bivariate analysis The examination of characteristics of more than one variable.

blinding A situation that occurs when neither the research subject nor the person assessing the outcome of the treatment is aware of the group to which the client belongs.

bracketing Setting aside the researcher's knowledge of the experience being investigated and approaching the data without preconceived ideas about the phenomenon being studied.

case control study Type of observational, nonexperimental research design.

central tendency An estimation of the center point of a distribution of values.

chain sampling A technique in which informants are asked to identify other informants who would be useful to the researcher and are representative of the community being studied.

champion In qualitative research, someone who is interested in the research and will either assist in recruiting participants or allow the researcher to use his or her credibility in the community to recruit.

cluster random sampling A type of sampling that is utilized when clusters or groups of potential participants, rather than individual subjects, are randomly selected.

cluster sampling A technique frequently used in nationwide research projects, because it randomly assigns research subjects to groups within a much larger population, and then research subjects within the assigned groups are surveyed.

codebook A book that contains all of the assigned category names in a master list.

coding A process in which the segments of data are marked with category names to further identify them during the data analysis process.

cohort A group of subjects who are followed over a period of time.

cohort study A study in which the researcher studies, over time, a specific group of individuals who typically experience the same significant event within a specific period of time.

compatibility thesis The idea that the quantitative and qualitative research methods can be compatible and can be used together in a research study.

complementarity A situation in which the researcher is striving to enhance, illustrate, or clarify the results that are achieved through use of results from both quantitative and qualitative designs.

conceptual framework Framework that creates a structure that guides the research project.

conclusions A section of a research article that should allow the researcher to evaluate and interpret the implications of the results presented in the previous section.

concurrent timing Timing method in which the researcher implements both quantitative and qualitative methods during a single phase of the research study.

confidence interval The extent to which the sample statistic deviates from the population parameter; for example, 95 percent confidence that the population mean is between 2.0 and 3.0.

confidentiality Protection of information so that researchers will not disclose records that identify individuals.

constant comparative method A study method in which data will be analyzed concurrently throughout the process of data collection as the researcher searches for a core variable that will be the foundation for formulation of the grounded theory.

content validity A situation that occurs when the instrument and its items are representative of the content that the researcher intends to measure.

context The subject's worldview that influences how his or her life is lived and interpreted and allows the subject to assign meaning to his or her life events, thoughts, experiences, and relationships.

contextual design A design in which the researcher samples cases within specific groups to accurately describe characteristics of the groups' contexts.

control group Research participants in an experiment who do not receive the treatment or intervention; it will be compared to the experimental group whose participants do receive the intervention.

convenience sampling   Type of sampling that is utilized when the researcher selects people who are most easily located or who are most available for participation in the research study.

core variable   The foundation for formulation of the grounded theory. The core variable that is sought by the researcher typically recurs on a frequent basis, links various data, has strong implications for development of formal theory, develops a great deal of detail, and includes people from various backgrounds.

criterion-related validity   The type of validity that requires the comparison of the measure in question with the best existing measure of the variable.

cross-sectional design   A type of study that gathers information about a target population at a specific point in time and essentially produces a snapshot of the respondents. *See also* cross-sectional study.

cross-sectional study   A study based on observations obtained at a single point in time. *See also* cross-sectional design.

data comparison   The comparison of data from both qualitative and quantitative sources.

data consolidation   Combination of quantitative and qualitative data, resulting in the creation of new sets of data.

data correlation   The element of data analysis that involves the correlation of quantitative and qualitative data for clarity.

data display   The element of data analysis that describes quantitative and qualitative data pictorially. This can be done using charts, graphs, and tables.

data integration   The element of data analysis that allows both quantitative and qualitative data to be integrated into a cohesive data set or to become two separate but equally important parts of an entire data set.

data reduction   **1.** A situation that occurs as information relevant to the topic is filtered and information not relevant to the topic is discarded. **2.** The element of data analysis that reduces the dimensions of qualitative and quantitative data. This can be accomplished through memoing, for example, for qualitative data, and descriptive statistics such as averages and percentages for quantitative data.

data saturation   A situation that occurs when data are collected until no additional new information can be located.

data transformation   The element of data analysis that allows quantitative data to be converted into narrative data that can be analyzed qualitatively and qualitative data to be expressed quantitatively using numerical coding and then statistics.

deductive reasoning   Thought process in which reasoning moves from the general to the specific, using a theory to produce a hypothesis.

dependent variable   The variable of interest in a hypothesis; the variable that is influenced by the independent variable (University of Maryland Medical Center, n.d.).

descriptive phenomenology   A form of phenomenological research design that proposes there are aspects to any participant's lived experiences that are common to anyone who has that experience.

descriptive statistics   A type of statistics used to provide summaries about the sample that was used and the measures that were used to describe that sample; they describe what the data that have been collected show.

descriptive study   Study that describes a specific population of research subjects (LoBiondo-Wood & Haber, 2002).

directional hypothesis   Statement that specifies the predicted direction of the relationship between the independent and dependent variables.

discussion   A section of a research article in which the findings are traced back in a logical manner to the research question or hypothesis that was investigated. The section should allow the researcher to evaluate and interpret the implications of the results presented in the previous section.

dispersion   The spread of the values around the central tendency.

disproportional stratified sampling   A sampling method that occurs when the researcher is not concerned with ensuring that the subsamples selected are in proportion to their sizes in the population.

distribution   A summary of how often values appear for a variable.

emic perspective   Research primarily concerned with how members of a culture being studied perceive their own world.

ethnography   Research primarily concerned with the need to learn about a culture from the people who actually are immersed in it every day.

etic perspective   Research concerned with the way that nonmembers perceive and interpret the behaviors of members of the culture.

exempt   Research involving human subjects that falls into a category that is not deemed necessary for review by an institutional review board.

expedited review   A review in which, usually, only one member of the IRB will review the project to ensure protection of human subjects; shortens the length of the review process.

experimental group   Research participants in an experiment who receive the treatment or intervention; it will be compared to the control group whose participants do not receive the intervention.

experimental study   A study in which research subjects are randomly selected to be in the experimental group and receive a new intervention or to be in the control group and receive either a standard intervention or no intervention at all.

exploratory study   Type of research design that explores a phenomenon in order to provide additional insight for the researcher.

external validity   The generalizability of results obtained to other populations.

fieldwork journal   Notes that can assist the researcher with the technique of participant observation, because it will record the capacity in which the researcher was present at the observation and the role he or she assumed.

frequency distribution   A summary of data developed when values are grouped into ranges, and then the frequencies are determined.

gatekeepers   The authority figures who control the researcher's access to the research participants.

global theme   A group of organizing themes that together present a position about an issue.

grand theory   Most abstract level of theory that establishes a knowledge base for nursing.

history   Type of threat to the internal validity of a research design; occurs when a specific event either inside or outside the experimental setting has an effect on the dependent variable.

homogeneity   The degree to which the individuals in a population resemble one another in regards to the characteristics being studied in a research project.

hypothesis   Statement of the proposed relationship between the dependent variable (variable of interest) and the independent variable (variable influencing the dependent variable).

independent variable   The variable in a hypothesis that influences the dependent variable (University of Maryland, n.d.).

inductive codes   Codes developed by the researcher as the data are examined during a research project.

inductive reasoning   Thought process in which reasoning moves from specific to general; used when the researcher collects data to address a research question or hypothesis.

inferential statistics   A type of statistics that allows the researcher to draw conclusions that reach far beyond a cursory examination of the data. It is typically used either to estimate the probability that statistics found in the sample are an accurate reflection of a parameter in the population or to test hypotheses that have been developed about a population.

informed consent   A situation that ultimately implies that the potential participant's ratio of risks to benefits has been clearly identified.

institutional review board (IRB)   **1.** An entity established within an agency to review research involving human subjects to ensure participants are treated within ethical guidelines. **2.** A group that reviews all research that involves human subjects either conducted at a facility or sponsored by that facility.

instrumentation   Threat to internal validity that occurs when there are changes in the way variables are measured or in the techniques used for observation that will cause changes in the measurements that are obtained.

intercoder reliability   A situation in which coding of the data is occurring consistently among a group of coders.

interim analysis   Data analysis that will be ongoing throughout the project until either the researcher exhausts the time and resources allotted to the project or a complete understanding of the topic being researched is achieved.

internal validity   The ability to infer that the independent variable in a research project is truly related to the dependent variable. A threat to internal validity means there are competing explanations for the results obtained in a research project.

interpretive phenomenology   A research design that proposes that the researcher cannot eliminate preconceptions about a phenomenon, and, in fact, it is those experiences that are used to interpret the experiences of other people.

interrater reliability   The type of reliability in which multiple readings of a measurement are assessed from several people for evidence of similarity.

interrupted time series with a nonequivalent no-treatment comparison group   A two-group pretest–posttest design using an untreated control group, but with the addition of multiple pretests and posttests.

interrupted time series with multiple replications   Interrupted time series that has the treatment intervention and removal of the treatment occurring multiple times according to a schedule. The design is strengthened when the researcher times these interventions and removals randomly.

interrupted time series with switching replications   Research design that uses two groups, each serving as either the treatment or comparison group on an alternating basis. This is accomplished through multiple applications of the treatment intervention and removal of the treatment.

interval   The level of variable that ranks objects or events on a scale with equal intervals between the numbers on the scale.

interview guide   A tool used as part of a life history research design; it should move in chronological order, including contexts that are particularly important to the participants, and it should include both open-ended questions and follow-up questions.

intracoder reliability   A situation in which each coder is coding the data consistently.

intrarater reliability   The type of reliability in which multiple readings of a measurement are assessed from the same person for evidence of similarity.

introduction   A section of a research article that should include the author's research question or hypothesis, which clearly states the population being studied, the intervention being proposed, the comparison that will occur, and the expected outcome (O'Sullivan & Rassel, 1999).

justice Ethical principle governing recruitment of research subjects. It mandates that research participants be selected from multiple groups rather than only from a pool of those most likely to be coerced, such as subjects with severe physical or mental illness or those who are economically disadvantaged.

key contacts In qualitative research, people who can suggest possible groups or participants who might take part in the study.

life history grid A tool that allows the researcher to organize the participant's life events, correlate events in the life history, and summarize the written record.

literature review An account of what has been published on a topic by researchers (Wooten & Ross, 2005).

longitudinal design A type of design that requires the researcher to ask the same questions of respondents at two or more points in time. *See also* longitudinal study.

longitudinal study A study designed to collect data at more than one point in time. *See also* longitudinal design.

maturation A threat to internal validity of a research design; refers to the natural developmental changes such as the aging process that would occur to research subjects over the course of time and are unrelated to the research project being conducted.

mean The average of a group of values.

median The score that is exactly in the middle of a group of values.

memoing Note taking in which a researcher records notes throughout each field day, giving his or her impression of what is occurring.

methods A section in a research article that should contain the author's description of exactly what was done in the research as well as how it was implemented (Lobiondo-Wood & Haber, 2002).

microrange theory Synonymous with *hypothesis*; considered to be concrete concepts that are linked so as to form a statement that can be examined in practice and research.

midrange theory Theory that incorporates nursing practice and research into ideas that are integral to nursing.

mixed method research A research method that occurs when both a qualitative phase and a quantitative phase are included in the same research study. *See also* mixed model research.

mixed model research A research method that is used when quantitative and qualitative approaches are mixed either within the research process or across the various stages of the process. *See also* mixed method research.

mode The score that occurs most frequently in a set of values.

mortality A threat to internal validity by way of the loss of study subjects from the time of administration of the pretest to the time of administration of the posttest. If the subjects who remain in the study are vastly different from the subjects who opt to remove themselves from the project, the results obtained will most likely be affected.

negative-case sampling A method of data interpretation in which the researcher attempts to locate and scrutinize cases that do not confirm his or her expectations and the tentative explanations that have been proposed.

nominal A level of variable that is used to classify objects or events into categories. The numbers that are assigned to the categories are only labels and do not indicate more or less of a quantity.

nondirectional hypothesis Statement that indicates the existence of a relationship between variables but does not specify the predicted direction.

nonrandomized clinical trial A type of study that is used when randomization is not feasible or ethical or when there is insufficient evidence to justify the difficulty and expense of a randomized clinical trial.

null hypothesis Statement that proposes that there is no relationship between the dependent and independent variables in a research study.

observational study A type of nonexperimental research design.

one-stage cluster sampling Type of sampling in which the researcher initially selects a random sample of the clusters or groups; the researcher then includes in the final sample all the individual names included in the chosen clusters.

operationalization   The process of defining how variables will be measured.

ordinal   A level of variable that ranks objects or events so that an object in a higher category can be considered to have more of a specific attribute than an object in a lower category.

organizing theme   A class of theme that organizes the basic theme into clusters of similar ideas.

panel study   A study in which the researcher opts to study how specific individuals are changing over time; the respondents will be surveyed repeatedly.

patterns   Recurring speech groupings that are noted as part of narrative analysis.

pilot test   A small survey that serves as a pretest to a major survey.

population   The full set of people from whom the sample is being drawn.

positivism   A school of thought that maintains there is an objective reality in the world that can be quantified in some way so that observation or measurement can occur.

pragmatism   The belief that a researcher should use any approach or combination of approaches that will function the best in a real-world situation, regardless of assumptions of paradigms or philosophies.

pretest–posttest design   A study in which the researcher looks at the outcome of interest before the application of an intervention and then after an intervention.

primary source   Source material that was written by the person who either developed a theory or conducted the research being reported (Polit & Hungler, 2000).

privacy   A person's ability to control other people's access to information about him- or herself.

proportional stratified sampling   A sampling method that occurs when the researcher makes certain that the subsamples that are selected are in proportion to their sizes in the population.

protected health information   Information about an individual's health status, the provision of health care, or payment for health care that can be linked to the person.

purposive sampling   A sampling method that occurs when the researcher specifies the characteristics of the population of interest and then locates individuals who match those characteristics.

quota sampling   A variation on convenience sampling; it involves setting quotas and then using convenience sampling to select participants to fill the quotas.

randomized controlled trial   The strongest design to provide healthcare professionals with information regarding the benefits of a specific healthcare intervention.

ratio   The level of variable that ranks objects or events on a scale with equal intervals between the numbers on the scale and the presence of an absolute zero.

reflexivity   A type of sampling in which the researcher uses self-awareness and critical self-reflection to better understand his or her personal biases and the way these may affect the research process and conclusions.

reliability   A characteristic that allows an instrument to be consistent and give the same results if the research is replicated.

representative sample   A sample that is similar to the population from which it was drawn in all areas except that it contains fewer people than the population.

research hypothesis   Statement regarding the expected relationship between the dependent and independent variables. Synonymous with *scientific hypothesis.*

research problem   Issue that will be investigated by the researcher and will generate either a research question or a hypothesis (LoBiondo-Wood & Haber, 2002).

research question   Most frequently used in an exploratory or descriptive research study; a research question rooted in an evidence-based practice problem identifies the patient group or patient condition, provides an issue or intervention that is being investigated, specifies a way for a baseline measurement to be made as well as a method for comparison, and indicates an outcome or result.

results   A section in a research article that presents the author's findings (LoBiondo-Wood & Haber, 2002).

sampling error   The possibility that the sample selected is not completely representative of its population of origin. Usually occurs because of an error in the sampling process.

sampling frame   A list of all of the potential participants who make up the population.

sampling interval   The population size divided by the desired sample size.

scientific hypothesis   *See* research hypothesis.

secondary source   Source material that was written by someone other than the person who developed the theory or conducted the research (Polit & Hungler, 2000).

segmenting   A process in which data are carefully reviewed and then broken into analytical units.

selection   Choosing of research subjects for a project results from the way in which research subjects were chosen for the project, particularly if precautions were not utilized to achieve a representative sample.

selection bias   A type of threat to internal validity resulting from the way in which research subjects were chosen for the project, particularly if precautions were not utilized to achieve a representative sample.

sequential timing   A timing method in which the researcher implements qualitative and quantitative methods in two distinct phases, using one type of data before using the other type of data.

simple interrupted time series design   A one-group pretest–posttest design that uses multiple pretests and posttests.

simple random sampling   The most basic type of random sampling; it allows everyone in the group from which the sample is being drawn to have an equal chance of being selected for the final sample.

snowball sampling   A sampling method in which each subject being used in the research study is asked to identify other potential research subjects who have the characteristics being studied. This technique is particularly effective with a population that is difficult to find and therefore has no sampling frame. *See also* snowballing.

snowballing   A sampling method in which the sample actually develops as the survey progresses, because as one person completes the survey, he or she is asked to recommend other potential research subjects who can be asked to participate. *See also* snowball sampling.

social network design   A study design that is used if the researcher is interested in gaining information on the relationships among individuals and organizations and the processes that link them.

Solomon four-group design   A type of study in which the researcher uses two groups that receive the intervention and two groups that do not. Only one treatment group will be administered a pretest, but all four groups will receive the posttest.

statistical hypothesis   *See* null hypothesis.

stratified random sampling   **1.** A sampling method in which a specific group is selected from the larger population and a random sample is then chosen from that specific group. For example, this would be used when the DNP researcher decides to survey nursing students at a college as the greater population, and then selects to random sample only the sophomore class from the larger population. **2.** The type of sampling that occurs when the researcher initially selects a stratification variable that is used to classify the sampling frame, such as gender or race.

systematic sampling   A sampling method in which subjects to be included in the sample are selected at specific intervals within the population—for example, every seventh person.

t-test for differences between groups   A test that is performed when the researcher is interested in comparing the performance of two groups on one measure to determine if a difference exists.

testing   A threat to the internal validity of a research design used in a research project; refers to the effect taking a pretest has on the subject's posttest score. The result of the differences between posttest and pretest scores may not be an outcome of the application of an intervention but may instead be the result of the experience gained through the testing process.

thematic networks analysis   A type of analysis that involves extracting basic and global themes from text and then representing those themes as web-type maps with the relationships between them illustrated.

themes   Sets of patterns.

theoretical framework   A structure that will serve to guide the research project.

time series   A research design that involves the collection of data over an extended period of time and the introduction of an experimental treatment during the data collection process.

trend study   A study in which the survey collects data on the same variables with a new sample of the same target population so the researcher is able to observe changes in the population overall.

triangulation   A mixed method design in which the researcher uses qualitative and quantitative methods in order to achieve corroboration of results achieved from the different approaches.

two-stage cluster sampling   The type of sampling in which the researcher selects a random sample of the clusters or groups just as would be done in one-stage cluster sampling. The second stage involves taking a random sample of potential subjects from each of the clusters that was selected in the first phase.

univariate analysis   A type of analysis that examines the characteristics of only one variable.

universal essences   Aspects to any participant's lived experience that are common to anyone who has that experience.

validity   A characteristic of an instrument in which it measures what it was intended to measure.

References

LoBiondo-Wood, G., & Haber, J. (2002). *Nursing research: Methods, critical appraisal, and utilization*. St. Louis, MO: Elsevier.

O'Sullivan, E., & Rassel, G. (1999). *Research methods for public administrators*. New York, NY: Longman.

Polit, D., & Hungler, B. (2000). *Essentials of nursing research: Methods and applications*. Philadelphia, PA: Lippincott.

University of Maryland Medical Center—Nursing Research Council. (n.d.). Retrieved from http://umm.edu/professionals/nursing/research

Wooten, J., & Ross, V. (2005). *How to make sense of clinical research*. Retrieved from http://www.modernmedicine.com/modernmedicine/article/articleDetail.jsp?id=142654

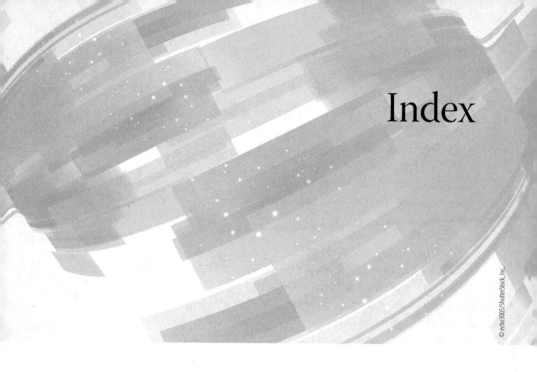

Index

Note: Page numbers followed by *f* or *t* indicate material in figures or tables, respectively.

A

a priori codes, 204
AACN. *See* American Association of Colleges of Nursing
Aboriginal Canadian Peoples (ACP), culture and chronic pain, 389
abstracts, 55
    critical appraisal of, 54–55
    in manuscript writing, 218
academia, 212
    qualitative research and, 103
Academic Center for Evidence-Based Practice (ACE) star model, 240
accounting in ethnomethodology, 111
accreditation, 453
ACE star model. *See* Academic Center for Evidence-Based Practice star model
across-stage mixed model research designs, 123
active participation, 162
activities of daily living (ADLs), 445

aesthetic knowing, 19
Agency for Healthcare Research and Quality, 241
aggregate focus, 16
AHA. *See* American Heart Association
AHA Target Heart Failure Program, 244
Alabama county public school system, 287
Alabama Department of Education, 286
alien
   and creature, 446–447
   fear of disability, 427, 446–447
American Association of Colleges of Nursing (AACN), 4, 16, 452–453, 460
American Association of Neuroscience Nurses, 18
American Heart Association (AHA), 234
American Indian/Alaska Native (AI/AN), 389
American Medical Association (AMA), 62, 394
analysis in survey administration, 180–181
analysis of variance (ANOVA), 201
appraisal in literature reviews, 50–51
assessment, 316
   care delivery processes, 326
   needs, 236–238
   organizational data, 324–325
   stakeholders, 326
associate degree nurse (ADN) curricula, 457
assumptions in ethnomethodology, 111
attrition, 58, 89, 90
autonomy, 62, 63

B

balance scorecard, 245
balanced participation, 162
basic themes, 205
beneficence, 62–63
Benner, Patricia, 374–378
bias, 85, 408
   collaboration and, 160
   in content analysis, 170–171
   convenience sampling and, 143
   interpretative phenomenology and, 107

bias (*Cont.*)
    IRBs and, 57
    observational methods and, 161–163
    quota sampling and, 143
    randomization and, 85
    with records/existing data, 169–170
    subjective data and, 103
    time series designs and, 92–93
bivariate analysis, 198
blinding, 85
body mass index (BMI), 288
bracketing, 106
briefing in survey administration, 179
BSN curricula, 457

C

capstone projects for DNP, 6–7
care delivery processes, 326
case control studies, 82, 89–90
Case Western Reserve University, 4
cause-and-effect relationships, 17, 101, 121
Centers for Medicare and Medicaid Services (CMS), 234
central concept type in literature reviews, 49
central tendencies, 199
chain sampling, 105
champions (of research project), 150, 151
chi-square statistic, 201
childhood obesity, 283–285
    background, 285–289
    BMI, summary of, 203, 204*f*
    data collection, 291–293
    implications, 297–298
    limitations, 296–297
    method, 290–291
    project overview, 289–290
    t-test, 293
    value propositions, 295–296
Children's BMI, for age preimplementation and postimplementation, 294*t*
Children's BMI Tool for School, 291–293

chronic pain, lived experience of nurse educators, 380–381, 400
    assessment, challenges, 383–389
    conceptual framework, 397–398
    coping, 410, 428–430, 447–448
    data analysis, 403–405
    data collection, 401–403
    definition of, 400, 410–411
    education and nursing pain curriculum, 389–397
    ethical considerations, 409
    experience, 370–372
    fear of disability, 410, 423–428, 445–447
    implication for nursing, 458–460
    introduction, 364–370
    management, 391–397
    measurement, 385–386
    methodology, 398–399
    need for pedagogical discourse, 410, 430–436, 448–449
    personal experience, 458–460
    philosophical perspective, 373–374
    physician/provider trust, 420–423, 442–445
    problematic, 382
    procedure/setting, interviews, 403
    protection of participants, 401
    sample demographics for participants, 405–407
    sample size, setting, and access, 401
    teaching, 411–415, 452–458
    theoretical framework, 374–380
    trustworthiness and validity, 407–409
    understanding and engaging, 411–415
    vulnerability, 410, 415–416, 440–442
chronological order type in literature reviews, 49
clinical practice guidelines, 6
clinical prevention, 11–12
clinical protocols, 22
clinical scholarship, 16–20
clinical trials, 82, 86–87
cluster random sampling, 142, 189
CMS. *See* Centers for Medicare and Medicaid Services
Cochrane Library, 240
Code of Federal Regulations, 65
codebooks, 75, 171, 203

coding, 75, 108, 131, 171, 180
cohort studies, 88, 191
Colaizzi data analysis, 403–405
collaboration, 10, 13, 160
Common Rule, 66–67
community case management staff nurses, 238, 243, 244
compatibility thesis, 120
complementarity, 122
compliance
  EBD, 337–338
  education for, 328
conceptual frameworks, 35–38, 51, 53, 55, 107
conceptualizations
  in content analysis, 171
  in survey development, 178
conclusion sections
  critical appraisal of, 58–59
  in manuscripts, 219
concurrent data collection, 172
concurrent timing, 130
confidence interval, 147, 148
confidentiality, 65–66, 74
confirmability, 408
consent. *See* informed consent
consistent education format, 241
constant comparative method, 108
contacts, key, 150, 151
content analysis, 170–171
  qualitative study using, 393
content validity, 158
context, 103
contextual designs, 190
control groups, 84, 91–92
  case control studies, 89
  in literature reviews, 57
  nonequivalent control groups, 87, 91–92
  pretest–posttest designs, 86
  in random assignment, 146
  randomized controlled trials, 84–85
  time series, 92–94
convenience sampling, 143, 189

coping, 410, 428–430, 447–448
core variables, 108
credibility, 407
criterion-related validity, 161
critical appraisal skills in literature review, 50–51, 54–59
critical-case sampling, 149
cross-sectional elements
   designs, 190
   studies, 87
   surveys, 82, 87–88
cross-sectional study, 87
culture (ethnography), 105
   and chronic pain, 388–389
Cumulative Index to Nursing and Allied Health Literature (CINAHL), 52
curricula inadequacies, 8

D

data
   comparison, 131
   consolidation, 131
   correlation, 131
   display, 131
   integration, 131
   interpretation, 107, 131
   reduction, 108, 131
   restricted, 67–68
   retrieval of, 245–246
   safety monitoring plan and, 74–75
   saturation, 108
   transformation, 131
   validation, 131
data analysis, 197–206, 246, 403–405
   childhood obesity, 293
   coding, 204
   descriptive statistics, 198–200
   EBD, 336–337
   inferential statistics, 201–202
   in mixed research process, 131
   narrative analysis, 204

data analysis (*Cont.*)
  qualitative research, 202–206
  quantitative research, 198–202
  thematic networks analysis, 205–206
data collection, 157–172, 401–403. *See also* Survey data collection
  appropriate method choice, 158
  childhood obesity, 291–293
  content analysis, 170–171
  focus groups, 167–168
  instrument development, 158
  interviews and questionnaires, 163–167
  literature reviews and, 158
  methods, 159–171
  in mixed method research, 172
  physiological measurements, 160–161
  in qualitative analysis, 100
  records/existing data, 169–170
  safety monitoring plan and, 74–75
data management, 244–245
  EBD, 334–335
data source collection, 52–59
deception in research projects, 72
decision making, evidence-based, 20–21
deductive reasoning, 33
delegitimation, chronic pain, 386–388
demographic characteristics, 56
demographic variables, 89
dependent variable, 32, 33
descriptive phenomenology, 106
descriptive research, 17
descriptive statistics, 198–200
descriptive study, 31
designs
  evidence, 339
  in survey development, 178–179
  in survey research, 190–191
developing research proposal, writing, 213–215
directional hypothesis, 34
discharge notebook, 246
  components of, 235
  development and implementation of, 239
  intervention, 244

discussion sections
    critical appraisal of, 58–59
    in manuscript writing, 219
dispersion, statistical, 199
disproportional stratified sampling, 142
distribution, statistical, 198
doctor of nursing practice (DNP) degree, 4–10
    benefits of implementing, 7–8
    capstone project, 6–7
    concerns over implementation of, 8–9
    faculty positions, 9
    job market demand for, 9
    program content recommendations, 9–10
    time line for development of, 4–5
    title upon receiving degree, 8
doctor of nursing practice (DNP) graduate
    as advanced practice nurse, 14–15
    aggregate focus, 16
    clinical scholarship/evidence-based practice, 16–20
    decision making, 20–21
    as healthcare advocate, 12–13
    information systems/technology and, 15–16
    quality improvement and, 10–12
doctor of nursing science degree, 5
document analysis, 100
dominant status design, 123
double blind trials, 85
Dreyfus model of skill acquisition, 376–377
drug seeking, 387–388

E

e-mail interviews, 164–165
EAU. *See* express admission unit
EBD. *See* evidence-based design
education
    for compliance, 328
    on red zone, 330–331
Educational Resources Information Center (ERIC), 52
effectiveness goal, 285

electronic submission of articles, 216

eligibility criteria for IRB review, 73

embedded designs, 126–127

emic perspective, 106

empirical knowing, 19

enlightened decisions, 62

environmental design, 313

environmental psychology, 339

equal probability selection method, 146

equal status design, 123

equity, 286

ethical considerations, chronic pain, 409

ethics in clinical research, 61–76. *See also* institutional review boards (IRBs)

    autonomy, 62

    beneficence, 62–63

    Common Rule, 66–67

    confidentiality, 65–66

    data and safety monitoring plan, 74–75

    data, restricted, 67–68

    in e-mail interviews, 164

    evaluation of research proposals, 69–70

    exempt reviews, 70–71

    expedited reviews, 70

    HIPAA compliance, 66–68

    informed consent, 63–64

    justice, 63

    multiple submissions of articles, 216

    participant rights, 64–65

    principles, 62–63

    Privacy Rule, 66–67

    protected health information, 67

    unethical situations, 88

ethics knowing, 19

ethnicity, 388

ethnography, 105–106, 111

ethnomethodology, 110–112

etic perspective, 106

evidence-based decision making model, 316*f,* 339

evidence-based design (EBD), 341

    acquiring, 317–318

    adopting and advancing, 338–339

evidence-based design (EBD) *(Cont.)*
   analyzing, 332–338
   appraising, 318–324
   assessment, 316, 324–326
   background and significance, 313–314
   catalyst, 315–316
   description, 311
   evidence-based practice question, 317
   evidence, critical appraisal, 322–324
   findings, 340–342
   goal of, 313
   impact of, 312–313
   implementation, 326–332, 339–340
   interruptions, 333–334
   outcomes and evaluation, 332–333
   PICO(T), 317
   population, 328–329
   potential barriers, 331–332
   process of, 327
   projects, 338
   proposed project, 314–315, 319–322, 319*f*
   small test of change *vs.* full implementation, 327–328
   theoretical framework, 315, 316*f*
   unintended consequences, 332
evidence-based medicine, 318
   intention of, 312
evidence-based model, 240
evidence-based practice
   clinical scholarship, 16–20
   decision making and, 20–21
evidence/critical appraisal, levels of, 241–242
ex post facto studies, 17
exempt reviews, 70–71
existing data/records, 169–170
expedited reviews, 70
experimental arrangement reactive effects, 94
experimental designs in quantitative research, 83–87
experimental groups, 84
experimental study, 83
experimental treatment/selection interaction, 94

explanatory designs, 127–128
exploratory designs, 128–129
exploratory study, 31
express admission unit (EAU), 237
external participation, 161
external validity, 94
    threats, 94–95
extreme case sampling, 149

F

faculty positions, 9
fear of disability, 410, 423–428, 445–447
Federal Policy for the Protection of Human Subjects (Common Rule), 66
field notes, 100, 162, 203
fieldwork, 100, 105
fieldwork journals, 203
financial resources for research project, 160
First National Pain Medicine Summit final report, 395
focus groups, 167–168
follow-up explanations model, 127, 151
format for manuscript, 218–219
frequency distribution, 198, 199*t*
"frequently" as problem word, 166
full-scope evidence-based design project, 334
full-time faculty, 400
funds for research, 126, 159

G

gap analysis, 237
gatekeepers, 150, 181
generalizability of results, 94
global themes, 205
Google Scholar, 240
graduate degree, 400
grand theory, 37
grounded theory, 108

H

Hawthorne effect, 322, 332
Health Information Portability and Accountability Act (HIPAA), 66–68
health teaching program, 290
healthcare advocacy of DNP graduate, 12–13
healthcare construction, in United States, 313
healthcare costs, for obese, 295
healthy weight, 288
Heideggerian phenomenological interpretive approach, 377–378
hermeneutic phenomenological method, 374, 378
    and human science approach, 378–380
hidden curriculum, 457
history (effect on research), 91
homogeneity, 146
    of sample selection, 149
hypotheses, 28
    appropriate use of, 32
    developing a testable, 32–36
    quantitative elements, 83
hypotheses development
    literature reviews and, 48, 50
    qualitative elements, 101
    quantitative elements, 101
    research designs and, 59

I

IBM SPSS Statistics Version 20 software, 293
IHI. *See* Institute for Healthcare Improvement
illegitimate curriculum, 457
implementation, of childhood obesity, 297–298
incentives for participation, 57, 148, 179, 181
independent variable, 32
Index Medicus (MEDLINE), 52
indexicality in ethnomethodology, 111
inductive codes, 204
inductive reasoning, 37
inductive research, 101

inferential statistics, 201–202
informed consent, 109, 403
   autonomy and, 62
   beneficence and, 62–63
   data collection procedures for, 165
   in e-mail interviews, 165
   IRBs' role in, 68–69, 151
   in literature review, 59
   participant rights and, 64–65
   in survey data collection, 188
   videotaping, 167
Institute for Healthcare Improvement (IHI), 234, 238
Institute of Medicine (IOM), 233, 285
   six aims of, 236
institutional review boards (IRBs), 66, 68–75, 242
   applications, 71–72
   conditions for approval, 69
   exempt reviews, 70–71
   expedited reviews, 70
   explanatory research designs and, 128
   informed consent responsibilities, 151
   interview guides and, 109
   in methods section appraisal, 57
   mixed method data collection, 172
   pitfalls, 72–73
   privacy reviews and, 66
   protected health information and, 67
   qualitative research and, 104
   reading level for, 72
   research proposal evaluations, 69–70
   review criteria, 61–62
   risk/benefit ratio assessment, 72, 74
   success with, 75
institutional review committee (IRC), 240
instructions to authors, 215
instrument development
   for data collection, 158
   model, 128–129
instrumentation, 91, 179
integration of practice change, 23

integration stage, 240

interaction of selection and experimental treatment, 94

intercoder reliability, 171, 203

interdisciplinary healthcare providers, constant barrage of, 342

interim analysis, 202

internal validity, 84

threats, 91–93

International Association for the Study of Pain (IASP), 367

definition of chronic pain, 367, 440

Internet

data authorization and, 67–68

e-mail interviews, 164–165

journal prominence in search engines, 215

questionnaires and surveys on, 87

representative responses from, 164

Web-based surveys, 179, 192

interpretive approach, 377–378

interpretive pedagogies, 459

interpretive phenomenology, 106, 107, 375

interrater reliability, 161

interrupted time series

with multiple replications, 93

with a nonequivalent no-treatment comparison group, 93

with switching replications, 93–94

interruptions, EBD, 312, 333–334

raw number of, 312*f*

statistical differences in, 313*t*

interval level of variable, 201

interval statistical measurement, 200

interview guides, 109

interviews, 163–167

intracoder reliability, 203

intrarater reliability, 161

introduction sections

critical appraisal of, 55

in manuscript writing, 218

IOM. *See* Institute of Medicine

IRBs. *See* institutional review boards

IRC. *See* institutional review committee

irrelevant replicability of treatments, 95

irrelevant responsiveness of measures, 94

J

job market for DNPs, 9
The Joint Commission Heart Failure Core Measure Set, 237
The Joint Commission standards, 342
justice, 63

K

key contacts, 150, 151
knowing patterns, 19
knowledge application, 17
knowledge in ethnomethodology, 111
Kolmogorov-Smirnov test, 201

L

legal capacity, 62
life history grid, 109–110
life history research design, 109–110
limitations, childhood obesity, 296–297
literature reviews, 47–59
    abstract sections, 54–55
    bracketing and, 106
    critical appraisal, 24, 50–51, 54–59
    data collection, 158
    data source collection, 52–59
    discussion/conclusion sections, 58–59
    introduction sections, 55–56
    in manuscript writing, 218
    methods sections, 56–58
    purpose, 48–49
    references sections, 59
    results sections, 58
    structure, 49–50
logs (record-keeping), 162
longitudinal designs, 190
longitudinal studies using cohorts, 82, 88–89

M

MADOS. *See* medication administration dispensing observation sheet
mail surveys, 165
maintenance of practice change, 23
Mann-Whitney U test for independent groups, 201
manuscript writing
    format, 218–220
    submission for publication, 215–216
maturation, 91, 92
maximum variation sampling, 149
mean, statistical, 199
median, statistical, 199
medical/nursing databases, 52
medication administration dispensing observation sheet (MADOS), 327, 333
medication errors, 314, 321, 334
medication therapy, side effects, 384
medicine, 312
MEDLINE, 52
member checking process, 408
memoing, 202
mentoring, 458, 460
meta-analysis literature reviews, 49
methods sections
    critical appraisal of, 56–58
    of manuscript, 218–219
microrange theory, 37
midrange theories, 37
mixed method capstone research projects, 119–132
    across-stage mixed model designs, 123
    advantages and limitations, 120–122
    approaches, 122–124
    data analysis, 131
    data collection, 172
    decision to utilize, 122
    design type selection, 129–130
    design types, 124–129, 125t
    embedded designs, 126–127
    explanatory designs, 127–128
    exploratory designs, 128–129

mixed method capstone research projects (*Cont.*)
   mixing, 130
   process stages, 130–132
   timing, 130
   triangulation designs, 124–126
   weighting, 130
mixed model research, 122–123
mixed purposeful sampling, 149
mode, statistical, 199
monitoring
   by IRBs, 69
   in survey development, 180
mortality, 91–92
motivational interviewing, 112–113
motivations for research participation, 202
multidisciplinary discharge process, 242
multiple healthcare providers, constant barrage of, 342
multiple-treatment interference, 94

N

narrative analysis, 204
National Center for Education Statistics, 235
National League for Nursing Accrediting Commission (NLNAC), 453
need for pedagogical discourse, 430–436, 448–449
needs assessment, 236–238
negative-case sampling, 132, 149
negative emotion, 447
nominal statistical measurement, 200
nondirectional hypothesis, 34
nonequivalent control group designs, 87, 91–92
nonexperimental designs, 87–90
nonrandom sampling types, 143–144, 189
nonrandomized clinical trials, 86
nonstructural environmental design, 313
null curriculum, 457
null hypothesis, 35
Nuremberg Code, 62
nurse educators, 8, 342

nurse faculty, 399–400
nurse interruptions, characteristics of, 320
nursing, 313
nursing intervention/patient care outcomes link, 22
nursing/medical databases, 52

O

obese, 288
objectivity, 106, 163
observational methods, 161–163
observational studies, 82
one-group posttest-only designs, 90–91
one-stage cluster sampling, 142
open-ended items in surveys, 166
operational curriculum, 457
operationalization, 158, 171
opportunistic sampling, 149
ordinal statistical measurement, 200
organizational data, 324–325
organizing themes, 205
outcomes
    vs. process, 100
    of quality improvement intervention, 244
overweight, 288

P

pain. *See also* chronic pain, lived experience of nurse educators
    assessment, 365–368
    curriculum, education and nursing, 389–397
    evolution of the concept of, 381–382
    management, 365–368
pain numeric scale (PNS), 386
pain-related fear, 445
panel studies, 191
paradigm emphasis, 123

participants. *See also* informed consent; populations for research studies
    characteristics, 56
    observation of, 161–163
    rights, 64–65
    selection model, 127
passive participation, 161
patient care, 312
patient care outcomes/nursing intervention link, 22
patient education materials, 242
patterns in narrative analysis, 204
PCPs. *See* primary care providers
PDSA quality improvement model. *See* plan, do, study, act quality improvement model
Pearson correlation coefficient, 201
pedagogical discourse, 410
    need for, 430–436
peer reviews, 13, 54, 206, 211, 218
percentiles, 288
performance measures, identification of, 245
periodicity, 141
personal knowing, 19
personnel resources for research project, 160
phases of project, 242–243
phenomenological research, 379
phenomenological themes, 404
phenomenology, 101, 106–107
physician/provider trust, 420–423, 442–445
physiological measurements, 160–161
PICOT, 29, 317
pilot reliability, 171
pilot tests, 22, 159, 188
plan, do, study, act (PDSA) quality improvement model, 238, 239
planning in survey development, 179
population health, 11
populations, 140
populations for research studies
    in cluster sampling, 189
    confidence intervals and, 148
    in convenience sampling, 143, 189
    definition of, 41, 56

populations for research studies (*Cont.*)
    description in manuscript, 219
    in disproportional stratified sampling, 142
    external validity and, 94–95, 131
    generalization of, 121, 131, 140
    homogeneity considerations, 147
    inferential statistics and, 201–202
    in mixed research designs, 128
    motivation for participation, 202
    participant observation and, 161–163
    in proportional stratified sampling, 142
    in purposive sampling, 143–144, 189
    in quota sampling, 143
    random sampling/random assignment, 146
    representative sample, 140
    response rate, 88, 190
    in simple random sampling, 141, 188
    size, 56, 146–148, 190
    in snowball sampling, 144, 189
    in stratified random sampling, 189
    survey data collection and, 190–191
    in systematic sampling, 141, 189
    vulnerable populations, 71
positive emotion, 447
positivism, 82, 101
potential risks/alternative strategies, 242
pragmatism, 120
preeducation assessment, 337
pretest sensitization, 86, 94
pretest–posttest designs, 85–86, 92
pretesting, in survey development, 179
primary care providers (PCPs), 235
primary sources, 54
privacy, 65, 74
Privacy Rule, 66–67
problem words in questionnaires, 166
process
    outcomes *vs.,* 100
    products *vs.,* 100
processing in survey administration, 180

programmatic research, 159
proportional stratified sampling, 142
proposal evaluations, 69–70
proposed project
    evidence levels for, 319–322, 319*f*
    purpose of, 315
    target population and location, 314
protected health information, 67, 169
Provision of Care, Treatment and Service (PC), 384
publication (of research paper), 215–216. *See also* research report, writing
PubMed, 240
purposive sampling, 143–144, 148, 181, 189
pursuit of knowledge, 378

Q

qualitative capstone research projects, 99–114
    advantages and limitations, 103–105
    data analysis, 202–206
    ethnography, 105
    ethnomethodology, 110–112
    grounded theory, 108
    life history, 109–110
    motivational interviewing, 112–113
    phenomenology, 106–107
    qualitative/quantitative research differences, 101
    qualitative sampling strategy, 149–152
    research designs, 105–113
    sampling designs, 148–149
    sampling strategies, 149–152
    selection, 113–114
    sensitive topic issues, 104–105
    types, 100–103
qualitative data, 244
    analysis, 245
qualitative design, 399
    chronic pain, 397–399
qualitative research, 389–391, 397–398
    project, 6

quality improvement, 238–240
  and DNP graduates, 10–12
  intervention, 234
quality improvement project, 238–240, 246, 284–286, 296, 298
  implementation of, 243
quantitative capstone research projects, 81–97
  advantages and limitations, 83
  case control studies, 82, 89–90
  cross-sectional surveys, 82, 87–88
  data analysis, 198–202
  differences, 101
  experimental designs, 83–87
  external validity, 94–95
  longitudinal studies using cohorts, 82, 88–89
  nonequivalent control group designs, 91–92
  nonexperimental designs, 87–90
  one-group posttest-only designs, 90–91
  pretest-posttest designs, 82, 85–86
  quasi-experimental designs, 90–95
  randomized controlled trials, 82, 84–85
  research types, 84
  sampling designs, 140–145
  subgroups of clinical trials, 86–87
  time series, 92–94
quasi-experimental designs, 87, 90–95
  external validity, 94–95
  nonequivalent control group designs, 91–92
  one-group posttest-only designs, 90–91
  time series, 92–94
quasi-experimental studies, 17
questionnaires, 122, 163–167
quota sampling, 143

R

race, 388
random sampling types, 141–142, 188–190
randomization
  clinical trials, 56, 86
  controlled trials, 84–85

randomization (*Cont.*)
    random number generator, 141
    selection *vs.* random assignment, 146
rating scales, 166
ratio statistical measurement, 200
reactive effects of experimental arrangements, 94
reading level for IRB application, 72
records/existing data, 169–170
red carpet, 327
red zone, 324
    education on, 330–331
    plan for measuring, 333*t*
    project, data from proposed, 340
references sections
    critical appraisal of, 59
    in manuscript writing, 219
reflective learning, 392
reflexivity, 111, 131
regularly as problem word, 166
reliability, 159
    assessment of literature reviews, 56
    in data analysis, 203
    in data collection, 159, 165
    in healthcare practice and outcomes, 17
    pilot reliability, 171
    in qualitative studies, 104
    types, 203
reporting, of content analysis results, 171
representative samples, 91, 140
representativeness, 88
research designs
    confidentiality and, 66
    hypotheses and, 59
    IRBs and, 74, 75
    in literature review, 57
    in manuscript format, 219
    mixed method research, 119–132
    qualitative research, 100, 101, 105–113
    quantitative research, 83–87
    quasi-experimental research, 90–95
research hypothesis, 34

research problem, 28
    selection of, 28–31
research proposal, writing, 213–215
research question, 28
    appropriate use of, 31–32
    development of, 28–31
research report, writing, 211–215
    journal choice, 215–216
    writing process, initiation of, 211–213
researcher participation levels, 161–162
response rate, 87–88, 180–181
results sections
    critical appraisal of, 58
    in manuscript writing, 219
Rights and Responsibilities of the Individual (RI), 384
rights of participants, 64–65. *See also* informed consent
risk/benefit ratio, 72, 74

S

sample recruitment, 181–182
sample size, 56, 146–148, 190
sampling, 139–152, 401
    in content analysis, 171
    decisions in survey development, 179
    error, 147, 189
    frame, 141
    interval, 141
    nonrandom sampling types, 143–144
    qualitative sampling designs, 148–149
    quantitative sampling designs, 140–145
    random sampling types, 141–142
    random selection *vs.* random assignment, 146
    recruitment techniques, 148
    sample size, 56, 146–146, 190
    stratification variable, 141
    during survey research, 188–190
    type comparison, 143–144, 145*t*
scholarship of practice in nursing, 16

scientific hypothesis, 34
secondary source, 55
segmenting, 203
selection bias, 84, 93
selection/experimental treatment interaction, 94
self-regulation questionnaire, 183*f*–187*f*
semistructured interviews, 164
sensitization, pretest, 86, 94
sequential data collection, 172
sequential timing, 130
simple interrupted time series designs, 92–93
simple random sampling, 141, 188
skeletons of research reports, 55
skill acquisition, Dreyfus model of, 376–377
small test of change, 329–331
    vs. full implementation, 327–328
snowball sampling, 144, 189
social network studies, 191
Solomon four-group designs, 86
stakeholders, 19, 101, 102, 180, 238, 326
statistical controls, 87, 90
statistical hypothesis, 34, 35
statistics, 198–200
stigma, chronic pain, 386–388
stoic, vulnerability, 419, 441–442
stoicism, 414
stratified random sampling, 141–142, 189
strengths, weaknesses, opportunities, and threats (SWOT) analysis, 237
structural environmental design, 313
structured interviews, 163, 165–166
structured observational methods, 162
studies evaluation literature reviews, 49
subgroups of clinical trials, 86–87
subjectivity, 103
sufficient understanding, 62
survey data collection, 177–191. *See also* data collection
    designs in survey research, 190–191
    example, 182, 183*f*–187*f*
    information gleaned, 178–181
    planning stages, 179

survey data collection *(Cont.)*
  response rate, 180–181
  sample recruitment, 181–182
  sampling during survey research, 188–190
  survey instrument content, 182–187
survey types, 165
SWOT analysis. *See* strengths, weaknesses, opportunities, and threats analysis
synthesis of evidence, 22
systematic sampling, 141

T

t-test, 293, 327
  for differences between groups, 201
taxonomy development model, 128, 129
telephone surveys, 165, 244, 245
testable hypothesis, 32–36
testing, 91
thematic networks analysis, 205–206
themes in narrative analysis, 204
theoretical approach, 107
theoretical frameworks, 34–38, 48
theory and rationale in content analysis, 170–171
threats to validity, 93
time order, 123
time series, 92–94
timeliness, 286
title pages of manuscripts, 218
topic guides, 168
total participation, 162
training
  in content analysis, 171
  in survey administration, 179
transferability, 408
translation stage, 240
treatment groups, 83, 85, 86
trend studies, 191
triangulation, 407
  designs, 122, 124–126
trustworthiness, 407–409

two-stage cluster sampling, 142
typical-case sampling, 149
typification in ethnomethodology, 111

U

underweight, 288
univariate analysis, 198
universal essences, 107
University of South Alabama Medical Library, 240
unstructured interviews, 164
unstructured observational methods, 162

V

validity, 159, 407–409
    content validity, 158
    criterion-related validity, 161
    in e-mail interviews, 165
    external threats to, 94–95
    internal threats to, 84, 91–93
value propositions, childhood obesity, 295–296
van Manen, Max, 378–380
van Manen's six activities for phenomenological research, 402
variables, 32
    ANOVA, 201
    in content analysis, 171
    core variables, 108
    demographic, 89
    dependent/independent, 85, 131
    in ex-post facto studies, 17
    measurement of, 160
    in mixed research, 128–129
    operationalization of, 158
    in qualitative research, 103, 149
    in quantitative research, 101, 198
    in quasi-experimental studies, 17
    in random assignment designs, 146
    stratification variables, 141

verification in survey administration, 180
videotaping consent, 167
visual analog scales, 166
voluntary (as term), 62
vulnerability, 410, 415–416, 440–442
vulnerable populations, 71

W

Wong-Baker FACES Pain Rating Scale, 385–386
writing process, initiation of, 211–213